PLAGUE
Revised Edition

PLAGUE

An Ancient Disease
in the
Twentieth Century
Revised Edition

Charles T. Gregg

UNIVERSITY OF NEW MEXICO PRESS
Albuquerque

Library of Congress Cataloging in Publication Data
Gregg, Charles T.
Plague: an ancient disease in the twentieth century.
Bibliography: p.
Includes index.
1. Plague—United States. 2. Plague—United
States—History. 3. Plague—History. I. Title.
[DNLM: 1. Disease Outbreaks—United States. 2. Plague—
occurrence—United States. WC 355 G819p]
RC176.A2G72 1985 614.5′732′00973 85–976
ISBN 0-8263-0807-4
ISBN 0-8263-0803-1 (pbk.)

Contents

Contents

Illustrations

Acknowledgments
for the First Edition

This book was begun in Berlin and finished (except for final revisions and updating) in Los Alamos, New Mexico, some two years later. Between these two points in time and space, contributions to the work have been made by many people—friends, colleagues, and librarians—in half a dozen cities in the United States and in Europe. I am deeply grateful to those who read the entire manuscript and gave me the benefit of their suggestions. They are Ernest C. Anderson, Ph.D., scientific advisor, Health Division, the University of California's Los Alamos Scientific Laboratory; Prof. T. H. Chen, M.D., School of Public Health, University of California, Berkeley; Prof. Dr. (med.) Diether Neubert, Pharmakologisches Institut für Toxikologie, der Frien Universität, Berlin; and Docent Dr. (med.) Boris Velimirovic, chief, Field Service, U.S.-Mexican border, Pan American Sanitary Bureau, World Health Organization (WHO), formerly regional advisor on Communicable Disease, WHO Western Pacific Regional Office.

All of these men gave generously of their valuable time and wide experience and have made substantial contributions to the merits of this book. For any errors, whether of fact or of interpretation, I am solely responsible.

I have learned much from discussions with Allan Barnes, Ph.D., chief, Plague Branch, the U.S. Public Health Service Center for Disease Control, Fort Collins, Colorado, as well as from Loris Hughes, Ph.D., director, Microbiology Division; Janet Mullins, former chief, General Microbiology Section; and Bryan Millar, former chief, General Sanitation Division— all of the Health and Social Services Division of the State of New Mexico; and from Jonathan Mann, M.D., New Mexico State Epidemiologist.

The quotations of Agnola di Tura and of the Catanians rebuking the archbishop are from translations by Philip Ziegler in his book *The Black Death* (New York: John Day Company, 1969) and are reprinted with permission of the author and his publisher. The lines from Albert Camus's novel *The Plague* are from the Stuart Gilbert translation published by Alfred A. Knopf and are used with the publisher's permission.

The drug company advertisement quoted in connection with the Los Angeles plague epidemic appeared in a paper by Arthur J. Viseltear, Ph.D., in the *Yale Journal of Biology and Medicine* (published by Academic Press, Inc.), and appears with the permission of the author and the publisher. Likewise, the remarks of Louis Weinstein, M.D., on the subject of multiple drug resistance are from *The Pharmacological Basis of Therapeutics*, fifth edition, L. G. Goodman and A. Gilman, editors (New York, Macmillan, 1975), and are used with the permission of the publisher and of Dr. Weinstein. The excerpt from the presidential address of Professor William Reeves is reprinted with the permission of the *American Journal of Tropical Medicine and Hygiene* and of Professor Reeves. The paragraphs from René Dubos are from his book *Man Adapting* (New Haven: Yale University Press, 1975) and are quoted with the permission of the author and the publisher.

Special thanks are due Susanne Kirk, my charming editor at Scribner's, who was consistently meticulous, demanding, and sympathetic, and to her erudite colleague, Robert Scott. Their help and support were essential.

Last, I want to acknowledge my considerable debt to Dr. A. L. Lehninger, DeLamar Professor and chairman of the Department of Physiological Chemistry, the Johns Hopkins University School of Medicine, who, by precept and example, first taught me to write (at least occasionally) a lucid English paragraph.

Acknowledgments
for the Second Edition

The draft for the second edition was carefully read by Dr. Walter Dowdle, director of the Center for Infectious Diseases, Centers for Disease Control, Atlanta, and by Dr. Ernest C. Anderson, formerly scientific advisor to the Life Sciences Division of the Los Alamos National Laboratory. I benefited greatly from their suggestions. As for the first edition, I received valuable information from Dr. Allan Barnes and Dr. Thomas J. Quan, chief and assistant chief, respectively, of the Plague Branch, Centers for Disease Control, Fort Collins, Colorado. The quality of this edition also benefited greatly from the careful scrutiny of Dana Asbury, my elegant and capable editor at the University of New Mexico Press. For any remaining errors of grammar, syntax, fact, or interpretation I am obviously responsible.

Preface
to the Second Edition

Donna Marie Delattre died just six and a half hours after her parents first learned that she was dreadfully ill, and only two and a half hours after they reached the hospital in Greenville, South Carolina. Dr. and Mrs. Edwin J. Delattre and Donna's younger sister, Lee, had said goodby to her six days earlier in Santa Fe, New Mexico, as Donna Marie left for a visit with her maternal grandparents in the little mountain town of Seneca, South Carolina. They planned that the family would reassemble in Seneca, drive to Virginia for a visit with her paternal grandparents, and then on to Annapolis, Maryland, where Donna would have started ninth grade.

They never saw her again. Instead, the family was reunited at Donna's graveside at ten o'clock in the morning of Friday, August 5, 1984, in Liberty, South Carolina.

Donna's death was only one of the tragedies of the 1983 plague season in the United States that ultimately claimed forty victims, by far the worst year for human plague in America since the Los Angeles epidemic of forty-one cases in 1924–25. The 1983 epidemic, which led to an unusual amount of publicity in the news media in America, was also the catalyst for preparing a second edition of this book.

PLAGUE
Revised Edition

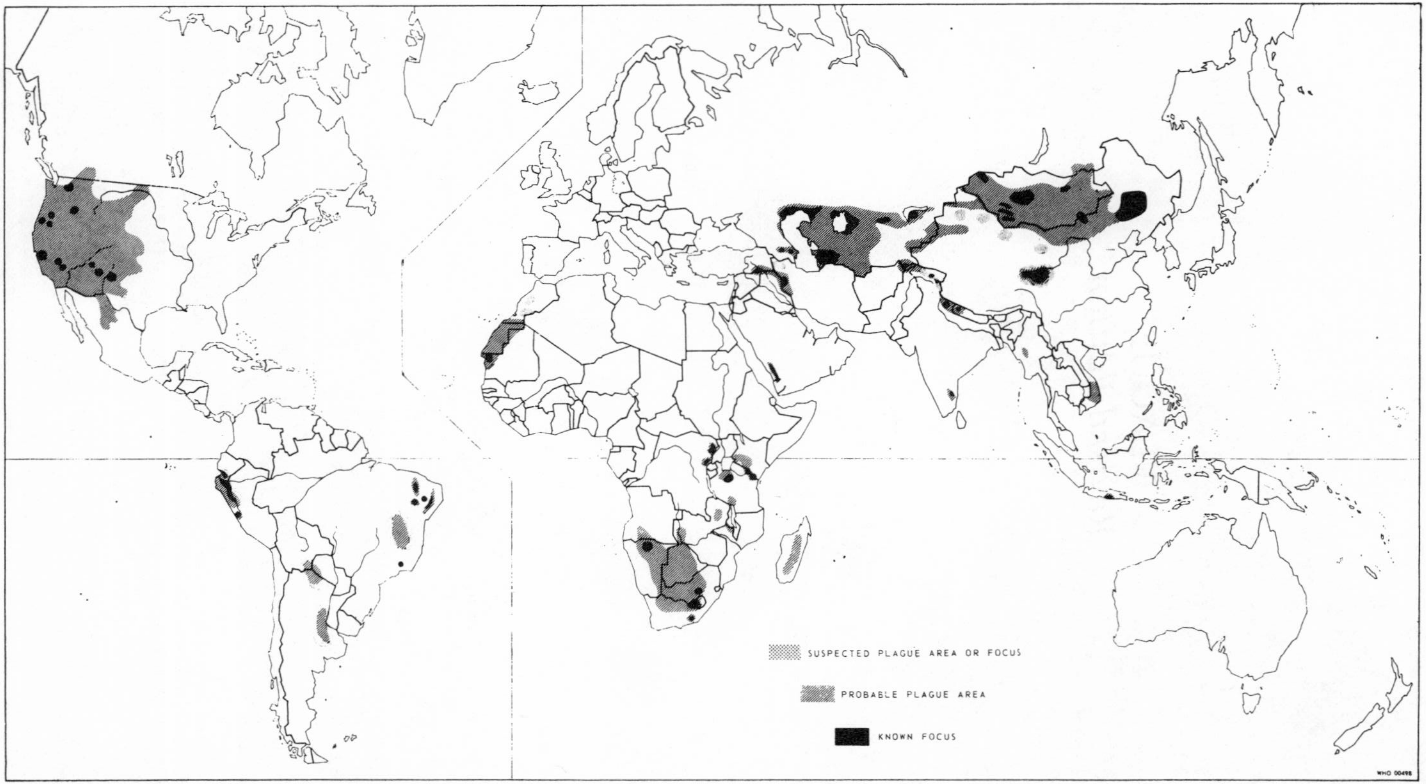

Figure 1   Plague Foci

1

The Past as Prologue

... rather it was come to this, that a dead man was then of no more account than a dead goat would be today.
—Boccaccio, *The Decameron*, 1353

Saturday, February 8, 1975, dawned cold and clear. By early afternoon, as eleven-year-old Danny Gallant and his friend Dale trudged over the foothills of the Sandia Mountains east of Albuquerque, New Mexico, occasional puffs of cloud were sharply outlined against the intensely blue sky. A breeze had come up. But the warmth of the sun took the bite from it, although frequent patches of snow still hid in shaded spots.

Just a short distance from Danny's house the boys reached open country. Passing a gigantic water tank painted an incongruous baby blue and officially named the Supper Rock Reservoir, they took a trail leading around the lower barren slopes and into a broad canyon from which other trails ran to the ridgetop some ten thousand feet above sea level. The two friends had no particular goal: just an ordinary Saturday search for adventure. Both were armed with sheath knives against the unexpected. It would soon appear.

The area has a wild beauty. The hillsides and canyons are studded with bare rocks, some the size of automobiles, juxtaposed with small junipers, piñon pines, and clumps of rabbitbush. Everywhere there are dead stands of cholla, the walking-stick cactus, whose bare branches claw enviously at the sky like the gnarled fingers of some imprisoned earth spirit.

Dale saw it first—and let out a whoop of delight and surprise. The coyote lay half hidden in a cluster of rocks, its limbs rigid in death. After examining the animal, Dale suggested they skin it. The boys set to work with great enthusiasm, although less skill, and eventually they succeeded. Soon it was late afternoon, and the two boys, like all successful hunters since the dawn of time, trudged homeward in triumph, bearing the ragged gray pelt.

The boys' families admired the skin they bore so proudly, and perhaps because Danny's mother was not home at the time, the hide ended its journey at his house.

At the Apache Elementary School on Monday, Danny described his adventure for friends and savored his celebrity. From the playground of the one-story brick school he could almost point out the place where he had found the animal. It was less than a mile away.

By Tuesday, the great adventure was fading into memory. But for young Danny an unpleasant sequel was beginning. He complained of a bad headache and felt listless and weak. Wednesday he stayed home from school, suffering from shaking chills and pain in his right shoulder. At 5:00 A.M. Thursday, Danny woke his mother to show her an egg-sized, excruciatingly painful swelling in his right armpit. Later that morning, Danny entered the Bernalillo County Medical Center. He was obviously a very sick boy, but not until some days later was the suspected cause of his illness verified: Danny Gallant had bubonic plague!

To those who think of plague as a medieval disease, the idea of this particular blight in the United States in the last quarter of the twentieth century may be shocking, but Danny's case was not unique. In fact the 1975 plague season in the western United States, which began with Danny Gallant's infection, was the worst in half a century—and much worse was to come. Besides the human cases, myriad wild animals perished from plague, and each wild animal death was a potential threat to domestic animals and to humans as well.

At this moment plague-infected animals infest at least 40

percent of the continental United States, from the Pacific Ocean eastward to a line (the one hundredth meridian) running through Dodge City, Kansas, and Abiline, Texas. Parts of Canada and Mexico are also infected. Ominously, the average number of cases per year has risen sharply since 1964. From 1965 to 1977 the average yearly number of cases was seven times higher than that of the preceding forty years; in the 1975–76 epidemic the average rose to eighteen times—and in the 1980 epidemic to twenty-two times—the earlier level. The 1983 outbreak was the worst in nearly sixty years; for the first time since 1924 there were forty cases of human plague reported in the U.S.

The dread disease is still capable of vicious outbreaks. One occurred in Vietnam concomitant with the large-scale American military incursion beginning in 1965. The result, in that rather small country, was twenty-five thousand reported cases of plague in a five-year period, and an actual number several times that.

Plague remains a threat. The threat is compounded by the dreadful certainties of overpopulation, famine, and war.

Where did it all begin? We can only guess. Certainly the plague bacillus and its insect and animal hosts were on the earth for hundreds of thousands—perhaps millions—of years before the emergence of man. The disease remains largely an affliction of small animals. Plague only occasionally spreads to humans, but such occasions can be catastrophic.

The first human cases may have occurred when the earliest hominids began to vary their diet by running down small game. A sick animal is more easily captured than a healthy one, but the captor risks taking disease as well as sustenance from his prey.

As man began to congregate in the earliest agricultural communities around 10,000 B.C., he became subject to true epidemics. Plague must have decimated some of these early settlements, but we know no more of this than of the songs of cavemen.

The first plague epidemic for which there is reasonably good evidence was that which befell the Philistines in the twelfth

century B.C. The urbane Philistines defeated an army of the
nomadic Hebrews at Eben-ezer, captured the sacred Ark of the
Covenant, and carried it triumphantly to Ashdod, a city near
the Mediterranean Sea. In the sonorous language of the King
James version of the Bible, the prophet Samuel tells us (1 Sam.
5–6) that the triumph was short-lived, for "the hand of the
Lord was against the city with a very great destruction: and
he smote the men of the city, both small and great, and they
had emerods [swellings] in their secret parts" (1 Sam. 5:9).

From Ashdod, the Philistines hastily bore the Ark of the
Covenant inland to Gath. Plague broke out there. The Philistines removed the ark to Ekron, where, apparently, plague
followed. Terrified, they implored their priests to tell them
how to lift the vengeful hand of the Hebrew God from their
tormented cities, and it was done as the priests directed. The
ark and golden trespass offerings to the people of Israel and
their mighty lord were placed on a cart, newly made, and
drawn by two milk cows. If the cattle—unguided—drew the
cart toward the Hebrew border town of Beth-shemesh, their
action would signify that the Lord of Israel had smitten the
Philistines. If the cattle went some other way, it would mean
that the suffering in the Philistine cities was only by chance.

Thus, one day, the farmers of Beth-shemesh straightened
from the task of harvesting their wheat, wiped the sweat from
their eyes, and watched astonished as the newly made cart
creaked into the field of the Beth-shemite Joshua and stopped
beside a great stone. Exulting when they discovered its contents, the farmers put the ark and the golden offerings on a
stone and then burned cart and cattle as an oblation to the
Lord.

Throughout the land of Israel there was wild rejoicing that
the sacred ark had returned. But in Beth-shemesh the songs
became sobs, for plague came there as well: "And He smote
the men of Beth-shemesh, because they had looked into the
Ark of the Lord, even He smote of the people fifty thousand
and three score and ten men: and the people lamented because
the Lord had smitten many of the people with a great slaughter" (1 Sam. 6:19).

The plague of the Philistines probably invaded the town of Ashdod from a stricken ship rather than with the Ark of the Covenant and then infected the crowds that conveyed the ark to the other afflicted cities. Had the plague begun in Israel there should have been accounts of it in the Old Testament, but Samuel mentions the disease no more.

Ever since the wails from the Philistine cities rose to heaven, plague has regularly marred the history of civilization, most often as isolated outbreaks affecting only a single city or a small region. Three times, however, vast plague pandemics have ravished nearly the whole of the inhabited world.

Plague's normal state is as an infection of animals—field mice, gerbils, squirrels, marmots, guinea pigs, hamsters, prairie dogs, and others. Periodically, the disease explodes in its animal hosts. Meadow and plain are carpeted with corpses of little animals dead of plague. This is an epizootic: the disease is no longer only *in* the animal poulation (enzootic) but *on* them, as a burden and a curse. An epizootic usually precedes an epidemic in humans. Then, when epidemics spread over much of the world, they became pandemics involving, in the literal meaning of the word, all the people.

The first of the three great pandemics began in the fifteenth year of the reign of the Roman emperor Justinian I. There were threatening signs. A great comet (Halley's) lit the night sky for twenty days in A.D. 531. Plague followed quickly. It struck the great Egyptian port of Pelusium (twenty miles, or thirty-three kilometers from modern Port Said) the following year. In October 541, probably aboard grain ships from Egypt, plague entered the city that was still called Byzantium (it had been officially named Constantinople over a century before and is now Istanbul), the capital of the Christian Roman Empire.

Our knowledge of what followed comes largely from the pen of Procopius, the observant secretary of Justinian's great general, Belisarius. In *De Bello Persico* he noted that

> the bodies of the sick were covered with black pustules or carbuncles, the symptoms of immediate death. . . . Those who were without friends or servants lay unburied in the streets or

in their desolate houses. . . . Corpses were placed aboard ships and these abandoned to the seas. . . . Physicians could not tell which cases were light and which severe, and no remedies availed.

It is a dirge we shall hear again.

Plague swept most of the lands that were then, or had been, part of the Roman Empire. In the spring of the second year, the disease reached a pinnacle of ferocity. The historian Edward Gibbon wrote, in *The Decline and Fall of the Roman Empire:* "I only find that, during three months, five and at length ten, thousand persons died each day at Constantinople."

For over half a century the disease surged across western europe. Pope Gregory the Great headed a procession to Saint Peter's to pray for relief from the pestilence that struck Rome in 590. As he crossed the Tiber on the Bridge of Hadrian, the pope saw the Archangel Michael standing on Hadrian's mausoleum, sheathing a bloody sword. In that instant the plague ceased. The event is commemorated by a chapel atop Hadrian's tomb, called Saint Michael's in the Clouds.

But divine intervention was intermittent, and nearly half the inhabitants of the former empire writhed and died under the lash of plague. The Plague of Justinian, according to a contemporary chronicle, "depopulated towns, turned the country into a desert and made the habitations of men to become the haunts of wild beasts."

Minor eruptions of the disease, springing from seeds scattered by the First Pandemic, took a century to disappear. Then the world was free of widespread plague for six hundred years, a pattern that we now know to be typical. Plague erupts with pandemic intensity, scourges humanity for years or centuries, and then disappears as mysteriously as it comes.

When plague did return to East and West in the fourteenth century, its impact was spectacular. This was the Second Pandemic that we now call the Black Death.

Portents of its coming abounded. A series of disasters struck China beginning in 1333. There were droughts, then floods, earthquakes, then clouds of locusts blotting out the sun. Plague exploded somewhere in the East, probably in the present Kirgiz Soviet Socialist Republic, part of the primordial plague reservoir of central Asia. From there, near the present Soviet-Chinese border, the Black Death spread leisurely south and east to China and India and then west to Turkestan and the shores of the Caspian Sea. By 1346 the seaports of Europe were abuzz with rumors that a plague of insatiable ferocity was sweeping the East. But the wealthy shipowners of the Italian city-states never let rumors interfere with business.

In 1347, in the Crimean trading port of Kaffa (now the southern Soviet city of Feodosiya) a group of Genoese traders had been trapped in the city when it was besieged by the Janibeg Kipchak khan. The siege lasted several years, while the Kipchak Tatars waited for the stroke that would decide the outcome.

That stroke was the Black Death.

In their crowded and unsanitary encampments, the long-limbed warriors of the khan fell to the plague, mowed down as grass before the scythe. Furious and fearful, the Janibeg khan prepared to decamp, but before doing so he ordered that plague-infested corpses be catapulted over the walls of Kaffa so that he might share the pestilence with his enemy. The siege was ended as the remnants of the khan's stricken army hurried away from their unburied dead. The Genoese traders quickly sailed from their homeland. The great galleys winched up their anchors, loosed sails from yardarms, and bore off to the western seas bearing cargoes of jewels, nutmeg, rich cloth—and the Black Death.

The ports of Sicily and mainland Italy took the first blows (plague comes from the Latin *plaga,* meaning a blow). Later, the disease moved inland to cities such as Florence, then one of the greatest in Europe. Florence had troubles even before the Black Death—floods, droughts, earthquakes, and famine. Then came plague to slay the people and perplex the physicians. Boccaccio echoed in *The Decameron* the sad words of Procopius of eight centuries before: "These . . . maladies seemed to set entirely at naught both the art of the physician and the virtues of the physic; indeed, whether it was that the disorder was of a nature to defy such treatment, or that the physicians were at fault, . . . almost all died." He went on to complain that, besides qualified physicians, "there was now such a multitude both of men and women who practiced without having received the slightest tincture of medical science and, being in ignorance of its [the plague's] true causes, failed to apply the proper remedies."

There were, in fact, no proper remedies, nor would there be for six more centuries. The ignorant knew exactly as much about the Black Death as the learned, and the cure rate of the unlettered healers was as high as among those appropriately "tinctured" with medical sciences.

Throughout Europe, the Black Death lacerated all levels of society. Siena's situation was typical. This city, some thirty miles (fifty kilometers) south of Florence, was in a frenzy of creative activity in 1348. The Duomo, a striking building of Byzantine motif in black and white marble, was to be tripled in size. It would be larger, even, than St. Peter's in Rome, the greatest edifice in Christendom. For two years a steady stream of workmen and material had climbed the steep road to the mighty cathedral that looked down over the red brown walls of the city. The transept was completed; the foundations of the nave and the choir had been laid. In the city below, the fame of the Sienese school of art was burgeoning under the inspiration of Ambroglio and Pietro Lorenzetti.

A year later, the once-vibrant city of Siena had become a sepulcher. Lorenzetti, Ambroglio, and most of their students were dead. The great cathedral would never be finished; both the will and the workers had been swept away by pestilence. And not only art and architecture suffered in Siena. As described in the *Cronica Senese:* "Father abandoned child; wife, husband; one brother, another. . . . And so they died. And no one could be found to bury the dead for money or for friendship. . . . And I, Agnola di Tura, called the Fat, buried my five children with my own hands, and so did many others likewise."

Monastic communities were decimated by the Black Death with serious consequences for the church. The Franciscan monastery near the southern French seaport of Marseilles was wiped out; all 150 monks perished. Farther north, in Avignon, the English Austin Friars met the same fate.

What did these cloistered men feel as their numbers grew visibly smaller each day? At first there must have been much surreptitious counting under lowered eyes as they met for food and prayer. Later, numbers no longer mattered. Those left alive spent every waking hour tending the sick, burying the dead, and waiting for the Black Death to embrace them as well. What of the last man? Did he wander, delirious, through the cold and empty halls, chanting, calling to his friends, until he himself lay down to die? What sights met the eyes of the first curious townfolk who entered the silent monastery?

The decimation of the monastic communities in England had, arguably at least, another important consequence. In the mid-fourteenth century, a cultured Englishman spoke in French and wrote in Latin; he learned these languages from the monks. After the Black Death, with so many of the monasteries depopulated, this learning was greatly curtailed, and it became acceptable to speak and write in the native language of the island kingdom. Thus modern English literature was born.

In June 1348 the Black Death reached Paris. Its citizens, although they lived in terror for months, at least knew the root of their troubles. Philip VI ordered the medical faculty of the University of Paris to determine whence the pestilence had come. These learned men quickly found the answer in that durable quackery, astrology.

As they solemnly reported to His Majesty, there had occurred, on March 20, 1345, at 1:00 P.M., a conjunction of Saturn, Mars, and Jupiter in the house of Aquarius. In case the king was unable immediately to see that this caused the Black Death, the learned physicians hurried to explain that the conjunction of Saturn and Mars notoriously portended death and destruction, while the conjunction of Mars and Jupiter dispersed pestilence in the air. This was clearly so, because Jupiter, being warm and humid, drew up water and evil vapors from the earth, which Mars, being hot and dry, then kindled into infective fire. Obviously, the conjunction of all three planets could only presage a catastrophe gargantuan in scope.

Of course, some skeptics questioned whether a planetary conjunction could cause the disease to occur three years later, if, indeed, at all. But the attitude of most highly placed physicians was that expressed by one of Molière's *L'Amour médecin* three centuries later, who told the father of a rebellious patient, "Sir, it is better to die according to the rules than to live in contradiction to the Faculty of Medicine."

The medical faculty, having settled on the origin of the Black Death, next prescribed ways to avoid the disease. The eating of poultry, fatty meats, and olive oil was proscribed. The doctors recommended that sleep not be prolonged past dawn and opined that baths were dangerous and sexual intercourse possibly fatal.

At about the time Paris was stricken, plague swept down the valleys of the Rhine and the Moselle and also arrived in England, Denmark, Norway, and Sweden. Finally, in 1351, after four ghastly years, the main tide of the pandemic receded, although outbreaks spawned by the Second Pandemic caused intense local epidemics for another four hundred years.

No one can say with certainty why the pandemic ceased when it did, but it is clear that when the Black Death arrived, Europe offered it fertile soil. By the early fourteenth century, the population of the continent had risen rapidly, far more rapidly than the food supply. Soon bad harvests reduced the poor to eating dogs and cats, perhaps even their own children. Even before the Black Death, Europe was in the clammy grip of a vast depression, and the population had declined slightly. In England the population, already stagnant or declining at the beginning of the century, was reduced by three consecutive years of poor harvests in the second decade of the century. But starvation is a slow and clumsy corrective for overpopulation. Plague is fast and efficient. The Black Death slaughtered one of every four Europeans; subsequent epidemics raised the toll to one in three. The surplus population, for which there was little employment and less food, was efficiently consumed by plague. Unless gentler correctives for overpopulation are effective in time, the lesson of the Black Death may be repeated in this century.

Strategic military planners, who talk of "total assured destruction" and use merry words like *megadeaths*, assume that a country is helpless if one-third of its people are disabled or dead. It is hardly surprising that the Second Pandemic, which caused just such a mortality, aided in destroying that medieval society which the First Pandemic had helped create.[1] The effect was magnified by the later reverberations of what the Germans called "The Great Dying." One such local epidemic was the Great Plague of London.[2] It too was preceded by harbingers of evil and hallucinations born of fear.

In late December 1663 a comet appeared, rising in the east and then disappearing below the southwest horizon in the early morning hours. In March of the next year, a still brighter comet came into view. It rose two hours after midnight and remained visible until dawn. There were murmurings about plague in Holland. People saw coffins in the air and flames and heard sounds of distant cannon, although there were none.

Just before Christmas 1664, two men died of plague in Drury Lane, and there were scattered cases throughout that winter. But it was bitterly cold, and the icy winter slowed further progress of the disease.

In March the frost lifted. By May London was warm. Five months of warm, sometimes hot, weather followed under beautifully blue and cloudless skies. There was a day or two of rain in August and a brief period of torrential rain in September. But, on the whole, it was a lovely summer in London— but not for the people.

As summer advanced, so did the plague, and the wealthy quickly retreated. The president of the College of Physicians set an example by leaving early; by late June the college was bereft of faculty. The Royal Society suspended meetings, and the legal inns were empty. King Charles II, odious man, fled the city in early July.

Ministering to the mounting flood of sick was left to apothecaries and a handful of courageous physicians. Most physicians took the advice offered by a candid member of the profession who had written in a London epidemic forty years before, "I may not take upon me to cure the Sicke, because I meddle not with the Sicknesse (for to practice on the Plague now would prove a plague to my Practice hereafter) but I must labour to preserve the sound; because by profession I am a Physition."

Apothecary William Boghurst was one who worked tirelessly to aid those stricken with plague. He had his own preservatives against the disease in which he placed great faith, but tobacco smoking was not one of them. At this supposed remedy Boghurst drew the line. As he later wrote, "I never took a pipe this year, nor ever do, nor ever will do. How many thousands of tobacco smokers, think you, died this year?"

This eccentric view was not common. Even children were encouraged, and sometimes forced, to smoke to protect themselves against plague. A young Eton student reported that all the boys smoked on order, and that the worst whipping he ever received was as punishment for not smoking when told to do so.

Physician Nathaniel Hodges also remained in London to do his duty. His account mirrors those of Procopius and Boccaccio, as he describes the difficulties of treating the disease: "Many patients were lost when they were thought in a safe Recovery; and when we thought the Conquest quite obtained, Death ran away with the Victory; whereas others got over it, who were quite given up for lost, much to the disreputation of our Art."

Physicians treating the disease continue to this day to echo Dr. Hodges's complaint, as we shall see later on.

As one delightfully sunny day followed another that summer in London, the death toll mounted to hundreds, then to thousands, a week. In the last week of August, at least seventy-five hundred persons died in a city that, by then, contained only some three hundred thousand. Samuel Pepys noted in his diary for August 31,

> In the city died this week, 7,496, and of them, 6,102 of the Plague. But it is feared that the true number of the dead is near

10,000, partly from the poor that cannot be taken notice of, through the greatness of their number, and partly from the Quakers and others that will not have any bell ring for them.

Shortly after, the clanging bells for the dead, which had become an almost continual din, stopped altogether. In the five weeks ending September 26, 1665, more than thirty-eight thousand Londoners were swept away by the pestilence, one of every seven or eight who remained. As Dr. Hodges wrote, "Who would not melt with Grief to see the Stock for a future Generation hang upon the Breasts of a dead Mother? Or the Marriage-Bed changed the first Night into a Sepulchre, and the unhappy Pair meet with Death in their first Embraces."

Still, the tide was turning. October was better. November better still. By February 1, 1666, the mortality rate declined so markedly that even the king returned to London. But the toll had been frightful: close to a hundred thousand dead.

The churchyard of Saint Giles in the Fields was, and is, among the largest in London. In June 1665 the rector asked his sexton, John Geere, to have dug a pit to receive the flood of plague victims that was already too vast for individual burial. Geere hired men for one shilling and sixpence for a twelve-hour day. He paid out four pounds and nine shillings. That means the work took nearly sixty man-days. What a pit it must have been! When Sexton Geere looked into the great hole that he had caused to be dug, he could only pray it would be the last. It was the first of five.

To this day, the graveyards of old London rise above the surrounding ground in mute witness to the time when they so gorged on the dead that they could never return to their former level. But since 1666, London has never experienced another serious plague epidemic.

Although there were paroxysms of plague for more than a century after 1665 and Malta, Marseilles, Moscow, and Vienna were engulfed by the disease, it became apparent that plague was withdrawing into the East whence it had come.

A long interval without epidemic plague always introduces a sense of complacency about the disease. An example is the opinion of a select committee of the British House of Commons that reported in June 1819 that

> the Plague is a disease communicable by contact only.... It appears from some of the evidence that the extension and virulence of the disease is considerably modified by atmospheric influences; and a doubt has prevailed *whether, under any circumstances,* the disease could be received and propagated in the climate of Britain (italics added).

The committee did admit that there was some evidence that the disease had been "received and propagated" in Britain in years past. It was to return to England less than a century after the committee's report was issued.

The word *plague* evokes images of the Great Plague of London, the Black Death, or sometimes the Plague of Justinian—all visions of a distant past shrouded in romance and mystery. Curiously, the Third Pandemic, which followed the Plague of Justinian and the Black Death, is virtually unknown, yet it began in the 1850s and ended, perhaps, about 1959. The Third Pandemic introduced permanent plague into lands across the great oceans from its ancestral homes in Africa and Asia.

Before the Third Pandemic, the only two permanent foci of plague were in central Africa and in central Asia. The former spawned the Plague of Justinian. In the latter were cradled the Black Death and the Third Pandemic. The Third Pandemic created a third region of permanent plague in the western United States as large as that of central Asia and much larger than the African focus.

The Third Pandemic led to plague epidemics in San Francisco, Berkeley, Seattle, Los Angeles, New Orleans, Pensacola, and several Texas ports, as well as in other coastal cities around the world. In recent years, besides cases in areas of chronic infection, there have been imported cases of plague in Dallas, San Francisco, Cambridge, Massachusetts, Nebraska, and North Carolina. In all but one of these cases the infection originated in the state of New Mexico.

This book is an account of the Third Pandemic—the story of modern plague. The pandemic phase of the Black Death lasted only four years; the Third Pandemic spanned more than a century. The Great Plague of London took a hundred thousand lives in about six months; the Third Pandemic killed as many in a few weeks and continued month after month, year after year, until more than thirteen million were dead.

The horrors of the Black Death and the Great Plague of London are softened for us by the mists of time; we comfort ourselves with their antiquity. Yet nearly all who read these words are survivors of the Third Pandemic, although they may never have known of its passage.

Plague is now neighbor to us all; for many only minutes or hours away, at most a day's journey distant. Plague is a willing handmaiden to famine and war; these threaten us still, perhaps more than ever. The plague bacillus and its hosts show increasing resistance to antibiotics and pesticides. This raises the specter of our most potent weapons splintering in our hands at that moment when they are most needed.

Albert Camus's great novel *The Plague* tells of a fictional epidemic. When it is over there is great rejoicing. But the doctor, Rieux, is less optimistic.

And indeed, as he listens to the cries of joy rising from the town, Rieux remembered that such joy is always imperiled. He knew what those jubilant crowds did not know but could have learned from books; that the plague bacillus never dies or disappears for good; ... and that perhaps the day would come when, for the bane and enlightenment of men, it would rouse up its rats again and send them forth to die in a happy city.[3]

2

Plague Sociology
and Superstition

'Tis the Destroyer or the Devil that scatters Plagues about the
World.
—Cotton Mather, *The Wonders of the Invisible World,* 1693

As expected of such a terrifying phenomenon, plague has inspired a substantial body of folklore as well as monuments,
both cultural and architectural, to its passing.

In Vienna plague was said to be carried by the Pest Jungfrau,
or Plague Maiden, who was seen as a blue flame emerging
from the mouths of the dead. Perhaps for the same reason, the
French spoke of plague as *la morte bleue* ("blue death"). In
Lithuania the Black Death was also carried by a young woman
who waved a red scarf through the door or window of a home
to infect its inhabitants. In one threatened village, a brave
man deliberately waited, sword in hand, by the open window
of his home until the Plague Maiden thrust in her arm. Then
he cut it off. He died, but his home and village were spared,
and a scarlet scarf was long preserved in a local church as a
sacred relic.

Many people believed that the swellings of plague were the
result of wounds from arrows shot by God's avenging angels.
Saint Sebastian (condemned to death by a firing squad of arch-
ers for preaching Christianity to the soldiers of the emperor
Diocletian) was a natural ally to invoke for protection against
the heavenly missiles, especially since he, although pierced

19

by many arrows, survived his wounds. That Diocletian later had Sebastian beaten to death and his body thrown in a sewer failed to detract from his popularity as a plague saint.

Saint Roch's claim to miraculous powers against the disease was more direct. He tirelessly tended the plague-stricken in Italian cities in the fourteenth century and was credited with many spectacular cures. But when he caught the disease he was expelled from the city of Piacenza and left to die in the woods. He was saved by a nobleman's dog that daily brought him bread. Saint Roch recovered, only to die in prison in his native Montpelier, in the south of France.

In 1414, an effigy of Saint Roch was said to have halted an outbreak of plague in Constance, and his posthumous fame waxed large. Venice, lashed repeatedly by the pestilence, began to take a lively interest in the saint's relics. In 1485 the Venetians spirited his body away from Montpelier and installed it in their own city within the great Church of San Roco. Every year, on August 16, the doge of Venice knelt before the relics to implore Saint Roch to protect the republic from plague.

According to one contemporary account, the Black Death arrived in Messina, in Sicily, in October 1347, with a fleet of thirteen Genoese galleys. Only after the disease was well entrenched ashore did the inhabitants of the town drive the plague-stricken ships and seamen from their harbor.[1]

The distraught Messinese sought help where they could. Humbly, they petitioned the patriarch archbishop of neighboring Catania to allow the relics of Saint Agatha to be taken to Messina to help assuage their sufferings. The patriarch generously agreed, but the Catanians emphatically did not. They argued that Saint Agatha, or what was left of her, must remain on duty in her own cathedral. They matched fiery word with fiery deed: "They tore the keys [to the cathedral] from the hands of the sacristan and stoutly rebuked the Patriarch, saying that they would rather die than allow the relics to be taken to Messina."

The archbishop, a kindly man, now proved himself to be clever and courageous as well. Accepting the mob's decision, he persuaded them to let him dip some of the relics in holy water, which water he then personally carried to the plague-swept port. Whether this aqueous extract of Saint Agatha was as effective as the original relics is uncertain; the doughty patriarch unfortunately died of plague soon after his return home from Messina.

The origin of plague remained a mystery. An ancient view, dating from Hippocrates, was that plague came from poisonous clouds—miasmas—from swamps, battlefields, or graveyards. The defenses against miasmas were running away, or as the popular Latin phrase went, *Fuge cito, vade longe, rede tarde* ("Flee quickly, go far, return slowly"); staying inside with doors and windows fast shut; or interposing suitable fumes, such as those of tobacco, to turn aside the poisonous vapor. The special leather suits worn by some medieval plague doctors were adorned with great beaks containing aromatic spices to purify the air. More humble persons contented themselves with sweet-smelling elixirs and plague waters. Eau de cologne originated in this way.

One of the liveliest, although sometimes inaccurate, accounts of the Great Plague of London is that of Daniel Defoe. His *Journal of the Plague Year* bore the legend: "Being observances or memorials of the most remarkable occurrences, as well public as private, which happened in London during the last great visitation in 1665. Written by a Citizen who continued all the while in London. Never made public before."[2]

Purporting to be a narrative of a middle-aged and middle-class saddler of Calvinist bent, and written in an often clumsy style, it is, in fact, a novel of great art. Only five years old at the height of the epidemic, Defoe wrote his fascinating account of the Great Plague when he was past sixty. Defoe tells of worthless nostrums against the pestilence that were industriously peddled by the unscrupulous as the Laetriles of the day. "An Italian gentlewoman just arrived from Naples, having a choice secret to prevent infection, which she found out by her great experience, and did wonderful cures with it in the late plague there, wherein died 20,000 in one day." And again, "An experienced physician, who has long studied the doctrine of antidotes against all sorts of poisons and infection, has arrived to such skill as may, with God's blessing, direct persons how to prevent their being touched by any contagious distemper whatever. He directs the poor gratis."

The direction was, of course, that the poor must buy the physician's secret medicine, naturally at a price few could afford.

After the plague victims in a particular house had died or recovered, there was the problem of disinfecting the dwelling. The recipe of an anonymous physician from an earlier London plague advised the tenants to "take large Oynions, pale them and lay three or foure of them upon the ground, let them lie ten daies, those picled Oynions will gather all the infection into them that is in one of those Roomes, but burie those Oynions afterwards deep in the ground."

On a larger scale, when an epidemic passed from a city, there was often disagreement as to why the disease had ended. In the London plague of 1625, a series of general fasts were proclaimed in hope of lifting God's scourging hand from the city. As one clergyman pointed out, the plague disappeared after the seventh general fast, just as the walls of Jericho had fallen after the seventh blast of the trumpet. However, others noted that the disease began to abate only after a proclamation banning the Jesuits.

Another cultural monument to plague is sometimes said to be the well-known nursery rhyme

> Ring a ring of rosies,
> Pocket full of posies,
> Achoo, Achoo,
> All fall down.

The verse allegedly describes the habit of wearing garlands of flowers in plague time, to ward off miasma. The last lines suggest that the effort was in vain and plague-slain people, gasping their last, all fell down. The verse only appeared in Mother Goose in 1881, however; an earlier version deals with an ancient corn spirit instead of the spirit of plague.[3]

On the other hand, the legend of the Pied Piper of Hamelin (Hameln) may be a plague story in disguise.[4] Plague ravaged the German town in 1348 and probably again in 1361, at a time when the rat population was rising all over Europe. Dating from the fourteenth century, the story was immortalized in Browning's poem and is depicted in murals adorning the walls of the ratcatcher's house in present-day Hameln. According to the story, the village officials, their town inundated by rats, hired the Pied Piper, whose magic notes charmed the rodents into flinging themselves into the River Weser. Then, when the mayor refused to pay the price agreed upon, the Piper piped another tune, and, enchanted, the village children frolicked behind him until an immense door opened in the side of Koppelberg Hill into which the Piper and children vanished, never to be seen again.

Perhaps the reality was only slightly different. An army of rats invaded Hameln. The town corporation hired an itinerant ratcatcher, gaily dressed, by way of advertisement; shortly afterward the rats began to die. The ratcatcher demanded his fee, the corporation offered a pittance, and the ratcatcher angrily departed, swearing revenge. Meanwhile, the children of the town busily gathered the rat corpses that littered the crooked streets and threw them into the swift-flowing Weser. Then the children, exposed to the plague that had killed the rats, began themselves to die. Finally, the bodies of the young victims were interred in a new cemetery dug on the side of Koppelberg Hill.

It's an interesting story. It may even be true.

The destruction of Sennacherib's army, as described in 2 Kings 19:35 and in Lord Byron's lilting poem, may be a plague story, too, although the evidence for this is even flimsier than for the Pied Piper legend.

Another kind of plague memorial was the unfinished cathedral of Siena. There are many such monuments to the Black Death across Europe, among them the plague columns. One of the best known is in the Viennese street called the Graben. At its beginning, Vienna was a Roman fortress built to defend the Danube from the eastern barbarians. Sixteen centuries later it still played that role. While beset with plague, the city was besieged by the Turks. The Austrian emperor Leopold I led his people through these twin catastrophes and, in 1687, raised a baroque monument to commemorate the city's deliverance from plague. The column is crowned with figures of the Father and the Son and a dove representing the Holy Ghost. Below that are clouds, multitudes of angels, and still lower down a figure of Leopold praying to the Trinity above him to save his people from the pestilence. On the lowest tier of this incredible pyramid, the figure of a woman holds the cross over the prostrate figure of an old hag, symbolizing the victory of faith over the plague. The old hag presumably represents the Viennese Plague Maiden prematurely aged by defeat. Unfortunately she was restored to girlish vigor all too soon.

The Brotherhood of the Holy Trinity, whose influence is reflected in the Viennese plague column, was founded in Austria in the middle of the seventeenth century to minister to the plague-stricken and to promote worship of the Trinity. But it is the growing influence of the Jesuits, the "shock troops" of the Counter-Reformation, that is apparent in later plague columns scattered throughout Austria and Bavaria. The Jesuits' patron saint was the Virgin Mary. She appears at the bottom of the earlier columns; later she is floating halfway up; and finally the Virgin is on top of the column, while the Trinity is relegated to the bottom or sometimes banished altogether.

The villagers of Oberammergau tried another tactic against plague. They vowed to present a religious performance at intervals forever if the dread hand of the pestilence was lifted from them. It was. The Passion Play, first given in 1634, is still performed in Oberammergau today.

One of the few defenses against plague in the fourteenth century was imposed isolation of travelers or ships coming from plague regions. On July 7, 1377, the Great Council of the Republic of Ragusa (now the Yugoslavian city of Dubrovnik) voted to require all persons from an infected area to remain at one of two stations distant from the city for a period of thirty days. Later the time was extended to forty days, or *quaranta giorni*, from which comes our modern word *quarantine*.

Why forty days? It may have been taken from the period of Christ's sufferings in the wilderness. More likely, it reflects the Jewish laws (Lev. 12–15) requiring a forty-day period of ritual cleansing following the handling of corpses or other things considered unclean.

Quarantine was always controversial. The shutting up of infected people in their houses during the Great Plague of London drew strong criticism from both William Boghurst and Dr. Nathaniel Hodges. Boghurst wrote, "As soon as any house is infected all the sound people should be had out of it, and not shut up therein to be murdered." Dr. Hodges concurred: "I verily believe that many who were lost might have now been alive, had not the tragical mark on the door drove proper assistance from them." The "tragical mark" was a red cross and the words "May God have mercy on us."

An anonymous tract put it even more strongly: "This shutting up would breed a Plague even if there were none. Infection may have killed its thousands but shutting up hath killed its ten thousands."

The event that led Defoe to write his *Journal of the Plague Year* was the epidemic that began in Marseilles in the spring of 1720. The origins of the infection illustrate the weakness of quarantine as well as the usual search for scapegoats in time of plague.

The ship *Great St. Antoine*, Captain Chataud commanding, had sailed from Port Said bearing cotton, muslin, and silk. Plague broke out in Syria while the ship was at sea, and she may have touched at other infected ports on her way to Marseilles. Captain Chataud attempted to anchor in the harbor of Cagliari, on the island of Sardinia, but his ship was driven away by the port authorities. She sailed on to the northern Italian port of Leghorn. By then the ship's surgeon, six of the crew, and a Turkish passenger were dead of plague. Later, with a new surgeon, the *Great St. Antoine* sailed on to Marseilles and doom.

On May 25, 1720, Captain Chataud anchored his vessel in

the harbor of Marseilles. He pointed out to the port authorities that seven deaths had occurred under suspicious circumstances. What happened then is incomprehensible. The ship should have been ordered to quarantine at the isolated Ile de Jarre, to remain there with passengers and crew until the quarantine period had passed. Instead, only routine shore quarantine was required.

A guard was put on the ship, and the passengers, crew, and cargo were detained at the Lazaretto on shore, only a short distance from the city. Quarantine was to last fourteen or fifteen days; even this was laxly enforced. The sailors smuggled goods from the ship into the city before they began to die. The cabin boy died. The quarantine guard on the *Great St. Antoine* died. The last cases among the seamen had bubos (swelling of the lymph nodes characteristic of bubonic plague), but the port surgeon refused to diagnose plague. The deaths, he said, were caused by bad food.

Five of the porters who had opened and aired the bales of cotton stored in the Lazaretto died early in July, and the Lazaretto surgeon soon followed. Other ships with dubious papers meanwhile arrived from the Levant and received equally careless treatment. Then the epidemic ignited into the city itself. Before it was over, forty thousand had died in Marseilles, out of a population of about ninety thousand, and as many more perished in the neighboring regions of Provence and Languedoc.

Belatedly, to say the least, the authorities in Marseilles took alarm. The *Great St. Antoine* was burned to the waterline and ignominiously sunk. Her cargo was taken to the quarantine station and burned, and Captain Chataud was arrested and imprisoned in the dungeons of the frightful Chateau d'If, where he remained for years.

Many other failures of quarantine occurred before and after the epidemics in Marseilles. Equally terrifying was the search for scapegoats and the vengeance taken upon them. Scapegoating may have underlain the attack of the Tatars on the Genoese in the Crimea in 1347. English invaders were blamed for the Black Death in France, while the Italians blamed the

French, and the Spanish accused the Portuguese. Lepers were popular targets, but they were few in number.

There were, however, plenty of Jews, and they were nearly everywhere. Sometimes Jews and lepers were linked with a convenient third party. In Languedoc the lepers were accused of poisoning the wells (the usual allegation) after being bribed by the Jews, who were, in turn, said to be in the pay of the king of Grenada.

Usually such convoluted reasoning was unnecessary. The disease of anti-Semitism, that miasma of the mind, was as virulent and irrational as the plague itself. In May 1348, during the Black Death, the Jewish communities in three cities of southern France were exterminated. Aged and newborn, healthy and infirm, men, women, children—all were savagely murdered.

These isolated acts of barbarism acquired a new focus when, during a trial in Chillon, Switzerland, in September 1348, a Jewish physician confessed, after brutal torture, that he and all other members of the Jewish community had poisoned the wells. This "evidence" ignited persecutions all over Europe. Some 60 large and 150 small Jewish communities were wiped out in 350 separate massacres.

The Jews were often said to be in league with Satan, but sometimes he personally took over the necessary administrative work. In Milan, during the severe epidemic of 1630, the French and the English were first accused of poisoning the people. But they were soon upstaged by that old scene-stealer, the devil. His Satanic Majesty was said to have opened an office in the city for the distribution of the poison his minions were spreading. And he had been seen in a coach-and-six driving through the cobbled streets. He was described as a figure of imposing proportions, as one would expect for the spiritual leader of most of the world, with burning eyes and a flaming forehead.

At this level the rumors in Milan were relatively harmless. Then, on the morning of June 1, 1630, one Guglielmo Piazza, a commissioner of health, was making an inspection tour through the city. Taking notes as he went, he dipped his pen in an inkhorn at his belt. Periodically he wiped his ink-stained fingers on the walls of the houses as he passed. He had always done so. But he would not again.[5]

The ignorant women of the neighborhood accused Piazza of smearing the walls of the houses with plague poison. On order of the council he was to be tortured to obtain the truth. He was stripped, his head was shaved, and he was purged. Then the torture began. If Piazza survived three repetitions (degrees) of the ghastly sequence, God had obviously interceded in his behalf. He must be innocent. Stout Piazza's faith sustained him through two rounds of the torturer's repertoire. On the third degree he broke. Yes, he sobbed, he had smeared the houses with the noxious poisons of plague. With another turn of the screw, he implicated the barber Mora as the man from whom he had obtained the deadly paste.

Bewildered Mora yielded to the first application of the tortures and admitted to every crime his torturers suggested. Nor did it end there.

Piazza and Mora were sentenced to death. Death could only have been a welcome release from their sufferings, but it was no simple death. Their flesh was torn with red-hot pincers. Their right hands were cut off, and their bones broken with the wheel. They were afterwards stretched on the wheel for six hours and then burned alive. Their ashes were thrown into the river, their possessions sold, and Mora's house was burned to the ground. A "column of infamy" was erected on its site.

The Milanese were right. The devil had been at work in their city. But not in the way they thought.

3

Portrait
of the Pestilence
as a Young Pandemic

China's Yunnan (now Guang-dong) province is bordered on the south by Burma, Laos, and Vietnam. Plague smoldered among wild rodents in western Yunnan for at least half a century, causing only occasional human cases, a situation like that in western America today.

Then, in the 1850s, a Muslim rebellion erupted in Yunnan, and Chinese troops were sent to suppress it. As usual, innocent civilians became the principal victims of a clash of arms, and, also as usual, plague flourished on the misery of the people. The flight of frightened refugees spread the disease. Yunnan is a mountainous province, and the roads were poor. Slowly plague moved toward the provincial capital (now called K'un-ming) and entered the city in 1866. It then moved lethargically southward, as if unsure of itself and intimidated by the bold talk then fashionable in Berlin and Paris of the "conquest" of infectious disease.

The seaports of South China proved to be efficient exporters of the disease to the hitherto uninfected portions of the globe. The port of Pakhoi (now Pei-hai) in Kwangtung province was stricken in 1882 and again twelve years later, when the disease also arrived in Canton. On January 16, 1894, a missionary physician, Dr. Mary Miles, treated the daughter-in-law of a Chinese general for plague. The peak of the epidemic in Canton was reached in May. By July the disease had passed, leaving behind one hundred thousand dead. Many of the terrified citizens of Canton had fled meanwhile to Hong Kong, some 90 miles (150 kilometers) away. By May the disease has invaded that great port. Eventually nearly a hundred thousand died.

Farther west, in India, plague was no stranger. There had been regular epidemics between the eleventh and seventeenth centuries, and occasional outbreaks thereafter. Bombay, free of plague for two hundred years, was the next great port to be infected after Hong Kong. In late summer of 1896, the disease appeared in an area near the Bombay docks and then spread through the city. In 1896 two thousand plague deaths were recorded in Bombay, eleven thousand the next year, and nearly seventeen thousand the year after that.

The existence of plague in Bombay was first denied and concealed. But the people of the city knew what was happening, and ultimately nearly half of them fled into the interior of India, carrying the disease with them.

Calcutta, on the opposite side of the subcontinent from Bombay, was also affected. On November 3, 1896, a death in Raja Rajbullub Street was reported as caused by "ordinary non-venereal buboes, . . . enlarged glands, fever, bronchitis, and intestinal obstruction." The report might more simply have said plague, for that was what it was. Nor was it the first case. There had been ten more in the preceding year, retroactively admitted and conveniently blamed on the British soldiers of the Shropshire regiment that had been transferred to Calcutta from plague-ridden Hong Kong. No cases were acknowledged as plague in 1896; only eleven were recorded the next year. Then, in quick succession, the tolls rose from two thousand to between seven and eight thousand, where the yearly plague deaths in Calcutta remained for all but one of the first five years of this century.

The apparent death rates of confirmed plague victims in Indian cities were appallingly high, over 80 percent, while the number of plague cases reported was falsely low. Deaths due to confirmed plague took place most often in plague hospitals to which sufferers were taken only when they were terminally ill and too weak to resist. These hospitals had an unsavory reputation, and the people avoided them except as a last resort. The approximately equal number of plague victims who recovered unaided never appeared on the doorstep of the plague hospitals, and most of these cases were probably never reported.

In rural India the situation resembled that of London three centuries before. As Defoe had written, "They died in heaps and were buried in heaps," and no very accurate account was made.

The Third Pandemic continued to spread over the world. Thailand was infected by a plague ship in 1904, as was Burma the year after. Egypt, free of the disease for nearly fifty years, reported plague in 1899. Tunisia had been free of plague for even longer—eighty-five years—before the pestilence was reintroduced in 1907. The large island of Madagascar off the east coast of Africa had apparently never had the disease. Then, in November 1898, a ship from India laden with rice brought both rice and plague. There have been deaths from plague on the island every year since.[1]

Clearly a plague outbreak anywhere in the world is a potential menace to everyone, everywhere. It was unequivocally demonstrated in the last century when steamships carried the disease. It is even truer in the days of jet aircraft.

Plague also journeyed eastward from the Orient, and, like many a traveler before it, stopped in Hawaii before continuing on to the New World. Two ships from Hong Kong arrived in Honolulu in November 1899, both carrying human plague.

On Tuesday, December 12, 1899, Dr. George Herbert of Honolulu was called in to see a seriously ill patient who subsequently died. Dr. Herbert suspected plague; the diagnosis was subsequently confirmed. Four other deaths in early December were attributed to plague; three were bacteriologically confirmed.

Because most of the victims were Chinese, authorities ordered a *cordon sanitaire* around Chinatown and a house-by-house search for other victims. Buildings where plague occurred were burned, and strict quarantine was instituted. Steerage passengers were refused space on ships going to the continental United States, and one liner would accept only first-class passengers. No Asiatic passengers, baggage, or freight were shipped for several months. Some ships even refused to carry mail.

On December 19, the official quarantine against Chinatown was lifted, and three days later, Honolulu was declared "free of plague." Unfortunately, the disease has never shown much respect for official pronouncements. An average of one plague death in the "plague-free" city occurred on each of the last eight days of 1899. Drastic measures were employed, and the authorities began to move people out of Chinatown into detention camps. But, by the beginning of the third week in January, there had been forty-four cases and thirty-six deaths, three-fourths of them in the new year and in a "plague-free" city. Then, on January 20, the burning of an infected house in Chinatown got out of control, and a major part of the quarter was destroyed. Some five thousand persons lost their homes and possessions. Nevertheless the epidemic continued for several more months, ending only on March 31 after a total of seventy-one cases and sixty-one deaths.

An interesting feature of the Honolulu epidemic was that rats were suspected of a role in the disease. Years ahead of its time, the suspicion perhaps reflected the large Oriental population of Honolulu, whose folklore implicated the rat in plague transmission. As the *Maui News* put it near the end of the epidemic, "There seems but one thing left to Honolulu, in order to rid herself of plague, and that is to rid herself of rats . . . as long as sick rats are left to run along the telephone wires from one end of Honolulu to the other, just so long will the yellow flag [of quarantine] fly on her housetops."

But the epidemic continued. Human cases appeared at regular intervals in Oahu and later spread to all the other Hawaiian islands. On Maui, too, the earliest victims were Asiatics, and the result was the enforced depopulation of Chinatown and the destruction of the infected areas by fire—thus forcing rats to migrate into previously uninfected regions.

To make matters worse, plague continued to reenter the islands by ship. On June 10, 1899, a soon-to-be famous plague ship, the S.S. *Nippon Maru,* arrived in Honolulu with two human cases and three infected rats.

In the New World, South America was struck first. Plague was carried far inland on an infected steamer that landed at Asunción, Paraguay, in April 1899. The disease then spread back down the Paràna River, reaching Buenos Aires, Argentina, by the end of the year. Plague-infected ships steamed into harbors in Trinidad, Venezuela, Peru, and Ecuador during 1908. Bolivia and Brazil were infected somewhat later. The first permanent plague focus outside of Asia and Africa had been created; parts of it are slowly enlarging even today.

Completing the circle of the globe, South Africa was infected in a roundabout way. Because of the Boer War, forage was imported into South Africa from plague-infested ports of South America, and plague came with it. The railroads did the rest.

Plague also hit "down under," when the citizens of Sydney, Australia, received an unusual Valentine in 1900: plague-infected rats. During the next five years the island continent had about fifteen hundred plague cases, all in eleven towns and cities on the eastern coast. One of these outbreaks occurred in the small port city of Maryborough, some 170 miles (270 kilometers) north of Brisbane.[2]

Wednesday, May 24, 1905, was Empire Day. Dr. Crawford Robertson of Maryborough received a call to attend a sick child at the home of Richard O'Connell, whose wife had died a year and a half before, leaving him with seven children, ranging in age from three to eighteen. Such a responsibility would have been a burden for a man of substance and position. Richard O'Connell, an alcoholic waterfront laborer, had neither.

The O'Connell home was a pigsty. The children depended for food and clothing on neighbors' charity and on what they could scavenge from ships and from garbage cans. The playground for the younger O'Connells was an open sewer that led into the river.

When Dr. Robertson arrived at the O'Connell home, he found his seventeen-year-old patient lying on a makeshift bed of bags. The bags had been discarded a month before by a freighter from Hong Kong and then brought home by the elder O'Connell and put on the children's beds.

John had been severely ill for five days. He had a high fever, pain in his chest and abdomen, and a blinding headache. He was vomiting and coughing up large quantities of watery sputum onto the bed and the floor around it.

What Dr. Robertson did while in the O'Connell home is unclear. What he did not do is clear enough. He did not arrange for the immediate admission of the desperately ill boy to the hospital.

At 3:45 the next morning, one of the O'Connell children knocked on the door of the Edwardses' home across the street to plead for help. Mrs. Edwards dressed quickly and went to do what she could. She stayed with John, trying to clean up both the boy and his surroundings until he died, just ninety minutes later. Then, with the help of a family friend who was never identified, Mrs. Edwards laid out the boy's body for burial.

The medical establishment of Maryborough continued not to distinguish itself. The boy's father could not afford a funeral. Incredibly, his son's body lay in the bed where he died for a day and a half before the Health Department of Maryborough arranged for burial. During this time other children shared the bed with their brother's corpse. There was nowhere else to sleep.

The following Sunday, five days after the first call, Dr. Robertson returned to the O'Connell home to find four of the remaining children ill, a result that might have been avoided if John had been removed to the hospital, and the children from the house, after Dr. Robertson's first visit. James O'Connell, fifteen, and Ellen, seven, had symptoms as severe as John's; Kate, eighteen, and May, nine, were much less ill.

This time Dr. Robertson arranged for all four sick children to be hospitalized in quarantine. The two remaining siblings, Ritchie, ten, and Johanna, three, were taken in by the family friend who had helped Mrs. Edwards prepare John's body for its belated burial. On this same day Mrs. Edwards became ill.

Plague was, or should have been, suspected. Two people had died of it in Maryborough a year before, and there had been a case in Childers, forty miles away, just two weeks earlier.

On Monday, Mr. O'Connell asked that the two children not yet in the hospital also be admitted.

Wednesday was the eighth day since Dr. Robertson had first been called to the O'Connell home. On that day James O'Connell and his sister Ellen died in the hospital and Mrs. Edwards died in her home. Dr. G. P. Dixon had been called to the Edwards home when Mrs. Edwards first became ill. Knowing the history of the case, he refused to certify the cause of death until a postmortem examination could be done—and government officials were notified of the probable presence of plague.

Here the Maryborough drama took another amazing turn. When the government medical officer and Dr. Dixon assembled to do the autopsy, they found that Mrs. Edwards had already been buried. Permission for a postmortem examination had been refused, presumbly by her husband, and the sexton of the church had illegally permitted burial to take place without a death certificate.

The next day ten-year-old Ritchie O'Connell died, the fourth death in the O'Connell family. On that same day, Dr. Baxter Tyrie, a plague specialist from the Australian government, arrived in Maryborough. An autopsy was immediately carried out on Ritchie O'Connell, and tissue samples were sent to the government laboratory in Brisbane.

The following day, Saturday, June 3, eleven days after Dr. Robertson had first attended John O'Connell, Johanna, John's younger sister, died. An autopsy was performed on her with the same result as on her older brother Ritchie—no evidence of buboes (swollen lymph nodes) but severe lung involvement.

Dr. Tyrie, meanwhile, inspected the O'Connell dwelling. His verdict was immediate: whether plague was involved or not, the O'Connell house must be burned down. The time set was 3:00 P.M. Saturday. With five of the O'Connell children and the Good Samaritan, Mrs. Edwards, dead in the short space of eleven days, the Maryborough incident was in need of comic relief. The burning of the O'Connell house provided it.

Spectators began to assemble at noon; by the appointed hour it seemed as if the entire community were there. Precisely at 3:00 P.M. the superintendent of the fire brigade solemnly advanced on the house, followed by a fireman with a lighted torch. Mr. Rhule, the superintendent, opened a window, threw in two bags of wood shavings, a bucketful of kerosene, and then the burning torch. The room burst into flame and burned brightly for a few minutes, but the flames guttered out. Consternation! True, the fire brigade was trained to put out fires, not start them. And the O'Connell house, although it had fallen on evil days, had been built by careful Australian craftsmen in the days when careful craftsmen still existed. But it was humiliating just the same.

After a conference, the firemen repeated the procedure at another window. A lovely blaze ensued. And died just as quickly as the first. Finally, firewood was piled up against a corner of the house, shavings and kerosene were added and the pile set alight. This time the stalwarts of the fire brigade were successful; the little home on the corner of Pallas and Sussex streets burned to the ground. The comedy was over.

Cecilia Elizabeth Bauer, a nurse at Maryborough General Hospital, was on holiday at her home in Blackmount during the early period of the Maryborough tragedy. A handsome, black-haired, and buxom girl of twenty-two, looking forward to marriage, she received a letter from the medical superintendent asking that she return to help during this terrible time. Her family tried to dissuade her. They feared the unknown illness wreaking such havoc in Maryborough, but they knew better than to express such fears to Cecilia. Instead, they stressed how much remained to be done in preparation for her wedding. Nevertheless Cecilia Bauer returned to duty as the night nurse in charge of the ward where the O'Connell children lay. On the day Johanna O'Connell died, on the day the O'Connell home was burned, on that day Cecilia Bauer fell desperately ill with the now familiar symptoms.

Two days later, another nurse who had ministered to the O'Connell children also fell sick.

Monday, June 5, was the thirteenth day of the Maryborough epidemic, and two nurses specially trained in the care of plague victims arrived in Maryborough. They had received antiplague serum before coming to Maryborough, and they continued to receive it during their stay there. None of the Maryborough nurses ever received the serum. The antiplague serum was of minimal effectiveness in any case, but the Maryborough nurses should have had the option of receiving it.

The next day, Nurse Cecilia Elizabeth Bauer died, the seventh victim of the as-yet undiagnosed Maryborough disease. The day she died the report came from Brisbane, four and a half days after the specimens had been sent: the Maryborough sickness was the dreaded pneumonic plague, the most difficult of the several varieties of plague to diagnose and cure and the only highly contagious form. Six days later it claimed its last Australian victim, Nurse Rose Adelaide Wiles, age twenty-eight, who had become ill the day after Nurse Bauer.

When the two nurses were to be buried, the same sexton who had previously allowed Mrs. Edwards to be interred without a death certificate now insisted that the two bodies be buried far away from the other graves. Although the Wileses had a family plot in the cemetary, Nurse Wiles could not be buried there. The suddenly zealous sexton also demanded that the graves be dug half again as deep as usual and that lime be scattered beneath, around, and on the coffins. But the nurses' graves at least had headstones. The five forlorn mounds marking the last resting place of the O'Connell children were marked only with numbered iron pegs.

It later emerged that the Maryborough General Hospital carried life insurance policies on its staff physicians who could certainly have afforded their own. The poorly paid nurses had none. A plaque in their honor was erected in the hospital, however, and is there still.

One question remains unanswered and unanswerable. Where did plague come from? There were no reports of dead rats on the wharves or elsewhere. There were no other cases in Maryborough, then or later. The most reasonable explanation centers on the discarded bags that O'Connell had brought home for his children's beds. The bags on John's bed must have contained a plague-bearing flea or fleas. John developed secondary pneumonic plague, as do a certain percentage of plague victims after they are bitten by an infected flea—especially if they are ineffectually treated—and thus began the chain of infections that led to the deaths of eight persons.

So ended the only outbreak of pneumonic plague on Australian soil, merely an incident in the infamous history of plague—only eight deaths. Still, up to now, we have spoken just of numbers, a hundred here, a hundred times a hundred there, a million somewhere else. But the victims of plague are people, not numbers. Perhaps a detailed account of one small episode will help to give the greater numbers their true human perspective.

4

Plague
Discovers America

On Tuesday, June 27, 1899, the S. S. *Nippon Maru* sailed through
the Golden Gate, ending a voyage from Hong Kong via Honolulu. She was to play a central role in a bizzare little drama,
prelude to a far greater one.[1]

Two cases of plague had occurred on board *Nippon Maru*
after leaving China, and she carried plague-infected rats on
arrival in Honolulu seventeen days later. Thus, although no
passengers were ill, the ship was quarantined in San Francisco.
On inspection of the vessel, officials discovered eleven Japanese stowaways. The next day, when the crew moved to the
quarantine station on Angel Island, two of the stowaways were
missing. Their corpses, wearing life preservers from *Nippon
Maru*, were later fished from the bay. Both sodden cadavers
contained plague bacilli.

This macabre incident led to no demonstrable spread of the
disease, ashore or afloat, although infected rats from the ship
may have been the tinder that ignited the epidemic in San
Francisco nine months later.

On Tuesday, March 6, 1900, the body of a Chinese man was
carried from the basement of the Globe Hotel at 1001 Dupont
Street (now Grant Avenue) in the heart of Chinatown. Since

the death was unattended, an autopsy was required. The physician who performed it noted the great swellings in the victim's groin and reported his suspicions of plague to the city health officer. Dr. W. H. Kellogg, bacteriologist for the San Francisco Board of Health, found organisms in the body resembling those of plague.

Thus began, on the thirty-fifth day of the Chinese Year of the Rat, the incredible story of the first plague epidemic in the United States. It was one of the most scandalous events in the history of U.S. public health.

Dr. J. J. Kinyoun was the federal quarantine officer for San Francisco and a qualified expert on plague. Two days after the body was found, he inoculated tissues from the buboes of the dead man into rats, guinea pigs, and a monkey.

The day after the autopsy, the Board of Health, headed by Dr. J. M. Williamson, ordered that the twelve square blocks of Chinatown be cordoned off, and a search began for more corpses among the twenty-five thousand inhabitants of the largely unsanitary and rodent-infested buildings. In Washington, Dr. Walter Wyman, the surgeon general of the Marine Hospital Service (now the U.S. Public Health Service), received a telegram warning of the probable presence of plague, and he suggested control measures in his reply. America's first plague epidemic had, *so far*, been handled with calm and competence.

At the turn of the century, San Francisco was a city dominated by conservative business interests representing the railroad, shipping, and lumber industries. These business leaders greeted with cold fury the suggestion that plague stalked the streets of San Francisco. The newspapers of the city, excepting those of the Hearst chain, launched a vicious and unprincipled attack on every effort to control the epidemic. The *San Francisco Bulletin* ridiculed Dr. Kinyoun in bad verse:

> Have you heard of the deadly bacillus,
> Scourge of a populous land,
> Bacillus that threatens to kill us,
> When found in a Chinaman's gland?

Then, some lines later, referring to the inoculated animals:

> Well, the monkey is living and thriving,
> The guinea pigs seem to be well,
> And the Health Board is vainly contriving,
> Excuses for having raised the deuce.

It was execrable poetry and worse science. Within two days, one rat and two guinea pigs had died and the monkey had become seriously ill. Autopsy of the animals and bacteriological studies confirmed plague.

But the political pressure was unrelenting, and the quarantine of Chinatown was lifted after sixty hours. Guards were then placed at exits from the city to examine people (especially Chinese) attempting to leave. Further house-to-house inspection of Chinatown was ordered, along with cleansing and disinfection of unsanitary premises.

The choosing of sides continued. The *Occidental Medical Journal* (called the *Accidental Medical Journal* by its detractors) supported the Board of Health, as did San Francisco's Mayor James D. Phelan. The *Pacific Medical and Surgical Journal* supported most of the newspapers.

After the death of the inoculated animals (the monkey died two days after the smaller creatures), Mayor Phelan asked the leaders of the Chinese community to cooperate in the anti-plague drive. They refused, and the bodies of Chinese dead were hidden from the inspectors. Nevertheless, the remains of two more plague victims were found.

On Wednesday, March 21, an Associated Press dispatch picked up from the Hearst papers told the world that plague threatened San Francisco. The next day, Dr. Williamson, speaking as an individual, declared that plague existed in Chinatown, that local newspapers were suppressing the news, and that the Chinese were concealing cases of the disease.

On April Fool's Day, 1900, Texas instituted quarantine measures against goods and persons from California. New cases continued to be discovered. On May 17, the Editors' Association, the San Francisco Board of Health, and (briefly) the Merchants' Association accepted most of the recommendations for combating the epidemic that were suggested by Surgeon General Wyman. Two days later, the San Francisco Board of Health officially announced that the disease was present in the city. It was five weeks after the first case of plague had been bacteriologically confirmed. The house-to-house searches began again. This time the resistance of the Chinese was palpable. Shops and houses were locked, and access to them was impossible for several days.

On May 21, Wyman asked President William McKinley for authority to pass antiplague regulations. It was granted. Wyman promptly proposed steps that, although generally sensible, were unconstitutional in part. One rule prohibited transport on trains, streetcars, and ferries of Orientals or "members of other races particularly susceptible to the disease."

Along with its other distinctions, San Francisco was a hotbed of anti-Chinese feeling, of which the residents of Chinatown were painfully aware. When possible, they kept to themselves and let the leaders of the Chinese Six Companies speak for them to the white community.

On Thursday, May 24, the secretary of the Six Companies sought a restraining order against the federal government, and four days later, it was granted by Judge William W. Morrow of the U.S. Circuit Court. He ruled that only the city Board of Supervisors had power to restrict movement within the city. That same day, Colorado instituted a quarantine against California.

That evening, the Board of Supervisors grasped the nettle and established a cordon around Chinatown. The California Board of Health approved (in a move that was to be its undoing) and asked Governor Henry T. Gage for help. His reply set the pattern for the subsequent behavior of this incredible man— Governor Gage declined to aid or to cooperate with the authorities of San Francisco in any aspect of the antiplague campaign.

The struggle went on. The city Board of Health planned to remove the Chinese to detention camps at the Angel Island quarantine station and to demolish Chinatown. On June 7,

Judge Morrow ruled that such plans were illegal, and a week later, he ordered that the quarantine of Chinatown be lifted.

The Neanderthals among the conservatives still took the position that plague did not exist if they said it didn't, and they sent their champion, Governor Gage, into the lists to joust against reality. He somehow made an investigation without consulting the available evidence and concluded that "plague did not nor ever did exist in California." He then sacked the three members of the state Board of Health, including the state bacteriologist, who kept insisting that the Black Death was indeed black and living in San Francisco, replacing them with new members who were prepared to swear that it was white and that it did not exist—at least not in California.

Dr. Williamson soon found out the truth of the well-known observation that courage and honesty are often political liabilities. The San Francisco Board of Health, of which he was head, soon found its budget so shriveled that its biennial report could not be published, and some of its inspectors had to work without pay. Gage's new state Board of Health failed even to mention plague in its 1900–1902 report, although by June 1901 there had been sixty-one deaths from the disease and probably an equal number of unreported cases.

The polarization of opinion was complete even earlier. Governor Gage, in his 1901 message to the legislature on Monday, January 7, condemned "the plague scare." He then made the absurd allegation that the plague bacillus had been isolated by Dr. Kinyoun, not from victims of the disease, but from imported cultures. The governor clearly believed that anything worth doing was worth doing well. Since he had already made a fool of himself, he went on to propose that the transportation of plague cultures without permission (presumably his) should be made a crime punishable by life imprisonment and that it be made a felony to broadcast the presence of plague!

The lines were distinctly drawn. The city Board of Health and most of the city government admitted the existence of the disease, as did much of California's medical profession, especially those in the university medical schools, along with the San Francisco Medical Society and the U.S. Marine Hospital Service.

On the other side, the governor, the reconstituted state Board of Health, the Merchants' Association, most San Francisco newspapers and residents, the Chinese, and the railroad and shipping interests denied that plague existed in California, as did the San Francisco Clinical Society. The latter organization was a group of physicians who had strongly supported the governor at the time of his election. They subsequently agreed that plague could not possibly be in San Francisco since an infected ship could not reach the Golden Gate without having a human case on board, and this had not happened. The case of *Nippon Maru* and its plague-infected stowaways was conveniently forgotten.

The conflict had to be resolved at a level above that of the state government. On January 19, 1901, Secretary of the Treasury L. J. Gage (no relation to the governor) appointed a commission of experts to resolve the question of whether plague existed in San Francisco. The commission consisted of Professors Simon Flexner and L. F. Barker, formerly colleagues at the Johns Hopkins Hospital, and, as the commission's bacteriologist, Professor F. G. Novy of the University of Michigan. It was an experienced and highly qualified group. They were charged by the surgeon general to keep in close touch with him, to keep their final report secret, and to avoid all unnecessary publicity. By Sunday, January 27, the commission was hard at work in the "City by the Golden Gate."

Surgeon General Wyman was inclined to act with little regard for the sensibilities (and sometimes the rights) of others. He did not tell Governor Gage about the commission, but the governor soon heard about it from California's Senator George C. Perkins and immediately wired President McKinley politely expressing his displeasure. Other telegrams from Sacramento were to follow.

Doctors Flexner, Barker, and Novy met with Mayor Phelan and the Board of Health on January 29 and were offered a laboratory in the Department of Pathology of the University of California's medical department. That same day they requested an appointment with Governor Gage to pay their respects, but the meeting was delayed several weeks. Meanwhile, the governor worked diligently to thwart and harass the commission.

On January 31 a bill was introduced into the legislature, at Governor Gage's behest, to stop the work of the commission, but it failed to pass. Undaunted, the governor forced the University of California to evict the commission from the laboratory made available to them. The San Francisco Board of Health then gave them a small room, from which they continued their work, supplementing studies there with interviews at the Occidental Hotel where they lived.

Belatedly, some of the more astute businessmen of the Bay Area began to have a change of heart. It was becoming clear to them that it was in their best interest to have the matter of plague cleared up once and for all. One by one, they trooped to the Occidental Hotel to pledge the commission their support. The word quickly reached Sacramento. Among the first results was the rejection of Gage's bill directed against the Flexner commission.

The governor and the commission went on as before. Gage wired the president and then the Treasury Department, proposing ingenious schemes to protect his own interests and subvert most everyone else's. The commission completed its investigation and wrote its report. Near the end of its labors it met with the governor, apparently amicably, and on March 6 its report arrived at the Treasury Department—exactly one year after the body of the first plague victim had been dragged from the basement of the Globe Hotel.

Beginning on April 8, 1901, Chinatown was cleaned up as never before. Every house in the district, except for those of the well-to-do, which were already clean, was scrubbed from roof peak to basement with strong caustic and then sprayed with mercuric chloride. Household goods were removed and aired for several days, and dark rooms and basements were whitewashed. Houses where plague had appeared were fumigated by exposure to sulfur dioxide fumes for forty-eight hours. Other items were sterilized by either steam or disinfectant. Nearly twelve hundred houses and fourteen thousand rooms received treatment.

Governor Gage, meanwhile, continued to oppose all control measures; he refused to permit inspection of other cities where the disease might exist; and he stated publicly that the disease in San Francisco was "syphilitic septicemia found in the Chinese." The misdiagnosis of plague as venereal disease when it occurs in despised minorities was to become an American tradition.

San Francisco's Mayor Phelan had taken a courageous position based on the evident facts and had thereby infuriated the politically powerful of the city. The bosses sought a more suitable candidate for the upcoming election and found one in the unlikely person of the former first violinist of the San Francisco Orchestra, E. E. Schmitz. Schmitz won the election handily and immediately began to play in harmony with the strange melody wafting over from Sacramento. He started to dismantle the city Board of Health, as Gage had done with the state board, but was blocked by an injunction obtained by Dr. Williamson. Williamson saved the board, of which he was head, but he was powerless to stem a near-fatal hemorrhage in its budget.

The situation changed slowly. In January 1903, retiring Governor Gage, in a farewell speech to the legislature, still denied that plague existed in California. He went on to boast that he had saved the taxpayers' money by using only three hundred pounds of sulfur to disinfect an area that the experts said required two hundred times as much. At this point, deaths from plague stood at ninety-three, and Gage's antics had brought California to the brink of total quarantine by the other states of the Union and the rest of the world.

But reason was returning. California's new governor was George C. Pardee, M.D., Ph.D., a practicing physician and a former member of the Oakland Board of Health. His views were strikingly different from those of his predecessor. On January 19 Governor Pardee said publicly, "Whatever the Marine Hospital Service desires me to do in the way of public health preservation will be done." Three days later he enlarged on his earlier remarks:

> I want to say that I propose to act in complete harmony with the Federal authorities. . . . The medical authorities have emphatically declared that plague has existed and does exist in San Francisco, and that settles it as far as I am concerned. . . . What we want to do is to put an end to the suspicion with which California is regarded outside the State's limits.

Governor Pardee also rid himself of Gage's handpicked state health board. Gage had never bothered to have his nominations ratified by the state senate. Pardee simply withdrew the nominations and appointed a new and vigorous group.

On Sunday, February 29, 1904, a thirty-three-year-old woman died of plague in the town of Concord, California. She was the last victim of the first San Francisco epidemic. There had been 121 cases in the city and 5 elsewhere. Total deaths were 122, an apparent mortality rate of 97 percent. The oldest victim was sixty-two and the youngest four. The bulk of those stricken were between the ages of twenty and fifty, reflecting the age distribution in Chinatown. Only twenty-seven were women.

The sorry tale of America's first plague epidemic had ended. The refusal to admit the existence of plague in the face of overwhelming evidence and the political and economic interference with sound measures to protect the health of the community were old stories elsewhere, but the California epidemic marked their first appearance in America. Unhappily, it was not their last.

5

The Unholy Trinity

In the nineteenth century man lost his fear of God and acquired a fear of microbes.

—Anonymous

As the Third Pandemic began, humanity was no better able to defend itself against plague than at the time of Justinian, thirteen centuries before. The papal physician Gui de Chauliac had described the pneumonic and bubonic forms of the disease as they consecutively attacked Avignon in the spring and summer of 1348:

The mortality . . . lasted seven months. It was of two types. The first lasted two months with continuous fever and spitting of blood, and from this one died in three days. The second lasted for the rest of this period, also with continuous fever but with apposthumes (abscesses) and carbuncles on the external parts, principally on the armpits and groin. From this one dies in five days.

Beyond this, little more was known. The causative agent of the disease was an enigma; the means of transmission, mysterious. But the curtain of impenetrable ignorance was about to lift.

Dr. Shibasaburo Kitasato, a highly skilled microbiologist, had worked for six years in Berlin with the great Robert Koch and with Koch's skillful associate, Emil von Behring. Koch and Pasteur were the founders of modern microbiology. Kitasato was the first to isolate and grow the tetanus bacillus and, with von Behring, had developed a tetanus antitoxin. In 1892, at the age of thirty-eight, he had returned to Japan hoping to head a government laboratory. Now he was asked by the Japanese government to go to Hong Kong to investigate the plague outbreak there.

Kitasato was confident, well trained, and ambitious. He knew that in accord with ancient academic tradition, whatever he had accomplished in Berlin would be largely credited to Koch and von Behring, no matter how great his own contribution. He was anxious now to prove his mettle as an independent investigator, and he knew that immortality awaited the discoverer of the causative agent of plague. On Tuesday, June 5, 1894, he sailed from Japan, accompanied by Dr. T. Aoyama, a pathologist; two assistants; and two medical students. The Japanese team arrived in Hong Kong on June 12 and moved efficiently to assure themselves of material to study by contacting Dr. James A. Lowson, acting superintendent of the Government City Hospital.

At the outset of the Hong Kong epidemic officials set up three plague hospitals. There was a floating hospital for Europeans, a Chinese hospital with Chinese doctors, and Kennedy Town Hospital, a former police station, with English doctors. Dr. Lowson arranged that space and facilities be made available at Kennedy Hospital for the Japanese investigators and directed that all bodies of plague victims be accessible to them. The Japanese team had effectively cornered the market in plague-infected corpses, a valuable scientific resource.

Facilities at Kennedy Town Hospital were hardly palatial. There were no beds and no blankets. The building swarmed with insects, especially at night, and there were no mosquito nets. Mattresses were available only for Indians and Japanese; Chinese patients lay on the bare floor. What it meant for the Japanese team to begin working under these conditions can only be imagined. Dr. Kitasato and many others of the time believed that plague could be spread by mosquitos and flies, both of which were plentiful in and around Kennedy Town

Hospital. But neither the Japanese group nor the English physicians were wanting in courage. In fact, Dr. Aoyama and his assistant did contract plague in Hong Kong, probably while performing autopsies; both recovered.

Kitasato wasted no time. He examined autopsy material on Thursday, June 14, finding numerous bacilli in a groin bubo and in all the organs of the victim. The patient had died some eleven hours earlier, however, and Kitasato doubted that the bacillus he saw was really the cause of plague. Nevertheless, the Hong Kong papers of that day published accounts of Kitasato's discovery of the plague bacillus. Perhaps that was where the trouble started.

On the very next day, Dr. Alexandre E. J. Yersin arrived in Hong Kong by a circuitous route. Of all the great actors in the dramatic struggle against plague, Yersin was the least conventional of an unconventional group and one of the most interesting on a stage crowded with unusual personalities.

In 1883 Kitasato had ended his medical studies at the Tokyo Medical School, and Yersin, a Swiss had begun his in Laussane. Later, Yersin transferred to the medical school in Paris. He subsequently became an assistant to Émile Roux, in Pasteur's laboratory.[1]

At the end of three years in the laboratory, Yersin had a secure and distinguished career ahead of him. His thesis for the medical degree was outstanding, and the work he had done with Roux on diptheria toxin was admired around the world. He was now a citizen of France and, under the aegis of Pasteur and Roux, there was no limit to what he might achieve in science. It was a situation any young scientist might envy.

Instead of eagerly grasping the opportunity presented him, this enigmatic man sailed for Indochina as a ship's doctor and whiled away the long hours at sea learning navigation. Fortunately, Yersin left nearly 1,000 letters to his mother, and these have been recently made available.[2] They offer many important clues. For instance, he often spent his free days on the Normandy coast, and he wrote on September 15, 1889 "I miss the sea. In the stillness of the night I often think I can hear it surging." In Indochina he began a career as an explorer of the central highlands of what is now Vietnam, mapping the villages with his new skills and fighting off severe attacks of malaria and dysentery with his older ones. He wrote his mother from Saigon on August 28, 1891, "You must remember that it has always been my innermost dream to follow in the footsteps of Livingston." Yersin became a member of the French Corps de Santé, and in 1894 his superior in Saigon asked him to go to Hong Kong to investigate the plague epidemic. The corps did not entirely suit Yersin. He had written his mother shortly after entering it, "I have had to don a uniform. . . . What is very annoying is that those with less rank must salute me, and that I must salute all my superiors. . . . I have to constantly avoid getting lost in my own thoughts so as not to pass in front of a colonel or captain without noticing him." Yersin might have welcomed transfer to Hong Kong as a temporary relief from military etiquette.

In contrast to the large Japanese team, Yersin arrived in Hong Kong on June 15 with only a servant. He was given space on an open porch in one of the buildings of the Kennedy Town Hospital but was told that no autopsy material would be available because it was reserved for the Japanese.

Yersin paid a courtesy call on Kitasato, but it was unsatisfactory for both men, so different in so many ways. In the gloom of the autopsy room where they met, Yersin could see that Kitasato looked as much like a German stereotype as was possible for a Japanese. He was short, stocky, and round-faced, with a clipped moustache and hair close-cropped in the Prussian manner. Yersin was slender, with a short, full beard, and piercing eyes. Kitasato was the foremost Japanese microbiologist of his day. Yersin, eleven years younger, had turned his back on just the sort of academic career that Kitasato had espoused, to explore the jungles of Southeast Asia. They had no common language. Had an interpreter been present, the history of the discovery of the plague bacillus might have been different.

After meeting with the Japanese, Yersin set to work as best he could. He finally received permission to build himself a straw hut near a larger straw hut with the imposing name of

Alice Memorial Hospital. By June 20 he still had no official access to human material, but he was determined to examine the buboes of human victims. He wrote in his diary,

> With the help of Father Vigano, I try to persuade some English sailors, whose duty it is to bury the dead from the city and other hospitals, to let me take the buboes from the dead before they are buried. A few dollars conveniently distributed and the promise of a good tip for every case have a striking effect. The bodies before they are carried to the cemetery are deposed for one or two hours in a cellar. They are already in their coffins in a bed of lime.
>
> The coffin is opened. I move the lime to clear the crural (thigh) region. The bubo is exposed, within less than a minute I cut it away and run to my laboratory. . . . I see a real mass of bacilli, all identical. . . . From the bubo I inoculate agar tubes, mice and guinea pigs. . . . My bacillus is most probably that of plague but I am not certain.
>
> June 21 . . . I go on cutting and examining buboes. I always find the same bacillus, extremely abundant. My animals inoculated yesterday are dead and *show the typical plague buboes* [italics added].

On Saturday, August 11, 1894, *The Lancet,* a weekly British medical journal, printed an account of notes the editor had received from Dr. J. A. Lowson. Accompanying the notes were drawings of "the plague bacillus," some done by Kitasato, some made later by Lowson himself. Bacterial cells certainly existed in these preparations in large numbers, but the brief note in *The Lancet* gave few details.

The edition of August 25 was more satisfying. In it was a two-page article by Professor S. Kitasato entitled "The Bacillus of Bubonic Plague," translated into flawless English. Kitasato wrote that the bacilli were found in great numbers in the tissues, buboes, and blood of plague victims. When suspensions of the bacteria, or tissues containing them, were injected into mice, rabbits, or guinea pigs, the animals died at various times according to their size. Then came the three sentences that were to cause so much controversy for the next eighty years. "I am unable at present to say," wrote Kitasato, "*whether or no* Gram's double-staining method can be employed. I shall report upon this on a future occasion. The bacilli *show very little movement . . .*" (italics added). The animals Kitasato injected seldom showed the typical buboes of plague. He went on to describe the bacteria, the history of the disease and its symptoms, and measures to prevent and control it. He concluded, "All that I have described above must be regarded only as a short preliminary notice. The results of extensive study on the subject of the plague bacillus will be published by me at a later time."

Meanwhile, Yersin had sent a note to the *Annales de L'Institut Pasteur* that appeared in the issue of July 30. It described the plague organisms he had found as showing *no movement whatever* and *no coloration by the Gram stain.* The organism was, in other words, gram-negative. A subsequent note, published the following September, gave further details and clear photographs of the organism. He named it *Bacterium pestis*. In 1900 it was renamed *Bacillus pestis*, in 1923, *Pasteurella pestis* and, in 1970, *Yersinia pestis.*

Yersin left Hong Kong on August 3, 1894. Later, he settled in Nha Trang, in what is now Vietnam, and established the second branch of the Pasteur Institute in Indochina. He died and was buried there at the age of eighty, and one of the streets of the city bears his name.

Yersin, physician, explorer, cartographer, and scientist, had written his mother from Saigon in 1891,

> I find great pleasure in taking care of those who come to me for help, but I do not want to make a profession of medicine. That is, I could never ask a sick human being to pay me for the care that I have given him. I consider medicine a ministry, as is the pastorate. To ask for money for treating the sick is a bit like telling them, "Your money or your life."

Kitasato and his colleagues returned to Japan. Professor Kitasato had a long and productive life, becoming a baron in 1924 and dying, at the age of seventy-five, in 1931. The institute he headed is now named for him.

The question of who discovered the plague bacillus raged throughout the lives of both men and continued long after their deaths.[3] A curious split developed. Since Kitasato's results were published in an English-language medical journal of wide circulation, he became, for much of the Western world, the discoverer of the plague bacillus. Yersin's paper in a French research journal was less widely read. Yersin published further work in plague immunization for only two years after leaving Hong Kong, while Kitasato continued to take part in conferences on plague and to publish papers on the subject for another fifteen years. Oddly, Kitasato's Japanese colleagues accepted Yersin as the discoverer of the plague bacillus.

Kitasato stoutly maintained that his organism and the one that Yersin discovered were two different bacteria. His reasons for thinking so were convincing and were accepted by his colleagues in Japan, including Aoyama, who worked with him in Hong Kong.

Kitasato's subsequent research was published almost entirely in Japanese, but in 1901 he and a colleague contributed to an American medical encyclopedia an article that clearly spelled out the difference between the organism he had discovered and what by then was known as *Pasteurella pestis.* Then, two years later, a book by Tohiu Ishigami, Kitasato's student and assistant in Hong Kong, and revised by Kitasato himself, contained this surprising statement: "His [Kitasato's] investigations proved no doubt that the bacillus of bubonic plague is *identical* with the Yersin bacillus . . ." (italics added). Throughout the remainder of a long professional life, Kitasato never explained this change of opinion.

Kitasato undoubtedly saw the plague bacillus intermixed with others and, in his first account, reported on its isolation and partial characterization. Unfortunately, his subsequent work badly confused the issue. Either his cultures were contaminated, or he was studying the wrong organism. Since 1970 the official name of the plague organism has been *Yersinia pestis.*

More than two centuries before, another man with a microscope thought he saw, in the blood of plague victims, the minute worms he believed caused the disease. Dr. Nathaniel

Hodges, the seventeenth-century London physician, was aware of the claim of the contemporary Jesuit priest-scientist, Athanasius Kircher, and since the Great Plague of London provided plenty of material, Hodges, too, looked for the worms but failed to find them. Dr. Hodges was moved to write, "As for the Opinion of the famous Kircher, about animated Worms, I must confess that I never could come at any such Discovery with the Help of the best Glasses . . . but, perhaps in our cloudy Island we are not so sharp-sighted as in the serene Air of Italy." Hodges was right. With the lenses available to Kircher, the priest could not have seen the plague organism. But in a sense, Kircher was right too, because the organisms were there even if neither he nor Hodges could actually see them.

The discovery of the plague organism was an event of immense importance, but it did not answer the question of how the disease was contracted by man or how it spread, although Yersin had made some prescient comments in his Hong Kong diary. On Saturday, June 23, he wrote, "I search and find the organism in the corpses of dead rats and there are many throughout the city. . . ." Later, in a detailed account of his work in Hong Kong, he wrote, "Plague is therefore a contagious and inoculable disease. It is probable that rats are the principal vector [véhicule]." The term *vector* is often used to indicate a disease-carrying agent, such as an animal or insect.

The involvement of rats or mice with plague was mentioned in the Bible. Among the golden offerings of the Philistines to the Lord of Israel, there were images of "the mice that mar the land." Since ancient Hebrew had only a single word for both rats and mice, it is probable that rats were what marred the land during the plague of the Philistines. Similar suggestions of the rat's role in plague appeared in Arab and Byzantine literature before and during the Second Pandemic.

Farther east, folklore had long established the connection between plague in rodents and plague in man. A sacred work, the *Bhagavata Purana*, written in the twelfth century, advised the people of Hindustan to leave their home when rats began falling from the ceilings and dying. In the city of Chaochow (now Ch'ao-an), in China's Yunnan province, a talented young poet, Shih Tao-nan, plaintively expressed in 1792 the relationship between epizootics in rats and epidemics in man. In a poem entitled "Death of Rats," he wrote,

> Few days following the death of rats,
> Men pass away like falling walls.
> Deaths in the day are numberless,
> The heavy sun is covered with somber clouds.

Shortly after completing the poem, Shih himself died of plague.

In 1837 an epidemic of plague in the Pali region of India was accompanied by the death of large numbers of rats, and when Dr. Mary Miles reported in the Canton epidemic of 1894, she mentioned the widespread death of rats in houses of plague victims.

All this collective wisdom of centuries had remarkably little impact on the British authorities responsible for combating the epidemics in Hong Kong and in India in the last years of the nineteenth century. They took the view that *Y. pestis* entered the human body on contaminated food, or through minute cuts on the feet of the barefoot natives. Massive campaigns of disinfection were carried out to destroy the organisms in infected houses and districts. In Bombay, in 1897, fire engines pumped carbolic acid (phenol) solution onto the walls and floors of the houses of plague victims, and millions of gallons of disinfectants were pumped through the sewers each day. The result was to spread the infection even faster, since it dispersed the rats from their normal environment.

The fact that rats died from plague during epidemics was considered in the West to be because rats caught the disease from humans, rather than vice versa, so that the epizootics in rats and the epidemics in man were more or less simultaneous events. The folklore of centuries made it clear that the widespread death of rats preceded epidemics, as Shih Tao-nan had pointed out a century before, but this had no effect on Western majority opinion.

The first scientific link between plague-infected rat and plague-afflicted man was made by another Japanese physician,

Masanori Ogata, while studying the disease on the island of Formosa. Ogata published an article in a German scientific journal in 1897 suggesting that "one should pay attention to insects like fleas for, as the rat becomes cold after death, they leave their host and may transmit the plague virus directly to man." Ogata had also ground up fleas from plague-infected rats and injected the suspension into healthy rats, some of which died with the typical symptoms of bubonic plague.

Meanwhile a rather mysterious figure entered the arena. His work on plague has been justly described as one of the greatest single contributions to our understanding of the disease, yet much about the man himself is obscure. Dr. Paul Louis Simond was French, or at least he wrote in French and published his work in French journals. He had reported on plague in Indochina in 1894; four years later he was in Bombay. He may have been a medical officer, or a former officer in the French navy, since he published his article in plague in Indochina in the *Archives de Médecine Navale*, and one photograph shows him in a bemedaled uniform. Beyond that, he is a shadowy figure sometimes described as a missionary.[4]

The original ideas on plague during this period came from individuals working alone under difficult circumstances. Teams and commissions, of which there were many, contributed very little. Simond worked in a tent in Bombay throughout the monsoon season, with little equipment other than an open mind and a penetrating intelligence. The results of his work appeared in a sixty-two-page article, in which he clearly defined the relationships between human and rat plague and the role of the flea in transmission of the disease. His ideas were ridiculed.

Simond had noted in Indochina the relation between heavy rat mortality and severe plague epidemics in man. He also remembered a particular morning in Bombay when a cotton mill was found littered with the bodies of dead rats. Natives went to work at once picking up the furry corpses. Within three days many of these workers became, themselves, victims of the disease, while those who had not touched the animals remained well.

As the monsoon rains drummed steadily on the roof of his tent, Simond began his experiments. He found that sick rats had more fleas than healthy ones. Then he made the very important discovery that the rat fleas would bite man—an idea completely contrary to prevailing opinion. In some plague victims, the location of the flea bite was evident. From the vesicle marking the bite, plague bacilli could be recovered in the early stage of the infection.

Simond also studied fleas from an infected rat under his microscope and found organisms similar to *Y. pestis* in their digestive tracts. He repeated Ogata's experiment (of which he was probably unaware) by grinding up fleas from an infected rat and injecting the suspension into mice. All the mice died. Simond then put a rat from the home of a plague victim in a large glass jar to which he added fleas taken from cats. When the rat was near death from plague, a small cage containing healthy rat was put into the jar for a day and a half and then removed. Five days later, the healthy rat died of plague. Something must have carried the disease from the sick rat to the healthy one, because they were never in direct contact.

Simond also showed that an animal sick with plague could not transmit the disease to healthy animals if the sick animal did not have fleas.

On the basis of his studies, Simond recommended methods for controlling the spread of plague by ship and other means and studied the administration of antiplague serum to mice as a protective measure. Simond published his monumental sixty-two-page article in the *Annales de L'Institut Pasteur* in October 1898. All (or nearly all) the pieces of the puzzle were there for those discerning enough: the plague bacillus was found in the rat and in the alimentary tract of the rat flea; rat fleas would bite humans, and when such a bite was located early enough, it was found to swarm with plague organisms; plague-infected rats usually infected other rats only if fleas were transferred from the sick to the healthy animals. So must it be also with humans.

Despite Simond's evidence, British officialdom remained unimpressed at best and at worst hostile. It retained its view that *Y. pestis* entered the human body on contaminated food or through minute cuts on the feet of barefoot natives. The British Indian Plague Commission stated in its 1899 report, "There is *absolutely no evidence* that the disease has ever been carried from one country to another by plague-infected rats in ships" (italics added).

The English editor of the Indian Medical Gazette showed his customary astuteness in an editorial written in 1902 in which he described Simond's work as "worthless" and his hypothesis of the role of fleas in the transmission of plague as "completely demolished" by the work of others.

Not everyone was blind. Human plague broke out in Sydney, Australia, in 1900, and a careful investigation of that epidemic wholly verified the ideas of Simond and the earlier ones of Ogata on the roles of rats and their fleas in the transmission of plague.

In the summer of 1905, the new British Commission for the Investigation of Plague in India went to work in Bombay. The senior member was W. Glen Liston, a captain in the Indian Medical Service. The report of the plague commission investigations under Captain Liston's leadership was published in 1908. It completely confirmed and extended Simond's major conclusions of a decade before in such a convincing way that they have never been subsequently questioned. The rat, the flea, and *Y. pestis*, the unholy trinity of urban plague, stood clearly revealed.

Liston had published some of his work on the flea transmission of plague in 1905 in the *Indian Medical Gazette.* His results were nearly identical to those of Simond, with whose work Liston was familiar. But Liston hardly mentioned the older studies.

The following year, the same editor of the *Gazette* who had written so contemptuously of Simond's studies four years earlier, published another remarkable editorial hailing "Captain Liston's rat-flea theory" as a new and epoch-making discovery. Thus was Simond's immense contribution buried for decades by a sort of scientific imperialism. Like Yersin, Simond had published in French and was not considered a great authority on plague at that time. Like Yersin's, Simond's efforts went unrecognized in the West for many years.

Whether properly credited or not, the plague trinity was now unmasked. Plague was caused neither by heavenly arrows nor by miasmas steaming from corpse-sown ground. It was not caused by Jews (or lepers) poisoning the wells or by plague poison smeared on houses by minions of the devil. Tens of thousands of innocent people died horribly because of these superstitions. Yet the unromantic truth was that the disease was caused by a tiny bacillus and spread by fleas and rodents. One could do little against invisible arrows from the bows of avenging angels or against poison clouds, but defense against the vicious bacillus of plague and the creatures that spread it was possible, once each of them was better understood.

6

Plague Ecology:
Rats

Rats!
They fought the dogs and killed the cats,
And bit the babies in the cradles,
And ate the cheeses out of the vats,
And licked the soup from the cook's own ladles.
      —Robert Browning, *The Pied Piper of Hamelin*, 1845

We now know that plague is basically a disease of wild animals. In the vast plague reservoirs, the disease has persisted—for perhaps millions of years in the oldest foci—going through a cycle in which the plague bacillus infects fleas, the fleas infect animal hosts, and both fleas and animals die of plague, sometimes after transmitting the disease to other animals. Occasionally, a few humans become infected—a local epidemic may decimate a village or obliterate a family—but more often the carnage takes place only among the wild rodents and remains remote and unnoticed.

Still less often, sometimes only over the course of centuries, conditions grow ripe for plague to breach the barriers that guard the great cities, and the disease explodes in a densely packed human population. A major factor in transforming the plague of prairie, steppe, and meadow into the plague of cities is the rat.

The great, inexhaustible reservoirs of wild-animal plague seldom involve the rat. The rats that concern us are domestic (better called "commensal") animals, living close to the hu-

63

mans on whom they depend for food and shelter.[1] The term *commensal* literally means that they share our tables. This is figuratively true, although the image evoked may be unpleasant.

The role of the rat in human plague is that of a deadly messenger that carries the disease from infected wild rodents to the human habitat. Clearly, the rat has been effective and efficient, passing the disease over thousands of miles from the great plague foci of central Asia or Africa into India, Southeast Asia, Europe, and, finally, in the Third Pandemic, across the great oceans into the New World.

Two varieties of rat play major roles in the transmission of plague. One is the so-called black rat (which isn't always black) whose scientific name is *Rattus rattus rattus,* or *Rattus rattus* for short. The other is the equally misleadingly named Norway rat, or *Rattus rattus norvegicus.* For simplicity I shall call them the black rat and the Norway rat. Their histories are checkered and controversial.

As befits a phenomenon venerable of age and terrible of aspect, plague has a history in which fact, folklore, and mythology are intimately intertwined. The problem of distinguishing one from the other is sometimes insurmountable. One difficulty is to decide when rats first appeared in Europe. One version holds that the black rat arrived first, borne in the ships of returning Crusaders near the end of the eleventh century. This theory goes on to describe the displacement of black rats by the larger Norway rats some six centuries later. But how did the Plague of Justinian sweep over Europe in the sixth century if there were no rats?

Possibly the disease passed directly from human to human. This may happen with the highly infectious pneumonic plague, which spreads in the same way as does influenza. Another avenue of ratless transmission is by way of the so-called human flea (*Pulex irritans*) that could pass the disease from person to person. The third—and most likely—answer is that there were rats aplenty in Europe by the time of the Plague of Justinian (the First Pandemic) and that the disease moved from rats to humans in the usual way (although the human

flea and direct person-to-person transmission of the pneumonic variety of plague probably contributed as well). To eval-
uate these possibilities we need to know something about the
histories of those infamous creatures, the black and Norway
rats.

Both rodents apparently developed from animals native to
the Malay Peninsula and the Malay Archipelago, as did the
diminutive Polynesian rat, which later spread over the islands
of the Pacific. The warmth-loving black rat then traveled to
India and to the shores of the Mediterranean, while the hardier
Norway rat extended its domain north into China as far as
the Yangtse River.[2]

A subspecies of the black rat has been found in the stomach
of mummified sacred birds of the pharaohs, thus dating its
arrival in Egypt to at least 1000 B.C. By the first century of
the Christian Era, bronze statues of Roman origin clearly resemble both the slender, long-tailed, large-eared black rat and
the very different Norway rat. Thus, both species were probably peering myopically at the Mediterranean at least four
hundred years before the First Pandemic. Considering the vigorous traffic from Rome to the British Isles and the other
farflung outposts of the Roman Empire at the height of Roman
glory, it is reasonable conjecture that both species were as
widely dispersed over Europe as the goods and the soldiers of
Rome. In fact, black rat remains have been found in a filled-
in Roman well in York in the north of England. Roman arti-
facts and radiocarbon dating establish the date as the fourth
century or the fifth at the very latest.[3]

The library of a fifth-century Irish bishop was destroyed by
rats, according to Geraldus Cambrensis, the twelfth-century
Welsh scholar who in 1183 first clearly distinguished between
rats and mice. They were thought earlier to be simply large
and small versions of the same animal. In Ireland the rat was
called the "French mouse" in the same pejorative sense that
the French called syphillis the "Spanish disease" and the English called it the "French disease." Obviously, the French mouse
is no more French than the Norway rat is Norwegian.

It may be that the Norway rat was either rare or largely

wild in Europe and went generally unnoticed until it became commensal in the eighteenth century. This explanation is not as dramatic but is at least as likely as the other theories of its arrival.

One story has it that the Norway rat was introduced into Europe via Copenhagen in 1716, following a visit there of the Russian fleet. Another cites the report of the German naturalist Peter Simon Pallas that great hordes of Norway rats swam the Volga in 1727, signaling the invasion of Europe by that objectionable animal. A contemporary expert points out, however, that Pallas was not born until fourteen years after the event he so dramatically described and that, anyway, the rats were swimming the Volga in the other direction, that is from west to east. As another commentator wrote, "Naturalists persist in asserting that it [the Norway rat] did not reach Europe before the eighteenth century, and give figures purporting to be exact dates of the first arrivals of the brown [Norway] rats in different countries . . . as if they had actually stamped their passports."

This warning is important because a number of theories concerning the withdrawal of plague from Europe in the eighteenth century hinge on the idea that during this time the Norway rat, which was considered not to associate intimately with humans, replaced the black rat, which does. This theory suffers from the fact that plague declined in both central and southern Asia at the same time, in spite of a superabundance of black rats. It also overestimates the shyness of the Norway rat. In the United States it is the Norway rat that is usually involved in the fourteen thousand cases of rat-bite reported annually. This certainly implies as intimate an association of rats with man as one cares to imagine.

In the New World, rats from the colonists' ships almost destroyed the winter grain cache of the Jamestown, Virginia, settlement in 1609. These were probably mostly black rats. And although the arrival of the Norway rat in America is usually given as 1775, it is equally likely that both species arrived in Spanish ships long before. In any event, both were found in every state in the Union by the 1920s and had likely been there for many years. Norway rats are distributed throughout the United States, but the black rat most often exists within several hundred miles of the Pacific and Gulf coasts and along the southern Atlantic coast up to the Chesapeake Bay.

The black and the Norway rat are very different creatures. The smaller black rat is the traditional ship rat. Like the sailors of old, it climbs agilely but abhors water. It prefers moderate to hot climates and food suitable for human consumption. The black rat can run along telephone wires using its long tail to maintain balance, and it may enter buildings this way.

The Norway rat occasionally does the same thing, although it is the weightlifter of the rat world—powerful and thick-bodied, but clumsy and slow compared to its relative. It is an enthusiastic swimmer and eats anything that will let it. The Norway rat lives happily in sewers, in which it enjoys both food and drinking water. In these days of sink garbage-disposal units, the Norway rat dines at the best tables without ever going aboveground. Should it choose to, however, it can enter houses by swimming through the water seals in toilets and floor drains. The Norway rat is the larger and more prolific of the two species, although tales of its "driving out" its smaller relative should be taken with a large grain of salt.

Black and Norway rats do not usually mix. Both rats may inhabit the same building, with the "burrowing" Norway rat in the basement and the "climbing" black rat in the upper floors. Alternatively, one building may be infested with Norway rats, while the one next door is solidly held by black rats. In some parts of Texas, the black rats outnumber their larger relatives nine to one, while elsewhere in the American South, one community is infested with one species, while another town only a few miles away has exclusively the other variety.

In one survey of five hundred larger American cities (population ten thousand or more) 86 percent had Norway rats and 38 percent had black rats. Most cities that had black rats had Norway rats too. Under some circumstances, black and Norway rat get along peaceably together even under the most intimate conditions. Six males of each species will happily live in the same laboratory cage, sleep together in groups (as these gregarious animals usually do), and generally thrive.

It is well known in human society that males get on splendidly together. And so it is with rats. In both societies trouble begins when females are introduced. If six male and six female Norway rats are placed in a cage together, in a few weeks only the females, and the largest male, will survive. The vanquished do not die of wounds, since rats do not usually fight in the human sense, but rather they die of what, for want of a better term, is often called "shock."

As with humans, territorial as well as sexual problems foment murderous conflict. But even when rats compete for territory, food, and females simultaneously, the "victory" of the Norway rats over the smaller animals is seldom absolute. In a laboratory experiment, about one-third of the most aggressive black rats survived in a confined colony with Norway rats even though they were outnumbered nearly five to one and had no safe shelter from the larger animals.

Changes in housekeeping practices following the seventeenth-century plagues probably contributed to the population declines of black rats, since these creatures depend on man for food and, in cold climates, shelter. With reduced competition, the Norway rats flourished. Recently, however, in some parts of the world, the black rat is reconquering lost territory. Modern ratproofing of new buildings reduces access for the Norway rat, while the more agile black rat is less inconvenienced. In any case, the balance between black and Norway rats is more complex than it first appears.

Both the black and the Norway rats have numerous traits in common. Both gnaw incessantly since their incisor teeth grow some five inches (thirteen centimeters) a year. They can penetrate cinder block, unhardened concrete, and lead pipes, causing blackouts, fires, or floods depending on whether the pipe contains electrical wiring, natural gas, or water. Plastic, fiberboard, asbestos, and aluminum siding are easily penetrated.

Both species can squeeze through a hole large enough to admit an adult human forefinger, and the black rat readily climbs trees, any pipe (including smooth glass) it can reach halfway around, or larger pipes, if the surface is rough or if the rat can wedge its body between the pipe and a wall. Both species of rat are immensely prolific, destructive, and murderous. Like some humans, rats kill for pleasure.

For an epizootic to arise there must be a suitably high density of animals; this requires ample food, water (in some form), and adequate nesting places. In the late stages of a rodent population explosion, available harborage becomes intensely crowded, and one condition for an epizootic—overpopulation—is met. Overcrowding is relieved by migration, predation, starvation, or disease. Which mechanism prevails depends on circumstances.

The result of rodent overpopulation most likely to engage man's attention is migration. The lemming swarms in Norway, Greenland, and Canada are familiar. The migrations of rats and mice are less so, but they are not uncommon. In 1903, hordes of rats migrated over several counties of western Illinois. On a single farm that April, some thirty-five hundred were trapped. In South America similar population explosions, called *ratadas,* occur at intervals. In Brazil the interval between *ratadas* is about thirty years; in Chile, fifteen to twenty-five years. In South America *ratadas* are related to the ripening and decay of a dominant species of bamboo. Large quantities of it ripen over a period of a year or two, and the bamboo seeds provide so much food for the rats in the forests that they begin to multiply rapidly. When the bamboo ceases to ripen, armies of hungry rats descend on the cultivated areas, sometimes causing wholesale famine among the human population by consuming or destroying crops.

The same phenomenon occurs in Asia. In 1960 swarms of rats crossed the great Himalayas into the green hills of western Burma and India. For the first time in thirty years the bamboo was in flower, and as had happened thirty years before, myriads of starving rats came out of the eastern jungles. They first devoured the bamboo blossoms and then the peasants' crops. The 1960 plague of rats in Burma and India had another grim and unusual aspect. Of the animals killed by the farmers in a

vain attempt to protect their crops, an enormous proportion
were female. And those that were pregnant had unborn litters
of up to fifteen, twice as large as normal.

Rats continue to plague India. A report on March 5, 1984,
told of rats eating important government documents in New
Delhi consequent to a population explosion in the capital's
rats. Rats continue to destroy 25 million tons of food a year
in India, or approximately $2 billion worth.[4]

Both wild and commensal varieties of mice can also serve
as carriers of plague, and "mouse plagues" (in the sense of
population explosions) have a long history. Swarms of mice
appeared in Alsace at about thirty-year intervals between the
thirteenth and nineteenth centuries. They inundated Germany in 1348 and, again, in even greater numbers, two and a
half centuries later, when they also invaded England. Bavaria
was awash in mice in 1382, as was Poland a quarter-century
after. In 1611 swarms of mice arrived in Afghanistan concurrently with plague. In Ceylon (Sri Lanka) mouse swarms appear about every twelve years to feast on the ripe seeds of a
particular evergeen shrub.

Mice ravaged parts of Australia in 1903 and again in 1917.
So many were killed in 1917 that the corpses were measured
by tons (sixty thousand mice to the ton) rather than counted.
In one town in the state of Victoria during this mouse plague,
6.5 million mice were destroyed in a single night. In another
part of the same region, a six-week campaign netted six hundred tons of dead mice, or twice as many mice as there were
people on the whole continent.

Mouse plagues tend to end suddenly, and the population of
small rodents may even drop to subnormal levels. Infectious
disease is usually responsible. Bacterial or fungal infections,
or a combination of the two, cause mice to die by the millions.
Once a typhus epidemic slashed the swollen population of
Australian mice and caused some human cases as well. It
might have been plague.

In 1939 Australia suffered again, and the infestation was
repeated in 1970, when there was a wheat surplus and weather
favorable for mouse breeding. Barrels filled with water and

bait accumulated as many as a thousand drowned mice in a single night. Drivers reduced their speed to a comparative crawl because on the rippling, slippery carpet of mice that covered the roads, braking might cause an uncontrollable skid.

Such plagues are not unique to Europe or Australia. In the summer of 1968, officials carried out a vigorous antimouse campaign in Monterey County, south of San Francisco, an area with a long history of plague in small rodents and ground squirrels. Six aircraft, directed by radio-equipped spotters on the ground, dropped forty-six thousand pounds (about twenty thousand kilograms) of oats poisoned with zinc sulfide on an estimated population of fourteen million mice, a total number not far below the human population of the whole state. The mouse density averaged two thousand per acre (0.4 hectare). This determined antimouse campaign was carried out not to protect humans but rather the artichoke crop, which was rapidly being turned into mice instead of money.

Both rats and mice have been poisoned, bludgeoned, shot, starved, and cursed for centuries with little effect. The best that most modern cities can do is to keep the rat population within reasonable limits, usually one or two rats for every pair of people (with an equal number of mice), and to try to keep the commensal rodents separate from the wild rodent carriers of plague and from infected animals introduced from elsewhere in various kinds of cargo. The World Health Organization estimates (as of 1979) that the rat population of the world is at least four billion, and it's a reasonable assumption that there are at least as many mice. The smaller creatures worry some experts even more than the more fearsome rats. Dr. William B. Jackson, head of environmental studies at Bowling Green University in Ohio was quoted in the *Los Angeles Times* in October 1979 as saying, "Frankly, I'm more concerned about mice than rats. The rat may be in your basement but the mouse will be in your cereal box. Check those raisins in your cereal!"[5] As John H. Gedeon, a pest control operator trying to deal with Cleveland's burgeoning mouse population put it, "Mice have the greatest public relations man in the world—Mickey Mouse. So, a lot of people tolerate having mice around."[6]

Hardly anyone tolerates rats. In the spring of 1979 a woman in her thirties was attacked by brown rats near a vacant lot two blocks from New York's City Hall. The lot contained an estimated 200 rats. Bystanders helped beat the rodents from her clothing, and she left screaming in a car that picked her up. The lot was cleaned up the next day.[7] In Chicago, a year before, a UPI dispatch told of Bill Henderson, a twenty-four-year-old unemployed mechanic, lying awake in his West Side Chicago apartment with the lights on and a rifle in his hand. He finally shot a rat that got into his baby's crib. The family eventually left the rat-infested apartment and moved into a motel until their money ran out. Then they moved into their 1974 car and left their apartment to the rats.[8]

The rat population of the United States is between one hundred and two hundred million, with six to eight million rats in New York City alone. In an Associated Press report in October 1979, rats were reported swarming around the St. Moritz and Plaza hotels at night after being displaced from their normal habitat in Central Park because of construction.[9]

As of late 1970, in the Anacostia area of the U.S. capital, rats outnumbered people three to one; in Texarkana, which straddles the state line between Texas and Arkansas, there were fifteen rats for each human inhabitant; while in one district of Akron, Ohio, a control program killed an average of seventy-five rats in each dwelling, or about twenty-five rats per person. In 1954 a plague-infected rat was found in Tacoma, Washington; another was found in the Marina district of San Francisco in 1963; and plague-infected fleas appeared in Tacoma in 1971.

The message is simple. Plague-stricken rats and fleas still appear in urban centers, and many urban centers support vast rat populations. We depend, for the prevention of catastrophe, upon approximately equal measures of eternal vigilance and continued good fortune.

7

Plague Ecology:
The Fabulous Flea
and *Yersinia P.*

The rat is a creature unloved and unlovely, but its role in plague rests solely on its efficiency as a vehicle for transporting fleas into close proximity with humans. Fleas, plague-ridden or not, have been annoying man for millenia. As an anonymous poet once complained,

> Their number frights me, not their strength;
> I'd dare the Lion, Panther, Tiger or the Beare
> To an encounter, to be freed from these
> Relentlesse demi-devills, cursed Fleas.

Simond's work in Bombay on the role of fleas in plague transmission was only slowly accepted. One reason was the novelty of his ideas, but a major factor was the lack of information (or worse, the abundance of misinformation) on the habits of fleas.

The best-known plague-carrying insect (but by no means the only one) is the Oriental rat flea, *Xenopsylla cheopis*. As the name suggests, this flea probably originated on the grass rat of the Nile Delta. Then it was transferred to the black and the Norway rats who obligingly spread it around the world.

Adult *X. cheopis* is a very tiny creature—a large specimen

is about the size of an o. It is wingless, flattened laterally, and equipped on one end with an efficient syringe for extracting blood and on the other with a remarkable propulsion apparatus that allows it to leap enormous distances. For a man to make a comparable jump he would have to clear a sixty-story building, and land on his feet three times out of four. In addition to these accomplishments, a flea can walk straight up a vertical sheet of glass for some twenty thousand times its own length, a feat not even the athletic black rat can match.[1]

Under normal conditions X. cheopis lives about three months; a female lays three or four eggs a day during this time. The flea can, however, survive unfed for one to three months, so that under proper conditions it is capable of making long journeys by ship, rail, or plane or surviving the depths of winter in the burrow in which its plague-slain rodent host had died.

Rats and other animals often carry more than one species of flea, and since the adult fleas of dissimilar species do best under different climatic conditions, the density of the various species on a particular rodent changes with season. For example, in Marseilles, the European rat flea reaches a peak on the Norway rat in April, while the Oriental rat flea population peaks in August. This is one of many factors that gives plague its characteristic seasonal dependence in different parts of the world.

Rats differ considerably in the flea infestations they will tolerate. A larger animal has more fleas than a smaller one, and even a small rat has more fleas than a mouse. Most important from the standpoint of plague is that a sick rat is usually more heavily flea-infested than a healthy one. The ominous consequence is that a rat in the late stages of plague has many more fleas than normal, at a time when the concentration of plague bacilli in blood is highest and the fleas are more apt to become infected. This is probably true of wild rodents as well.

Even healthy rats can be heavily infested. In the late 1930s a Norway rat was trapped alive and removed from the basement of a building in San Francisco each day for ten days.

From these ten rats, 1,600 *X. cheopis* were removed, an average of 160 fleas per rat.

As both Simond and Liston found in Bombay, the Oriental rat fleas—contrary to the then-prevailing opinion—takes its dinner where it may. As a general rule, any starving flea will try to feed on any available host. In the case of *X. cheopis*, females elect to eat about half the time when offered a meal on a laboratory rat or guinea pig. If offered dinner on a human they accept about a third of the time, hardly a spectacular decline from the rate on their preferred host. Males are more gluttonous; they accept meals about two times in three from rats and about half the time from man.

In keeping with their catholic tastes and cosmopolitan distribution, Oriental rat fleas are also found on pigs, squirrels, monkeys, rabbits, and occasionally dogs and cats.

It was long part of plague mythology that the Norway rat was a poor host to the Oriental rat flea. This view conveniently dovetailed with the theory that the Norway rat drove the black rat from Europe in the eighteenth century. Since *X. cheopis* would have been driven out with its preferred host, the incidence of human plague should have fallen sharply, which of course it did.

Unfortunately, the facts are that *X. cheopis* infects both Norway and black rats at least equally heavily and may even have a slight preference for the former.

Although Simond convincingly demonstrated the role of the rat flea in the transmission of plague, the question of how this occurred remained unanswered for another eighteen years. Simond thought that since many fleas defecate while feeding, this was the probable route of infection. Feces containing *Y. pestis* would be rubbed into the wound when the bite was scratched. In this case, Simond was wrong, for *X. cheopis* and some other plague-carrying fleas do not defecate when feeding. And although there is some purely mechanical transmission of plague from contamination of a new bite by a tiny drop of dried blood carried on the flea's proboscis from a previous bite of a plague-infected animal, this mode of transmission is only important when large numbers of infected fleas are present.

The most effective mode of plague transmission is much more subtle and complex. It was discovered in 1914 by A. W. Bacot and C. J. Martin, using *X. cheopis* from a colony discovered living in the basement of Guy's Hospital, London.

The scientific name for fleas, *Siphonaptera,* aptly describes them as wingless siphons. When a flea bites, the insect takes in, in a few minutes, an amount of blood equal to its own weight. This blood is pumped through the flea's proboscis, then through a forestomach (called the proventriculus), and finally into the stomach (ventriculus). Once the flow is established, blood siphons from the victim's tissue to the flea's stomach. Should a flea feed again while its stomach is still partially filled, a valve in the proventriculus closes to prevent the stomach contents from being sucked back into the proboscis when the siphoning action is begun.

A terminally ill rat may have more than a *thousand million Y. pestis* in one milliliter (1/30 fluid ounce) of its blood. A flea biting such a rat may suck up half a million plague bacilli, and the flea immediately begins a battle for its own survival against the ingested plague organisms. About a third of the time, *X. cheopis* succeeds in destroying the invading bacteria; other fleas are more often successful.

The Oriental rat flea has a more particular problem that contributes to its unsavory reputation as *the* plague flea. Because of its proventricular structure, some ingested blood tends to remain in this organ rather than proceeding to the stomach. As soon as it finds itself inside the flea, wily *Y. pestis* releases an enzyme that coagulates the blood around it, forming a more or less solid clot that provides a safe and nutritious environment for bacterial growth. On the other hand, the stomach and proventriculus of *X. cheopis* produce another enzyme that dissolves the clots to make them easier to digest. Like feudal barons who have wagered their all on a joust between their champions, the lives of the flea and *Y. pestis* depend on which enzyme prevails in the contest. If the enzyme from the plague bacillus forms the proventricular clots more rapidly than they can be broken down by the flea, the mass of clotted blood blocks the proventicular valve and the flea's life is forfeit. In

X. cheopis, blockage, if it occurs, ordinarily takes place a week or two after the flea has bitten an infected animal.

Although *X. cheopis* is particularly susceptible, blockage of the proventriculus probably occurs in some degree in most fleas after a blood meal from an animal seriously ill with plague. The results for the subsequent transmission of the disease are serious. When a blocked, or partly blocked, flea next attempts to feed, the recoil of its suction apparatus may cause clumps of *Y. pestis* from either the proventriculus or the stomach of the flea to be regurgitated into the host on which the flea is trying to feed. This cannot happen when the proventricular valve is working, but in the blocked flea the proventricular valve cannot close because of the masses of *Y. pestis* and blood obstructing it.

The number of plague bacilli injected into the skin of its host by a blocked flea may be as high as a hundred thousand. Animals as large as monkeys have died from plague following injection of a single plague bacillus.

Fleas require substantial quantities of water, especially in warm, dry weather. The flea's blood meal supplies most of this need. But, if the proventriculus is blocked, the flea can neither drink nor feed. Starving and thirsty, the normally voracious flea tries, ever more desperately, to secure a meal. It bites again and again and may infect the same host in different places. It also remains much longer with its proboscis embedded in the skin of the host while it tries to dislodge the blocking mass of bacteria. All the while it may be pumping legions of *Y. pestis* into its victim. If the block is not cleared, the flea dies. It becomes, like the rat, a victim itself of the disease it transmits.

Other fleas (about a hundred species in all) are also involved in plague transmission. A plague carrier even more efficient than *X. cheopis* is its relative, *X. brasiliensis,* which inhabits the temperate regions of Brazil and of East Africa. The European rat flea, *Nosophyllus fasciatus,* has been widespread in Europe and probably helped spread the epidemics there. It is also usually the predominant rat flea in the northern United States. About one-third as efficient in transmitting plague as

X. cheopis, it may live twice as long, which partly compensates for its lower effectiveness.

The so-called human flea, *Pulex irritans,* is the predominant dog flea in such diverse places as North China and the Navajo reservation of western New Mexico and eastern Arizona. It is also common on deer. Fortunately it is not a very efficient transmitter of plague. The same thing is true of dog and cat fleas, although both are found on rodents. Cats and dogs are more likely to spread plague by bringing wild rodent fleas into contact with man. Of course, a heavy infestation with an inefficient plague transmitter may have the same result as a modest infestation with an efficient one.

The so-called stick-tight flea (*Echidnophaga gallinacea*) commonly exists on ducks, chickens, and other poultry, as well as on rodents, both wild and domestic. A single ground squirrel can carry over a thousand *E. gallinacea,* and these fleas are apparently efficient transmitters of plague.

Both the Oriental and European rat fleas are common in American cities, with the European flea generally dominant in cities north of the latitude of San Francisco, while the Oriental rat flea rules farther south.

The ancient Babylonians ascribed disease to tiny, sometimes invisible, insects that flew about the world bringing sickness and death. Their master was Beelzebub, the Lord of the Flies. For the transmission of plague to humans and other animals the Babylonians were close to the mark.

The third member of the unholy trinity of plague is the causative agent itself, the tiny bacterium now known as *Y. pestis.*[2] The other members of the plague trinity can be replaced. The rat's place can be taken by a chicken or a kitten, a mouse or a marmot. The flea's role as a transmitter of the disease can be assumed by a louse or even a bedbug, or the plague bacillus can spread directly from person to person without the intercession of any other creature. But plague is plague, if and only if *Y. pestis* is present. It is the unique and indispensable element in the disease.[3] The ancestors of *Y. pestis* were the oldest of all living things on earth. Insects and the earliest mammals existed as distinct species no more than about a hundred million years ago, while the oldest fossil bacteria (those of the Figtree formation in South Africa) date back three thousand million years.

Under favorable conditions the cells of *Y. pestis* multiply rapidly to a very high density. A culture of plague bacilli may contain, in a volume of one milliliter, five times as many cells as there are people in the United States. Half a dozen vigorously growing virulent plague bacilli will kill, in a week or ten days, 50 percent of the mice into which they are injected. This dirty half-dozen may multiply to more than seven thousand at the end of the first day inside the unfortunate animal; two days later the total number of plague bacilli may be some hundred million. At this point their miserable host is near to coma and death.

The vicious bacillus of plague is not especially rugged. Moist heat can destroy it, and it is susceptible to powerful disinfectants. Under some conditions, however, it remains alive and virulent (capable of causing disease) for long periods of time.

For example, a pneumonic plague victims coughs and spits continually to rid himself of the fluid gradually filling his lungs. His sputum is a nearly pure culture of *Y. pestis*, teeming with organisms. In tiny, dried particles of such sputum, the plague bacillus may remain alive and dangerous for more than five months. In dried rat feces the organisms survive even longer.

In moist earth the plague organisms remain infective for almost seven months. In infected tissue they live much longer. In Russia, half a century ago, the bodies of seventeen pneumonic plague victims were exhumed a year after burial. Although the bodies had been frozen solid in the depths of the Russian winter, infectious plague bacilli were recovered from six of them. Frozen animal tissue has yielded virulent organisms seven years later. Even after twenty years in refrigerator storage, nearly half the stored cultures of *Y. pestis* still killed guinea pigs within one week of injection.

There are various strains of the plague bacillus, but these different strains, whether isolated from a plague-struck man in Seattle or a stricken marmot in Siberia, are remarkably similar. The virulence, the major bacteriological properties, and the appearance of the organism under the microscope are nearly identical. There are differences, however. Some of these have been known for more than forty years; others are of very recent description. Still others, perhaps the most important of all, remain to be discovered, since the basis of the organism's lethality is not clearly understood.

One variety of Y. *pestis* is highly lethal to mice, but nearly innocuous to guinea pigs. This strain requires the amino acid asparagine for optimum growth. It grows well in mice, which have relatively high levels of asparagine in their blood, but does not grow at all in guinea pigs, whose blood lacks the amino acid. Had researchers assayed this strain for virulence in guinea pigs alone, as is frequently done, it might have been considered harmless—although it is capable of killing both mice and men.

Scientists have also isolated from fatal human cases other strains of the plague bacillus that show little virulence for guinea pigs.

The ferocious bacillus, Y. *pestis*, scourge of fleas, humans, and a great variety of other animals, is a potent foe, although there is nothing about its aspect under the microscope to inspire fear or awe. It is usually ovoid, about twice as long as it is wide, looking, when properly stained, like two black safety pins lying atop one another. The appearance, in the blood or tissues of man or other mammals, of these fattened cylinders with dark bodies at each end is often the first suggestion that the victim has plague.

But the properties so far described tell us nothing of why the plague bacillus is so spectacularly lethal. A survey of some of the more sinister characteristics of Y. *pestis* is in order.

A disease-causing organism is called virulent or pathogenic; the words are interchangeable. Such an organism must have three properties. It must penetrate the defenses of its victim. It must multiply within the victim, and it must derange its host's metabolism. The derangement (or derangements) leads to the symptoms of the disease for which the organism is responsible—anything from the runny nose and congestion caused by the common cold viruses to the prostration and sudden death of septicemic plague, in which the plague bacilli multiply wildly in the blood of their victims.

Some organisms are toxic but not invasive. Some produce symptoms by invading and destroying cells. The plague bacillus is usually both invasive and toxic.

The virulence of *Y. pestis* is measured in several ways, most commonly by determining the number of organisms that kill 50 percent of the animals to which they are administered. The so-called 50 percent lethal dose, or LD_{50}, depends on the species of animal tested, the strain of *Y. pestis*, the route of administration, and the natural resistance of the test animals. It also depends on the conditions under which the plague organisms were cultured before testing.

The yield of *Y. pestis* is highest at moderate temperature, while growth is reduced seven to ten times at human body temperature (98.6°F. or 37.5°C.). However, the virulence of *Y. pestis* is much higher at body temperature. For example, seven plague bacilli of a particular strain will kill fifty percent of the mice into which they are injected if the bacilli are grown at 26°C. Injection of one *Y. pestis*, if grown at 37°C., kills half the inoculated mice.

There are also strains of *Y. pestis* that are infective but not virulent. That is, they invade tissues and organs of the host and multiply to some extent, but they do not cause disease. An animal inoculated with such organisms does not have the symptoms of plague. However, the immune response is called into action. This is the basis of vaccination against plague, which is discussed later.

In reaction to the presence of *Y. pestis* in the tissues, certain body cells begin secreting rather specific proteins called antibodies. These antibodies may "coat" the bacterium and lead to its destruction through cooperation with other blood proteins, or they may facilitate the swallowing and destruction of the invading organisms by the body's defensive cells.

This mechanism has one great drawback: it is slow. Maximum response to a first encounter with plague organisms takes a week or more. Even on a second inoculation with an avirulent strain, several days are needed for maximum response. If antibodies against Y. *pestis* are present in the blood of human or animal, the mammal has some degree of immunity to plague. Since the presence of such antibodies is usually an indication of a comparatively recent exposure to plague, they also are valuable clues in searching for evidence of past disease in wild animals or in humans.

Massive doses of strains of the plague bacillus that cannot successfully invade a healthy animal or multiply within it can kill experimental animals. If the dose is high enough, death comes in a few hours. The corpses of plague victims may have no plague organisms in their liver or spleen, yet these organs show signs of serious damage. The tragic discovery that unborn infants carried by plague-infected women showed the same organ damage as their mothers even though no Y. *pestis* were found in any fetal tissues also suggested that the presence of the plague bacillus in one part of the body could damage tissue in another part from which the bacteria were absent.

These facts have a common explanation. An animal or human dying of plague is being fatally poisoned. The poison is brewed by wily Y. *pestis*.[4]

Most gram-negative pathogenic organisms produce a single toxin. Y. *pestis* makes a second. This toxin is bound loosely to the surface of the plague bacillus and is removed from it simply by washing the organism in dilute salt solution. Because of its location and properties, this substance is known as exotoxin or soluble toxin. It is highly lethal to mice and rats, but much less so for rabbits and monkeys.

The poisons common to Y. *pestis* and other gram-negative bacteria are complex molecules called endotoxins. These are firmly embedded in the bacterial cell wall and are made up of complex sugars and fatty acids (a combination called a lipopolysaccharide). The toxic activity is in the lipid fraction. Endotoxin is released into the surrounding fluid or tissue when Y. *pestis* dies. At high doses it kills mice, guinea pigs, and rabbits. The relative amounts of endotoxin required to kill a mouse or monkey are, however, almost exactly proportional to their respective weights, which is not so with the soluble toxin. Endotoxin is the cause of the spleen, liver, and lymph-node damage seen in man or animals dead of plague. Both toxins presumably play a role in the fatal poisoning characteristic of the disease.

Thus, virulent *Y. pestis* overcomes the defenses of its victims and grows and spreads throughout the body. The vicious bacillus of plague then releases toxins that travel to every part of their host's body, and the unlucky victim may succumb to massive poisoning.

8

Earthquake, Plague,
and Other Stories

At 5:13, Wednesday morning, April 18, 1906, the San Andreas
Fault slipped sideways over a length of 270 miles (430 kilometers). Forty seconds later, San Francisco was a twisted mass
of ruins. Fire followed, fed by gas hissing from wrenched-open
mains. Firemen had no water; the water pipes were shattered
as well. They used sewer water, five hundred gallons of wine
in one place, and finally dynamite to control the flames. Forty-
eight hours later it was over. Twenty-eight thousand buildings
were destroyed; more than a thousand people were dead, at
least thirty were suicides presumably, and quite reasonably,
convinced that it was the end of the world.[1] It was the most
destructive earthquake in North American history.

A year later, the city was still one huge refugee camp with
many inhabitants sunk in filth and squalor. There were over
five thousand stables in the city, many with wooden floors
built directly on the ground and without bins for manure.
Grain was kept in open boxes or in sacks on the floor. Chicken
yards, equally primitive, abounded. Under these conditions,
so did rats, and the climate favored a large flea population.

The refugee camps maintained by the Red Cross were usually in good condition. Speculators, however, seized the chance

to turn misery into money. They built large camps where the only latrines were reeking holes in the ground wreathed in clouds of flies. These camps had no provisions for garbage or rubbish disposal. Even where removal of trash had been contracted for with private operators, the refuse was often kept in uncovered wooden boxes or barrels. Those unwilling or unable to pay the collection fee dumped garbage in the many available vacant lots. Still other lots were dotted with the sheet-iron and scrap-lumber shacks of more refugees, most of whom had no sanitary facilities whatever.

A fourteen-year-old boy in East Oakland, across the bay from San Francisco, became seriously ill about the time of the earthquake. He recovered, and in all the turmoil, authorities never completely confirmed that he had plague. He probably did.

Some thirteen months after the catastrophe, a twenty-four-year-old sailor from the seagoing tug *Wizard* was examined at the U.S. Marine Hospital. He had lived on board his ship almost continuously for the previous month and a half, but at intervals he had tired of ship's cooking and had eaten at a waterfront boardinghouse at 247 Steuart Street, just off the Embarcadero near the present Bay Bridge.

On the same day that the young sailor entered the hospital his ship sailed for Oregon. On May 26 he died of plague. In a more superstitious age, *Wizard* might have been thought more likely to be under an evil spell than casting one; two days later she struck a rock off the coast of Oregon and sank within minutes. Fortunately, her crew was rescued and the men received thorough examinations on their return to San Francisco. No ominous symptoms were found.[2]

On Thursday, August 1, 1907, a fifty-year-old man became ill. After a long struggle he died of plague at the end of October.

A week after the older man fell ill, another young plague-infected sailor was examined at the Marine Hospital. He had not left his ship, the S. S. *Samoa*, for more than a fortnight, excepting only a single forty-five-minute period. Four days later he died. *Samoa* was fumigated and the crew quarantined, but no further cases were reported among them.

The warning trumpets had clearly sounded. Now plague

began to strike the city itself at widely separated points. Two days after the *Samoa* crewman's death, a woman came down with plague in a house northwest of Telegraph Hill, some blocks from the waterfront. Three other cases were reported about the same time. By September 4, 1907, twenty-five cases had occurred from August 1; about half were fatal.

The city's unsanitary stables and chicken yards supported a substantial rat population, and the conditions in the human settlements made San Francisco a rodent paradise. In its ruined and verminous state, the city was poised for an epidemic of awesome proportions. It only needed men like former governor Gage and his minions to ensure catastrophe.

The citizens of the Bay City, however, had had time to ponder the mistakes of the first epidemic. Now, with the ruined metropolis more vulnerable than ever, they did not repeat those errors.

On the day of the twenty-fifth case, Edward R. Taylor, mayor of San Francisco, wired President Theodore Roosevelt requesting that the federal government take charge of plague control. Passed Assistant Surgeon Rupert Blue of the Marine Hospital and Public Health Service was ordered to the city to take charge of the campaign. Dr. Blue was no stranger to the "City by the Golden Gate"; he had directed a similar effort in the first epidemic from June 1901 until the plague laboratory was closed nearly four years later.

By December 1907, twenty months after the earthquake, 1.4 percent of the rats trapped in San Francisco were plague-infected. The number seems insignificant. In fact, it is dangerously high. It is the level of infection commonly observed in some of the worst plague outbreaks of modern times, and a severe onslaught can be maintained with a level of rat plague far below one percent. Blue had reason to be worried. By the end of 1907 there had been 190 reported cases of plague, 96 of them fatal, scattered throughout the cities of the Bay Area including Oakland, Berkeley, Richmond, and Point Richmond.

Early in January of the next year, the president of the California Medical Society sent six hundred invitations to leading business and professional men asking them to meet with Dr.

Blue to consider antiplague measures. The apathy, antipathy, and ignorance of earlier years had not completely disappeared. Only sixty of the six hundred came, but they were enough; this group became the nucleus of a popular movement that was a paragon of civic cooperation and accomplishment.

On Tuesday, January 28, at a mass meeting on the floor of the Merchants' Exchange, the Citizens' Health Committee was formed to raise money and supervise antiplague measures. Soon, eleven new city ordinances were passed requiring that stables and chicken yards have concrete floors and be rat-proofed. Each family was required to have a covered garbage can, unsanitary housing was vacated, and rat-trapping began. In addition to a daily wage of $2.50, the ratcatchers got a 10-cent bounty per rat. Moreover, some seven million pieces of poisoned bait were distributed, usually in the form of arsenic and phosphorus paste on pieces of bread. The casualty rate among dogs, cats, and children was not recorded.

In an incredible six weeks, 162 meetings were held and seven hundred thousand circulars printed to enlist the help of various segments of the population in the fight against the threatened catastrophe. Organizers collected over $177,000, of which the Southern Pacific Railway donated $30,000. Things had obviously changed in San Francisco since the first epidemic. And, although the goal of $500,000 was never reached, the money collected was used so efficiently that 19 percent was eventually refunded to the original contributors.

The reactions of the citizens of the city, both high and low, were very different from before. By the end of June 1908, nearly seventeen hundred sick persons suspected of plague had been examined, along with nearly half the two hundred thousand rats trapped. Some eighty-two thousand notices to abate nuisances had been issued. That only a few hundred of these required further action reflected the changed attitude. Residents of the shattered city received nearly fifty thousand new garbage cans, and more than eleven thousand homes were disinfected.

The sewer system had previously served as both a home and a rapid-transit system for the enormous rat population.

Bond issues allowed rebuilding of the entire system. A plague hospital was set up where cases could be isolated, replacing the inadequate infectious-disease wards of the local hospitals. By late August 1907, vessels leaving the harbor for Canada, Mexico, Hawaii, or other U.S. ports were fumigated. One ship produced five hundred dead rats on the first fumigation; another yielded three hundred. By the third or fourth fumigation a ship was generally rat-free, at least for a while.

On Wednesday evening, March 31, 1909, a little less than three years after the earth opened beneath the city, a banquet was given at the Fairmont Hotel in honor of Dr. Blue, who received a gold watch. The second plague epidemic in San Francisco was over.

There had been a total of 205 cases in the Bay Area with 103 deaths. Although it was a much more intense epidemic than its predecessor and officially remains the worst outbreak in American history, it was remarkably light considering the circumstances under which it occurred. The fatality rate was 51 percent, in the usual 40 to 60 percent range for bubonic plague epidemics up to the middle of this century. About 4 percent of the cases were pneumonic; half that many were septicemic. The mortality rate was low compared to the previous San Francisco outbreak. The 97 percent rate reported for the earlier epidemic, however, was probably an illusion because nonfatal cases of the disease were simply not reported.

Although the widespread control program and extensive civic cooperation were the very model of a modern major miracle, what was really accomplished? In San Francisco itself there were twenty human cases in August 1907; sixty-one in September; and then thirty-one, forty-one, and eleven in the remaining three months of that year. In January 1908, the month in which the broad-scale civic movement was launched, there was only one case, in March another, and then no more for the remainder of the year. A cynic might argue that the epidemic was over before the massive antiplague campaign really got under way.

Whether this is true or not the campaign clearly carried out a number of measures long overdue to improve sanitation and public health and consequently reduced the risk of the citizens of San Francisco to a number of infectious diseases capable of flourishing in the deplorable conditions that existed before the plague outbreak. Characteristically, the prevention of disease is much less dramatic than the treatment of it, but it is at least as important, more humane, and far less expensive.

Most of the fleas taken during the second San Francisco epidemic were the European rat flea (*N. fasciatus*); about 20 percent were *X. cheopis.* Some districts had high levels of *P. irritans* and a common mouse flea (*Leptopsylla segnis*), which is usually found on rats.

Even before, and in the years between, the San Francisco epidemics, other American cities played host to plague. And the first San Francisco epidemic had a curious sequel that gave rise to a case of pneumonic plague in, of all places, Ann Arbor, Michigan.

Doctor F. G. Novy of the commission that investigated the first San Francisco epidemic was chairman of the Department of Bacteriology at the University of Michigan. In view of the tragic events in the Bay City, Dr. Novy thought it was advisable to begin production of a plague vaccine in the United States. This task was entrusted to a twenty-year-old third-year medical student, a Mr. C. B. (Ben) Hare of Boise, Idaho, who worked in Dr. Novy's department.[3]

Professor Novy returned from San Francisco to Ann Arbor in February 1901, bringing with him pure cultures of the bacillus, isolated from plague-ridden corpses, and he carefully directed Hare in how to make the plague vaccine from them. The preparation went smoothly for some three months. Then, on the first Saturday in June, Ben Hare came to the laboratory in midafternoon and announced that he was ill. A colleague, roommate, and fellow medical student, James G. Cumming, took Hare's temperature and then suggested that he return to his room. Cumming told Dr. Novy of Hare's illness, and Novy supplied two wide-mouthed sputum bottles to collect samples of anything Ben Hare coughed up. About ten o'clock Hare had a fit of coughing. Professor Novy at once collected the bottle containing blood-flecked fluid and took it back to his laboratory for examination and injection of the material into animals. The next day he confirmed the diagnosis of pneumonic plague.

About nine o'clock that evening, Ben Hare and James Cumming, who had volunteered to accompany him, set off in a horse-drawn ambulance for the pest house, a two-room structure with a toilet and a kitchen. All possible precautions were taken to prevent spread of the disease. Cumming himself used generous amounts of mercury chloride solution to prevent his own contamination with the plague bacillus. Dishes from the pest house were placed on the front porch and food was transferred to them by a nurse who brought it from the hospital kitchens. But in spite of all precautions no one in Dr. Novy's laoratory or the medical school gave either man much chance to leave the pest house alive.

On the fifth day of his illness, Ben Hare was delirious and his temperature reached 105.5°F. (41°C). Then, astonishingly, it slowly declined. By the end of the second week Hare's temperature was nearly normal. On the thirty-first day, Ben Hare and his courageous companion left the pest house, Hare on a stretcher and Cumming under his own power. Cumming never contracted the disease and went on to practice medicine for many years. Hare had a long convalescence. A week or so after he returned to his boardinghouse he walked just half a block away, but a carriage had to be sent to bring him home. For the rest of his life he required twelve hours of bed rest a day, the result of a heart permanently damaged by the toxins of *Y. pestis*. But he did finish medical school, and he practiced medicine in San Diego until his death at the age of fifty.

Doctor Hare had the unenviable distinctions of being the first (although not the last) victim of a laboratory-acquired plague infection in the United States, the first (and so far the last) plague case in Michigan, and the first known pneumonic plague victim in America to live to tell his story.

New York was the second U.S. city to be visited by a plague ship. In the fall of 1899, some months after the visit of *Nippon Maru* to San Francisco, the British vessel S.S. *J. W. Taylor* arrived off Manhattan from the Brazilian port of Santos. Plague was on board.

The disease had been officially declared to exist in Santos five days before the S.S. *Taylor* departed, and the ship's steward was treated ashore for what seemed to be eczema. A week after the ship had left Santos the steward fell seriously ill. A week later he was dead. At the same time, both the captain and the cook became ill. Although they were convalescent by the time the vessel steamed into New York harbor, both were later confirmed to be plague cases. Fortunately, the disease did not spread ashore into America's largest city as it had in San Francisco.

Then on Tuesday, January 30, 1900, the S.S. *Nanyo Maru* arrived in Puget Sound with a history of illness aboard. One person died in the quarantine station at Port Townsend, some fifty miles (eighty kilometers) from Seattle. Death was apparently due to beriberi, but a wary quarantine officer detained vessel, crew, and passengers until the cause of death could be confirmed. It was plague. This case was followed by sixteen additional cases among passengers and crew; two were fatal. Again, thanks to the alertness of the quarantine officer, there was no evidence of spread of the disease ashore.

There were certainly numerous opportunities for plague to spread into American ports during the early years of the twentieth century. What is surprising is not that there were so many incidents but that there were so few. The explanation may be that there were many cases not recognized as plague. One outbreak, belatedly identified, occurred in Seattle during the second San Francisco epidemic.[4]

Ernest C. Osborne, a twenty-seven-year-old policeman, was walking his beat in downtown Seattle on October 7, 1907. It was a miserable Monday, cool and humid, and he felt terrible. The gloomy surroundings of his skid road district did not help. As soon as he was off duty, Ernest went to the home at Twenty-fourth Avenue and Dearborn that he shared with his older sister, Lydia, and his brother and sister-in-law. On Tuesday, Patrolman Osborne was too sick to work.

Often during the next five days, his younger sister, Agnes,

and his brother's wife, Mary, stopped to see him. At the beginning of each visit they would ask Lydia how he felt. The answer was ever the same—worse. Six days after his illness began Ernest Osborne was dead. Forty-eight hours later, the faithful Lydia became ill. She died in four days. The assistant to the undertaker who embalmed Ernest sickened the day after Lydia and died in forty-eight hours.

Ernest Osborne's death was certified as typhoid. Lydia's death and that of the undertaker's assistant were listed as lobar pneumonia. No autopsies were performed.

Meanwhile, a forty-two-year-old Chinese, Leong Sheng, who lived in the part of Seattle that Ernest Osborne had patrolled, became sick four days after the young policeman. Leong was not hospitalized until Wednesday, October 16. He had been ill six days. At eleven o'clock Friday night he died. *Yersinia pestis* was found in the corpse, and Leong Sheng became the first confirmed case of plague in Seattle's history.

On Monday evening, October 21, two days after the death of her older sister, Agnes Osborne fell ill. The next day she had a temperature of 104°F (40°C), a cough, and bloody sputum. Her pulse and respiration rates and her temperature rose steadily. At 5:00 P.M. Sunday she went into convulsions and died. Agnes's lungs and spleen were riddled with *Y. pestis*. A sample of her sputum injected into a guinea pig caused the death of the animal from plague seventy-two hours later.

The very next day, Agnes Osborne's sister-in-law, Mary, had severe headache and low back pain. Because of a long history of menstrual difficulties she thought the symptoms signaled the beginning of her period. Within hours, however, a doctor was called. He found Mary Osborne with a weak and irregular heartbeat, headache, and an elevated temperature. Her tongue was coated, dry, and white. She coughed blood-streaked sputum. On Wednesday, October 30, Mary became delirious. She died at 11:00 P.M. Permission to perform a postmortem examination was refused, but Mary Osborne's sputum caused fatal plague in a guinea pig.

Agnes and Mary both died of pneumonic plague. In retrospect, it seems clear that the deaths of Ernest Osborne, Lydia, and the undertaker's assistant were from the same cause. That Lydia Osborne died of pneumonic plague was the opinion of the physician who attended both her and her younger sister. Their symptoms were identical; Agnes's death was unequivocally the result of the disease.

On Thursday, November 7, a month after Ernest Osborne was stricken, the first plague-ridden rat in Seattle was discovered at 5862 McKinley Place. A second was found the next day at 614 Main.

A vigorous program of garbage and rubbish collection began on November 9, and rat-killing campaigns were organized along with ratproofing and elimination of rat harborage. Between 1908 and 1917, U.S. Public Health Service personnel in the Seattle Health Laboratory on Maynard Avenue examined more than three hundred thousand Seattle rats. In all but two of these years, some rats were found to be plague-infected, but there were no more confirmed human cases. Then on Saturday, December 27, 1913, a thirty-one-year-old woman died from what a Public Health Service board concluded was probably septicemic plague. In that year, thirty-two plague-bearing rats were found in Seattle, more than in any year before or since.

From 1917 to 1933, authorities checked another 170,000 rats, but no further evidence of plague was found. Rats from Tacoma and Everett were investigated with negative results. At least for the time being, plague had withdrawn from Seattle and from the environs of Puget Sound.

To add a final note of symmetry to the first decade of American plague, in June 1910, our old friend, the S.S. *Nippon Maru*, returned to San Francisco and earned a second distinction in Bay Area history. A plague-stricken rat was found on board after the ship had been fumigated. It was the first plague-positive rat ever found on board ship in the United States and the only plague-infected rat ever found on a ship in San Francisco, despite the city's two major epidemics.

9

Metamorphosis:
Plague Goes Native

Out of the darkness, to the left toward the bay, looms the incandescent geometry of the Transamerica Building. Southward, pairs of headlights mark the Bayshore Freeway running down the penincula. To the right is the dark expanse of Mount Sutro, bordered by the lights of the University of California's San Francisco Medical Center, at the top of a street called Parnassas. Between Mount Sutro and the Bayshore Freeway is the dark mass of San Bruno Mountain, dotted with television and radio towers.

This mountain lies about halfway between the south window of the cocktail lounge atop the Mark Hopkins Hotel on Nob Hill and the San Francisco International Airport. It is the most intensively studied plague focus in America.[1]

San Bruno Mountain is some five miles (eight kilometers) long and thirteen hundred feet (about four hundred meters) high. It is covered with a mixture of grassland, low shrubs, and occasional willow thickets growing along the edges of small streams. The most important animals inhabiting it and the surrounding areas are the Norway rat, the brush rabbit, and four species of mice. On the lower slopes, in addition to commercial flower beds, there are several cemeteries and a golf course; housing developments crowd inexorably toward the summit.

San Bruno Mountain has probably been a plague focus since early in this century, although plague was not discovered there until 1942. Intensive study began on the southwest side of the mountain, near the town of Colma, in the spring of 1954. The California vole, or meadow mouse, is the dominant rodent and is host to three different species of plague-carrying fleas; two or more plague-transmitting flea species are found on other animals. In the first week of study, Y. pestis was isolated from a Norway rat and from 10 to 25 percent of the three species of meadow-mouse fleas. One of the plague-carrying fleas found on the meadow mouse was also found on three-fourths of the Norway rats and on a quarter of the common house mice in the area. The meaning is clear. In the San Bruno Mountain plague focus (and probably in plague foci generally), the disease could easily pass from the wild rodents in which it makes its permanent home to commensal rodents, which live more intimately with man.

Prior to the 1950s, it was generally thought that relatively large and conspicuous animals such as rabbits, prairie dogs, ground squirrels, and marmots were the principal reservoirs of plague in areas of permanent infestation. Since then, it has become increasingly clear that the tiny mice of field and forest are often the primary reservoir of the plague bacillus. The larger animals are frequently only secondarily infected.

Studies on San Bruno Mountain showed that the Norway rat also carried the efficient plague transmitter, the European rat flea. It was more surprising to find that three-quarters of the house mice carried the same flea, in addition to the fleas normally found on the meadow mice. Thus, there was extensive sharing of fleas among the meadow mice, house mice, and Norway rats, although fleas were more apt to go from meadow mice to commensal rodents than in the opposite direction. Unfortunately, this direction carries the plague-infected fleas of wild rodents into potential contact with humans.

The California voles on San Bruno Mountain showed incredible resistance to the symptoms of plague (an LD_{50} of more than ten million virulent *Y. pestis*), although their spleens, livers, and kidneys might teem with *Y. pestis*. The blood of a plague-infected vole might contain more than enough plague bacilli to infect a flea feeding on the wild mouse, but the little rodent itself showed no obvious sign of illness. This astonishing ability was inherited from either parent and was an immunity to disease rather than a resistance to infection. This is a phenomenon worthy of further study, both in the context of plague and in the generally important biomedical area of innate resistance to disease, since a clearer understanding of this process might make it possible to stimulate more effectively or enhance the body's natural resistance.

The resistance of the meadow mice to sickness and death from plague was not absolute: an epizootic in the spring of 1963 reduced their population about one-third. The deer mice on San Bruno Mountain, however, were cut to half their former number, and plague virtually exterminated the harvest mice.

By March 1963 all three populations were at their low point. But, in tribute to the amazing reproductive power of small creatures under favorable conditions, by late summer the vole population had increased sevenfold from its March low, and there were twice as many deer mice as before the epizootic. Even the harvest mice regained the level that existed before the disease struck, although they had been nearly obliterated.[2]

The most recent investigation in the area was reported in 1972. About 4 percent of the voles and deer mice were plague-infected, along with some 14 percent of their fleas. Nearly half the voles showed evidence of recent plague infection.

San Bruno Mountain has many of the characteristics of plague foci everywhere, although it is atypical in its proximity to a major city. The animal population shows the usual interchange of fleas between species; a mixing of both plague-resistant and plague-susceptible animals; and a multiplicity of both animals and fleas in the same area. The antecedents of the San Bruno focus go back nearly eighty years.

Saturday, August 5, 1908, was a red-letter day in the history of plague in the United States.[3] On that day a trapper caught a squirrel in Contra Costa County, California, a region across the bay from San Francisco that includes the cities of Oakland and Berkeley. The animal was an ordinary California ground squirrel. What was extraordinary was that it was infected with *Y. pestis*. It was the first native American aninmal ever found to carry the disease! And it signified the conversion of plague in the United States from an imported to an indigenous disease. The trapping was no accident.

Two plague deaths had occurred in rural Contra Costa County in the preceding month—one near the town of Concord and one near Martinez—and Dr. Rupert Blue, still involved with the second San Francisco epidemic, had put trappers to work collecting squirrels on the ranches near where the human cases were found. Searchers had found the infected squirrel on the same ranch where the first July case of human plague had originated.

The existence of a plague epizootic in rural Contra Costa County had been suspected five years before, during the first San Francisco epidemic, when there were three widely separated human cases. Two of the victims had hunted ground squirrels, and the other had eaten squirrels shortly before falling sick.

As if to emphasize the importance of the infected squirrel in Contra Costa County, on the same day it was trapped a boy was bitten by a ground squirrel in Los Angeles, 340 miles (550 kilometers) to the south, an area where plague of any sort had never been reported. The ten-year-old boy contracted the disease but recovered. A second plague-infected squirrel was found dead in the area where the boy was bitten.

The problem of plague in America suddenly took on a new and frightening dimension. Ground squirrels were generally infested with fleas known to bite man, at least one of which was an efficient transmitter of plague, in addition to the infamous Oriental rat flea and the stick-tight flea, both efficient plague transmitters. Moreover, wherever ground squirrels and rats intermingled, so did their fleas. The range of the California ground squirrel extended north, south, and east over an immense area, and the squirrels lived in intimate contact with other rodents to which the disease might spread. What would prevent plague from spreading "from sea to shining sea"?

What, indeed?

The response to the growing concern over the rat as a carrier of plague to humans had been a program of rat extermination by force and violence. Never very successful, the same approach was now employed against the ground squirrel. The goals were to create squirrel-free zones around cities, to eliminate the animal in areas where plague was found, and to survey California for the presence of the disease in squirrels. The last goal had some chance of being achieved.

It was a bad time to be a California ground squirrel. From 1908 through 1919 at least seven hundred thousand squirrels were killed, most of them in the first six years of the campaign. These enormous "body counts" induced the usual optimistic statements about the conquest of plague. In a federal report for 1914, officials announced that all discoverble plague in California would soon be eradicated and that the danger of its further spread had been removed. But the glow of accomplishment generated by the mountains of dead squirrels soon faded.

In the next annual report a more cautious statement appeared that pointed out that it would be unwise to predict that the disease had been completely wiped out in any county. There was, however, the 1915 equivalent of the "light at the end of the tunnel" about which we heard so much during the Vietnam War. The report went on to say that another year or two of work would eradicate plague in California.

The following year, a plague-bearing squirrel was found east of Berkeley, seven more were found near Richmond, and one near Hayward, all parts of the Bay Area that had been the subject of intensive efforts to obliterate the squirrel population by trapping, shooting, and poisoning. Such activities were vigorously resumed, but infected ground squirrels continued to turn up in awkward places, including inside San Francisco County.

Then, in 1934, came another milestone in the history of plague in America, one readily predictable—with the benefit of hindsight—from the discovery of the plague-infected ground squirrel in Contra Costa County. A sheepherder in southern Oregon came down with the disease and died in a Lakeview, Oregon, hospital on Monday, May 21. Investigation soon revealed that plague was enzootic in the ground squirrels of the area. This first report of wild-rodent plague outside California revived the fears of 1908 that the pestilence might spread over the whole United States.

In April 1934 a mobile laboratory set out to search for other plague foci. Soon public health officials in various parts of the West took an interest in the possible presence of the disease in animals in their own areas. In June 1935 plague-bearing animals were found in Wallawa County, Oregon, on the state's northern border with Washington and Idaho and more than 250 miles from Lakeview. In the next month three plague-infected squirrels were found in Montana. During the following year infected animals were discovered in Idaho, Nevada, Utah, and Wyoming; a year later in Washington; and in 1938 in Arizona and New Mexico.

As the search widened, so did the boundaries of the plague-infected area. Wild-animal plague was found in southern Canada in 1939, in Colorado in 1941, in Oklahoma the next year, and in Kansas and Texas soon after. In 1954 the disease appeared in the Mexican prairie dog in the northern part of that country. By the mid-1940s the roster of western states was complete; plague existed in every state from the shores of the Pacific east to the hundredth meridian, which runs through the center of Kansas and Oklahoma. How much farther east the disease may extend is unknown.

Squirrel eradication programs continued throughout California well into the 1940s. The luckless ground squirrels were getting it from both sides. On the one hand they contracted plague from the numerous plague-infected mice by interchanging fleas, and then, as a further insult, they were being shot, trapped, and poisoned to control a disease of which they themselves were victims.

Whatever its true hosts, the vicious bacillus *Y. pestis*, scourge of Europe, Asia, and Africa for millenia past, had clearly extended its beachhead in less than half a century from a few infected buildings near the San Francisco waterfront to infest nearly 40 percent of the area of the United States and had moved into Canada and Mexico.

Or had it? Perhaps it was there all along.

The marmot is a native of North America that migrated across the Bering land bridge into northern Asia. The native North Americans came the other way perhaps one hundred thousand years before Christ; plague may have come with them. According to this view, plague was entrenched in the wild animals of North America centuries ago; it was simply recognized for the first time during the early years of this century following the outbreaks in San Francisco and Seattle. There are some distinctly inhospitable areas between San Francisco and western Kansas—Death Valley, for one. Some scholars question whether wily *Y. pestis*, for all its low cunning, could have made the journey in such a short time by the slow transfer from one rodent host to the next most eastward one, in a sort of pestilential bucket brigade.

The question of the origin of plague may never be settled. The bulk of the evidence, however, seems to favor the older view that ship-borne infected rats introduced the disease in the last years of the last century or in the first years of this one.

Certainly there is abundant evidence elsewhere in the world for the rapid distribution of plague inland from seaports via train, truck, and bullock cart. There seems to be no reason to think that plague did not spread inland in North America in the same way. To say that the plague bacillus could not have made the journey from San Francisco to the Midwest in three or four decades is like saying that the disease could not have come to the West Coast from China in only a few months because the black rat is a slow swimmer. In both cases the role of man-made conveyances is ignored.

Whatever its origin, wild-animal plague in the other fourteen states thus far discovered to be infected mimics that in California in one way or another. In California, plague is carried not only by more than half a dozen varieties of ground squirrel but by chipmunks, flying squirrels, shrews, three kinds of rabbits, gophers, several species of wood rat, marmots, and a variety of mice. No other state can match this imposing list, but in all the other plague-infected states, the animals involved are either the same as in California or close relatives.

Some states have contributed new species to the long list of plague carriers. Kansas and New Mexico offer the cotton rat and the blacktailed prairie dog. New Mexico also adds two other species of prairie dog, while Wyoming supplies a third. In Oregon, badgers have been found carrying the disease. Badgers (like domestic dogs and cats) probably contract plague when digging up the burrows of plague-infected rodents, but they are not dangerous transmitters because they have little contact with humans, and their sparse, coarse fur supports only a small flea population.

Until the early 1960s, detection of plague in humans and other animals depended upon the isolation and identification of the plague bacillus in tissues or body fluids. In humans treated with antibiotics or in animals dead for some days, isolation of plague bacilli is difficult and frequently impossible. *Yersinia pestis* must be present in reasonably large numbers and competing organisms must be largely absent in order to give an unequivocal result. Because of the insensitivity of this method much plague infection was overlooked, especially in the early surveys for wild-animal plague. Then highly sensitive methods were developed that permitted detection of antibodies formed in response to plague infection, and these assays have been even further improved in recent years.

Unfortunately, most surveys of wild-animal plague in the American West were carried out before the more sensitive methods were available and before scientists knew that animals with no signs of illness could be plague-infected.

Although Texas had human plague in 1920, wild-rodent plague was not discovered until much later. In the summer of 1945, farmers and ranchers reported large numbers of dead prairie dogs, pack rats, and ground squirrels in the neighborhood of Brownfield, an aptly named community in west Texas near the New Mexico border. The nine plague-infected counties included nearly nine thousand square miles (an area larger than Massachusetts) that were home to twenty-two species of small mammals and eleven species of fleas. The principal animal victims of plague were the blacktailed prairie dog and the grasshopper mouse. Nearly two-thirds of all fleas from small mammals were stick-tight fleas, although the Oriental rat flea was also present. The predominant flea on the prairie dogs was the so-called human flea, *Pulex irritans.*

In Colorado, plague was first found in marmots and ground squirrels in 1941. At least nine other species later proved to be infected, and the distribution of the earliest reports suggests that the disease entered the state from New Mexico, where it had been found three years earlier. Of Colorado's four species of ground squirrels, two are involved in the maintenance of plague, the Wyoming ground squirrel and the Say's rock squirrel. Both the Gunnison prairie dog and the blacktailed prairie dog are host to fleas that are known plague carriers, but the latter animal has been driven to the brink of extinction by a federal organization recently renamed the Division of Animal Damage Control.

Marmots are found in the high mountains that run the length of Colorado. Typically a marmot has a dozen or more fleas, and all species of marmot fleas are known carriers of plague. In some parts of the Rocky Mountain National Park the marmots are so tame that they will climb onto the porch of a gift shop seeking food. The marmot colonies are widely separated, and the risk of an epizootic among marmots is small; but these animals do play a role in transporting plague across mountaines that are a barrier to other species.

Of the forty-one species of fleas found on wild rodents in Colorado, only fifteen to twenty play a role in plague ecology. These cause periodic epizootics that virtually obliterate the small-rodent populations over vast areas. In Park County a plague epizootic traveled across an area of 915,000 acres (366,000 hectares) at the rate of thirty miles a year between 1947 and 1949. When it had passed, 95 percent of the prairie dogs were dead, and in many "dog" towns the mortality was 100 percent.

The ground squirrels and the meadow and white-footed mice were also decimated.

Humans and their inventions have proved a great boon to the desire of *Y. pestis* to see the world. The iron steamship and the iron horse have played the predominant role in the Third Pandemic, although they may yield to the jet aircraft in the near future. But even the lowly pickup truck has done its part, especially in introducing plague into Colorado.

Ranchers often fervently dislike prairie dogs. This is not necessarily rational. Many of the same ranchers also hate coyotes, which are a major factor in keeping prairie-dog populations within limits. Perhaps the negative reaction is a response to prairie-dog infestations, which are often the result of the hallowed American tradition of overgrazing (prairie dogs will not establish burrows in thick grass), and thus a visible embarrassment. Whatever the reason, some ranchers will stop at nothing to get rid of prairie dogs.

There have been at least three known cases of Colorado ranchers driving as much as 250 miles (400 kilometers) to pick up prairie dogs dying "of some disease" in New Mexico and bringing the sick animals back to their own ranches to infect the animals there. In each case the disease that was killing the prairie dogs in New Mexico was plague.

In one incident a rancher's boy, apparently inspired by his father's entrepreneurial spirit, sold plague-infected prairie dogs to tourists as morbid souvenirs of Colorado.

A comparative newcomer to the list of plague-carrying rodents in Colorado and elsewhere is the Eastern fox squirrel. Introduced by humans into parks throughout the West, these animals have also followed the advice of some bushy-tailed Horace Greeley and migrated steadily westward to the western edge of the Rocky Mountains. The first report of a plague epizootic in city-dwelling Eastern fox squirrels was in June 1965 in Denver. Only a year before, an infected fox squirrel was found in Greeley, Colorado, some forty-five miles north of Denver (two years before that, an Eastern fox squirrel infected wth plague was found near the campus of Stanford University in Palo Alto, California).

Wild-animal plague in Colorado continues to erupt at intervals. In June 1974 disgruntled campers heard that they had to leave Morraine Campground in the Rocky Mountain National Park because the plague bacillus had been isolated from deer mouse fleas in the area. In August 1975 the campground was again closed for the same reason.

Rocky Mountain National Park is not alone among western recreational areas in playing host to plague-infected animals. Others include the popular Mount Shasta area in northern California and nearby Lava Beds National Monument; Lake Tahoe and Yosemite National Park farther south; and Bryce Canyon and Yellowstone national parks. Some of these infestations have led to human cases. It is reasonable to assume that plague-infected animals may appear in any part of the western United States, including all the recreational areas.

Wild predators, such as the badger, fox, bobcat, and coyote, also play a role in plague ecology. A human case of plague contracted from a coyote was described in the early pages of this book. Domestic dogs and cats (particularly the latter) are also predators and often play an essential role in the transmission of plague to man, as was grimly emphasized in recent plague seasons in America.

In May 1966 a program of plague surveillance began on the vast Navajo Indian Reservation located in the Four Corners area, where Utah, Arizona, New Mexico, and Colorado meet. A small blood sample was taken from dogs brought in for rabies vaccination and was examined for the presence of antibodies to plague, which would indicate recent contact with *Y. pestis.*

Dogs occupy a unique place in Navajo culture. The possession of dogs, especially males, is a status symbol; a family with ten dogs is not unusual. The relationship between dogs and master is different from that normally found outside the Navajo nation, since the dogs are neither fed by their owner nor allowed in his hogan. Thus, the animal becomes a predator, and, on the Navajo reservation, has an excellent chance of making a meal on a plague-infected rodent and acquiring plague-infected fleas in the process.

Of the dogs examined in May 1966, about one in twenty (5 percent) showed evidence of recent exposure to plague. A similar study in Vietnam about the same time revealed an infection rate of dogs there, in the midst of a plague epidemic, only twice as high as on the Navajo reservation.

That dogs and cats are sometimes victims of plague has been known for centuries, but, until relatively recently, there was little experimental data to support the ancient observations.[4] Now laboratory studies have demonstrated that dogs are readily infected with plague, either by injection or by eating the carcasses of plague-infected animals. They are also highly resistant to the disease. Dogs may become ill; some may develop a high temperature and have substantial quantities of plague bacilli in their blood; but even dogs in this latter state usually survive the infection if they were initially in good physical condition.

Like dogs, cats are readily infected either by injection of the plague bacilli or through the membranes of the throat and mouth when a plague-infected animal is eaten or even held briefly in the mouth. In cats, however, plague is a serious disease, and many infected animals die. One particularly dangerous aspect of plague in cats is the formation of abscesses on the afflicted creature. These may yield a thick, purulent material that is essentially a pure culture of the plague organism. Such boils may continue to drain for a week or two. An animal in this condition is a menace to anyone who touches it, as well as being in abject misery.

The blood of plague-infected cats, whether the cats succumb to the infection or not, is heavily infested with *Y. pestis*. Thus, the role of both dogs and cats in plague transfer to humans is multifaceted. The animals may bring plague-infected animals they have caught into close proximity to their owners. They may acquire plague-infected fleas either by killing and eating infected rodents or merely by exploring the burrows of such rodents long after their inhabitants have died of plague. Finally the dog or cat may be infected by eating a plague-infected rodent or by holding such an animal in its mouth. In either case, the dog's or cat's own fleas may become infected. Cats, especially, may infect those who handle them when their own disease is far advanced. They are also susceptible to the migration of the plague bacillus into their lungs. This results in a feline version of pneumonic plague that is as dangerous to humans in close contact with the animal as is the disease in man.

It is now clear that there is far more to plague ecology than the involvement of a few species of commensal rats. As early as 1895, Siberian marmots were found infected with plague, and evidence was accumulating, from California and elsewhere, that the Siberian experience was not an isolated one. In fact, some 230 species of mammals are involved in the perpetuation of the disease, along with a hundred species of fleas. In North America the situation is comparatively simple; there are a mere 37 species of animals to consider. Perhaps the most intriguing of unanswered questions concerning plague in the United States is how far east the permanent American plague focus really extends. The surveys date mostly from years before the highly sensitive methods now used were available. It would be interesting (and possibly frightening) to look carefully for plague antibodies in the blood of wild rodents or rural dogs on the eastern side of the hundredth meridian.

Although the United States and the Soviet Union contain the largest permanent plague reservoirs, those of Mongolia, Africa, South America, and possibly China also constitute a threat to humanity. All the foci are swept periodically by epizootics that may virtually eliminate the plague-susceptible species for a time and threaten passage of the disease to man.

Wild rodents play an essential role in plague ecology that early researchers did not even dream of. One might imagine the conquest of plague if only commensal rodents were involved, although even this would not be easy. But the immense, intractable plague foci in wild rodents make such a concept absurd. We must share our world with *Y. pestis* forever.

The concept of a plague reservoir, an enduring focus of wild-rodent plague lasting centuries, even millenia, is a more complicated notion than it may at first appear to be. Central to the notion of what the French call an inveterate focus is the fact that plague actively persists among the resident rodents for generations beyond number. Take, for example, a plague epizootic in a well-established reservoir in Kenya, Mongolia, or Montana.

The population of the focus has been increasing for some years because of abundant food and good weather. All available burrows are full, even crowded. New ones are being excavated, and the rodents in the focus must go farther and farther afield for food. As more young are born and weaned they are forced to seek new burrows elsewhere to make room for those to follow. The whole focus gradually expands. Because of the difficulties in obtaining food, and the stress of crowded conditions, the health of the rodent community is not as vigorous as it was earlier.

Plague breaks out. Only a few animals die at first, then more. Finally, most of the animals are swept away. Their dead bodies litter the now-empty burrows and the surrounding countryside, and the carrion-eaters wax fat. The fleas from animals that died in the burrows remain there, laying eggs on the putrefying bodies and waiting, although they may eventually congregate around the mouths of the burrows hoping that a new host, an inquisitive coyote or a curious child, will come by. Mostly they wait in vain. Although plague-infected fleas may live for months at low temperatures, most of the insects, inside the burrow or out, plague-infected or not, perish.

Some rodents survive the epizootic. If they did not, plague would usually die out in the area. For a region to be an inveterate or permanent focus some animals must always survive infection or the plague bacillus must live on in some corner of the environment.

Therefore, the usual minimal requirement for a plague focus is that it contain two populations of animals, one susceptible to plague and one resistant. Both may be of the same species—resistant and susceptible marmots, for example—or they may be different, with susceptible marmots sharing the region with resistant ground squirrels or gerbils. The role of the susceptible animals is to increase the level of virulent *Y. pestis* in the focus. The plague organisms in the bodies of the susceptible animals number hundreds of millions before the animal finally succumbs to the disease.

In the interval before its death, the flea population on the susceptible animal rises higher and higher because the animal can no longer effectively defend itself against its parasites, and the total number of infected fleas in the focus greatly increases. The dying animal excretes virulent plague bacilli during its life, and its putrefying body adds more organisms to the ground or to the bodies of predators that chance to feed on it.

Then the epizootic passes, and the stench of death hangs over the depopulated focus.

But the conditions that lead to overpopulation still exist. There is adequate food for many more rodents than survived the epizootic, and there is plenty of vacant nesting space. The survivors respond, as rodents always do under such circumstances, with a burst of fecundity. And the cycle in the focus begins anew.

After the epizootic there are always a few infected fleas or infected animals in the focus, but then none. For a long time, months or years, no infected fleas and no infected animals are found. Some fifty thousand fleas and nearly thirty-six hundred rodents are examined. None are infected. Wily *Y. pestis* has vanished into thin air.

But wait.

A dead animal is found near the focus. There are no fleas left. It has been dead several days but there are the unmistakable stigmata of plague, and the cause of death is confirmed by culture and reinoculation, by treatment of the isolated bacillus with a bacterial virus that under proper conditions only attacks *Y. pestis*, and by serological tests for the antibodies to the plague bacillus. There can be no doubt: plague has returned to the focus. From where? An imported case, perhaps? But no plague animals are found in the areas surrounding the focus. Now the number of sick and dead animals in the rodent community is increasing. Infected fleas are found as well. There is a Farsi expression used to describe a phenomenon that suddenly appears as if by magic, *Az zamine djouchide*—literally, "boiled from the earth." It was a phrase frequently heard in the conversations of the team from the Pasteur Institute, Teheran, that carried out some of the studies described here.[5]

Where did plague come from, when neither infected fleas nor infected animals could be found in the focus between the epizootics? The answer is that plague never left.

The plague bacillus, in the absence of rodents and in the absence of fleas, was isolated from the soil of burrows where infected animals had died as long as eleven months after the last animal's death. It probably remained there much longer. Rodents could be reinfected merely by burrowing in this contaminated soil. When the population began to recover from the effects of one epizootic and to reoccupy burrows left vacant, the stage was set for the cycle to begin again.

The conditions under which "burrow plague" exist do not always occur, but there is no doubt that the phenomenon is real. Work still in progress at the Pasteur Institute in Paris has shown that plague-infected soil in rodent burrows will maintain the infection and cause the reinfection of rodents for at least five years—in the total absence of fleas.

In 1894 the most learned medical historian in England published the second volume of his monumental studies on epidemics in Britain. In it he maintained, as he always had, that plague arose from contaminated soil and that the idea of an infectious agent of plague, other than the miasma arising from such soil, was nonsense. In the same year Yersin and Kitasato discovered *Y. pestis*, and no more was heard of miasmas. But Dr. Charles Creighton was not completely wrong after all, although it took nearly seventy years to find out. Yersin himself opined in 1897 that the plague bacillus was conserved in the earth, from which it could infect rats under favorable conditions.

Another important mechanism for preserving plague in permanent foci is the so-called hibernation plague. This results when an infective flea bites an animal about to hibernate. The plague bacillus grows very slowly at the low temperature—a few degrees above freezing—inside a hibernating animal. Only in spring, when the animal comes out of its winter sleep, does the plague infection flare up. Then, animals may begin to die of plague months after the last infected flea has been found.

The most compelling question about such epizootics is, what determines whether they will spawn a human plague epidemic as well?

Rodent populations can suddenly explode, as can their flea populations. But, besides its dependence on the number of hosts available, each flea species has its own cycle dependent on temperature, rainfall, humidity, adequate diet for the immature forms (such as larvae), and the level of predation by other insects, bacteria, and molds. Whether an epizootic triggers an epidemic depends upon myriad cultural, economic, social, and political factors (famine, population density, war, agricultural and public health practices, etc.), as well as events, such as earthquakes and floods, that may bring human and rodent into close contact when their native habitat is disturbed. In addition, human plague epidemics arise only within a comparatively narrow range of temperature and humidity; the ranges are different, depending on whether the dominant form of the disease is bubonic or pneumonic.

Events like the natural population cycles of wild and commensal rodents also play a role in plague ecology. If both peak simultaneously, the amount of contact between them obviously increases.

A plague epidemic is the result of a large number of more or less independent natural cycles falling into step with one another. A pandemic requires a much larger number of independent cycles to fall into synchrony. An example may make the idea clearer.

Waves in the open ocean result from the addition and subtraction of many independent wave trains, which fall in and out of step with one another. Statistically, one wave in twenty-three is more than twice the height of the average wave, one in nearly twelve hundred is more than three times average height, and one in more than three hundred thousand is greater than four times average. These "freak" waves, analogous to epidemics or pandemics, last a few minutes or less, and then the component waves are again out of step.

In the open Atlantic Ocean in summer, the average wave height is about eight feet (two and a half meters). For the small-boat sailor whose vessel is struck by a wave of thirty feet high, the fact that his experience is improbable may be cold (and wet) comfort. For a human population faced with a plague epidemic, the fact that such a thing is improbable is likewise little consolation. Seldom is not the same as never.

10

Human Plague

Every living thing is a sort of imperialist, seeking to transform as much as possible of its environment into itself and its seed.
—Bertrand Russell, *Philosophy*, 1927

We share our world, including our bodies, with a great variety of microorganisms: yeasts, molds, bacteria, and viruses. Our mouths usually contain organisms capable of causing pneumonic, staphylococcal, streptococcal, and other infections. The rest of the respiratory tract—excluding the deep lung—has smaller numbers of the same organisms. The lower intestine is packed with bacteria; they account for about one-third the weight of feces. A gram of fecal matter may contain a hundred million bacterial cells or more. Bacteria are commonly found in the nose and mouth, in the vagina (which also often contains fungi), and on the skin. The food we eat, no matter how carefully prepared, is contaminated with bacteria and other organisms, some of which enter the blood supply to the liver from the lower intestine. The air we breathe is frequently alive with tiny creatures, witness the rapid spread of colds and influenza from person to person.

Our continued healthy existence thus depends upon efficient control of potentially fatal infections the causative agents of which are frequently part of the normal flora of our bodies. Some properties of the responsible defense network are vital to the outcome of plague infections in man.

The system is a marvel of adaptation to a hostile environment. It is so sensitive and so finely tuned that it seems incredible that an invading organism could ever overcome such an intricately guarded fortress. But *Y. pestis* has evolved into a subtle and efficient killing machine.

To describe the course of the disease we will follow an imaginary miniepidemic. Although the setting is fictional the details are those of actual cases.

Michael Bailey walks wearily homeward, tired from a hard day's work on the New York docks and chilled by the biting wind making whitecaps on the river. He steps into a warehouse doorway to light his pipe away from the arctic blasts. On the other side of the door lies a rat—newly arrived on a ship from South Africa and newly dead of plague. Three of the infected fleas leaving the cooling body have hopped under the door. Now they leap toward the new arrival, guided by the vibrations of his steps, by his smell, or by both. Two miss their target; the third is more fortunate. It lands on the side of Mike Bailey's right shoe and its next jump takes it up under his trouser leg onto his sock. The hungry flea seeks to feed, but the sock is too thick for its tiny proboscis. Persevering, the flea moves upward, eventually reaching the bare skin, warm and inviting. The flea bites, and bites again, finally obtaining a tiny drop of blood as Mike Bailey walks, more briskly now, to the bus stop.

The flea injects into Mike's leg about fifteen thousand *Y. pestis*. Some of the skin cells in Mike's leg are killed by insertion of the flea's proboscis, others by the irritants injected by the flea to stimulate local blood flow. Chemical messages sent from the invasion point alert his cellular armies, and the defensive cells closest to the tiny wound (those called histiocytes) begin moving toward the injury, guided by the increasing concentration of chemical messengers as they near the beachhead of the bacterial invasion. As the histiocytes migrate, they swell to two or three times their former size to become cells called macrophages. These "big eaters" can engulf as many as one hundred ordinary bacteria and destroy them before they in turn perish.[1]

But *Y. pestis* is not an ordinary bacterium. The histiocytes migrating into the area of the flea bite engulf some of the invaders but cannot destroy them. The result: a large proportion of the plague organisms originally injected multiply freely in the tissue and inside the macrophages. They also move away from the site of injection, borne on tiny currents in the tissue fluids generated by movement of Mike Bailey's body, the pulsing of his arteries, and external pressures, as when he crosses his legs while sitting on the crosstown bus.

At home, Mike has dinner, reads the paper, talks with his wife and teen-age daughter about the events of the day, and then watches television for a couple of hours. Occasionally he scratches absent-mindedly at his right ankle. By now, there are three plague bacilli for each two the flea injected. A tiny spot on his leg contains some twenty-two thousand *Y. pestis*.

The chemical messages formed by reactions between *Y. pestis* and components of the blood have now reached every point of Mike's body. In response to the alarm, like soldiers rushing to the battlefield, other defensive cells and proteins move from the blood vessels surrounding the bite. Some of the chemicals released from damaged cells cause the walls of the tiny vessels near the injury to become more porous so that cells within them can migrate into the damaged tissue and join the fight against the invaders. About two-thirds of the white blood cells (leukocytes) are the type called neutrophils; each can gobble up five to twenty plague bacilli before dying itself. A single drop of blood may contain a hundred thousand neutrophils.

As Mike Bailey watches television, the neutrophils try to stem the invasion while the forces of *Y. pestis* are still in disarray. If they succeed, Mike will never know he was a plague victim. Usually they fail. They do, however, reduce the number of *Y. pestis* to below that originally injected by the flea. By the time the eleven o'clock news is over, the tide of battle seems to run against the plague bacilli.

Other things are going on in Mike Bailey's body. Proteins leak from the blood vessels around the original injury and form clots, in an attempt to seal the invaders behind an impenetrable wall. The plague bacilli counter by secreting enzymes that dissolve the clots here and there, and Y. pestis may escape the trap and invade the surrounding tissue.

Iron is essential for the growth of Y. pestis, as it is for other organisms. In response to bacterial invasion, the body reduces still further the iron level in the blood, already low compared with that in mice or guinea pigs. But this clever defensive move also fails, since virulent plague bacilli can extract iron from the body's iron-storage compounds. In the presence of unusually high blood levels of iron, a fatal human infection may result from a very small injection of virulent plague bacilli or even from the large inoculation with certain vaccine strains. Such elevated iron levels may result from severe protein deficiency (kwashiorkor), malaria, sickle-cell disease, or several varieties of blood and lymph disorders such as lymphoma, leukemia, or Hodgkin's disease.[2]

Like a contested city, the site of the struggle between the foreign invaders and the defenders is soon a mass of ruins. The magnificent architecture of cell and tissue is a shambles. Healthy tissue is destroyed and replaced by the viscid soup called pus—debris and dead cells, both bacterial and human. Substances released from the dead defending cells will soon cause Mike Bailey's temperature to rise. The increased temperature is another defensive measure, inimical to many invading organisms.

The cell contents are acid, or become so when the cells die. Consequently, the entire infection site turns more and more acidic as the battle rages, and the neutrophils, most numerous of the defensive cells, die quickly in an acid environment. Fortunately, when the neutrophils leave the blood vessels to join battle with Y. pestis, they are accompanied by a much smaller number of white cells called monocytes (this is the name given to blood-borne histiocytes). In the early hours after their release into the tissues, the monocytes are slowly transformed into another batch of the voracious macrophages, and these cells survive acid conditions.

The next morning, Mike Bailey kisses his wife and daughter and goes to work. It is a pleasant day. The wind has dropped and it's warmer. He feels fine. The struggle within his body, of which—although his life may depend on it—he is completely unaware, is now a battle at the inoculation site between *Y. pestis* and the newly formed macrophages.

While he was sleeping, the invasion of the plague bacillus had triggered a call to mobilize the defensive cell reserves. For such emergencies, the bone marrow contains thirty to one hundred times the number of white blood cells circulating at any one moment. Since the number always on duty is some thirty billion, or six times the human population of the world, the reserve forces are truly immense. Simultaneously, like armament factories abruptly placed on a war footing, the manufacture of white cells in the bone marrow accelerates. It remains high as long as body cells continue to be destroyed.

The human response to bacterial infection is awesome, but *Y. pestis* owes its fearsome reputation to the fact that it has some further tricks of its own.

The organisms growing at the low temperature inside a flea make little or none of three important proteins: the capsular antigen called F-1, and the two virulence antigens, V and W. When the organism finds itself inside a warmer body, it promptly begins to make the antigens. By three hours after infection, *Y. pestis* has begun to surround itself with capsular antigen and to make V antigen as well. A few hours later it has all three.

The effect is controversial. Apparently the result is that within some six hours after the flea bite both neutrophils and macrophages become largely unable to engulf *Y. pestis*. Even plague organisms swallowed by the defensive cells are not killed. They not only survive inside the defensive cells but multiply, and in this protected environment, they are also safe from many antibiotic drugs. Under the microscope, macrophages are found filled to bursting with *Y. pestis*, while earlier they contained only a few of the invaders. Chains of plague bacilli are seen snaking out of the neutrophils, apparently unscarred by the weapons of this important defensive cell.

Still other important events are taking place. Normal serum contains antibodies and other serum proteins (the properidin and complement systems) that stick to invading bacteria and speed their ingestion by the white blood cells. Some bacteria can be killed by the complement and properidin systems without the aid of white blood cells, but *Y. pestis* is apparently not one of them.

In any event, this ability of serum is greatly reduced as the plague infection progresses. There is also an apparent general paralysis of cellular defenses in the presence of large quantities of *Y. pestis* or its toxins. The endotoxin of the plague bacillus stops the migration of defending white cells toward it. Besides, white cells from an animal with plague frequently will not engulf *Y. pestis*, in part because of its surface antigens; but neither do they attack other bacteria that ordinarily would be rapidly engulfed and destroyed.

Wily *Y. pestis* has gained a firm foothold in Michael Bailey's leg. To spread quickly, it must penetrate one of the fluid transport systems, either the great superhighways of the blood vessels or the slower, but extensive secondary roads of the lymphatic system. Usually it is the latter. Blood vessels are nearly impermeable to bacteria (except in the lower intestine) while the ends of the lymphatic vessels permit, and are expressly designed to encourage, bacteria or large particles of cell debris to enter them. The scavenging ability of the lymphatics is essential to life. Deprived of it, we would die in twenty-four hours.[3]

The arrangement is ingenious. The terminal lymphatics have walls constructed of overlapping cells laid side by side like shingles on a roof. Each cell is anchored so that external pressure, like that caused by a bacterium borne on a miniscule current in the extracellular fluid, causes it to bend inward permitting the organism to enter the vessel. But pressure from inside the lymph channel only presses one cell wall more firmly against its neighbors. The bacterium, once in, cannot get back out. This "check valve" arrangement allows the lymph system to perform its major function of collecting debris and bacteria from the intracellular spaces.

The lymph system drains every part of the body. The walls of the lymph vessels are lined with cells that can engulf and dissolve invading materials, including bacteria. It is sometimes easy to follow the battle between bacteria in the lymph vessels and the defending cells. The substances released from the dying cells irritate and inflame the vessels and the surrounding tissue. The progress of the infection is clearly seen by the bright red streaks marking the site of the lymph channel and the path of the "blood poisoning," which has nothing to do with blood.

No such local reaction to the plague organism usually occurs. Having penetrated a lymph vessel, *Y. pestis* is borne quietly to the body's next line of defense, that bristling fortification known as a lymph node.

A week has passed since Mike Bailey stopped in the warehouse doorway to light his pipe. Deep within him a fierce struggle has raged; now the results begin to demand his attention. In the past week millions of his defensive cells have died in the battle. Little islands of plague bacilli here and there have multiplied wildly and then died as their food supply was exhausted and they were overcome by body defenses. With the dissolution of the plague organisms, toxins were released, and they, combined with substances from his own dead cells, begin to affect Mike Bailey's sense of well-being.

His work seems harder than usual. He arrives home irritable and tired. Later that evening, he is sipping a beer and watching television. Mrs. Bailey leans over the arm of her husband's favorite chair and gives him an affectionate kiss on his balding head. His skin is much warmer than usual, and so she fetches the thermometer from the medicine chest. Mike is distinctly feverish; the mercury in the thermometer comes to rest a little above 100°F (38.6°C). The next day Mike stays home from work.

Several million *Y. pestis* have arrived at the lymph nodes in Mike Bailey's thigh into which the lymph fluid drains from his foot and leg. Here they encounter a vast labyrinthine sponge composed largely of defensive cells, whose role it is to destroy them before they can reach the vital organs. If Mike Bailey had handled a plague-infected animal, the responsible lymph nodes would probably be those under his arm. If plague-infected fleas are killed by crushing them between the teeth, the lymph nodes under the jaw receive the brunt of the attack. But in rat-borne plague, the lymph nodes in the upper thigh or the groin are usually involved.

When the plague bacilli reach the convoluted maze of the lymph nodes, a terrible contest begins. *Yersinia pestis* attempts, with toxins, antigens, and enzymes, to paralyze the macrophages of the nodes, to render them unable to engulf or destroy the bacteria, and to coagulate the blood and seal off the sources of the armies of white blood cells rushing into the struggle against it. Millions of cells die, and the lymph nodes swell and merge into a formless lump, tiny at first and excruciatingly painful.

The first day Mike Bailey stays home from work he sleeps late and then wanders apathetically around the house. After lunch, he takes more aspirin for his agonizing headache and goes back to bed. When his wife wakes him for supper, he is a very sick man. His head aches horribly. As he gets out of bed, he grabs the edge of the dresser to keep his balance. The room reels as if he had just gotten off one of the violently spinning rides in the Coney Island amusement park. His back and legs ache. He eats only a little and promptly vomits.

Back under the covers he shakes with cold. His temperature has risen to 103°F (39.5°C). Mrs. Bailey calls the family doctor, who suggests that her husband come into the office the next day if he does not improve. He also telephones in a prescription for a penicillin-like drug.

The next morning, had anyone taken a sample of Mike's blood and cultured it properly, plague bacilli would have been found. There were not many, and the blood-cleansing organs—liver, spleen, and bone marrow—quickly trapped and destroyed most of the brief shower of *Y. pestis* that appeared in the blood. Where did they come from? Most of the lymph fluid, after passing through the chain of tortuous lymph nodes, empties into the bloodstream high in the chest. Perhaps the first bacteria to arrive at the lymph nodes in the thigh were not effectively filtered out. The defense was caught, as it were, unaware. Or the plague bacillus may have penetrated directly into the damaged blood vessels near the flea bite. However *Y. pestis* reaches the blood the results may be serious. That afternoon, Mike Bailey is in the hospital.

By now his temperature has soared to 104°F (40°C), he staggers, his coordination is poor, and he speaks like a drunken man, his words hesitant, indistinct, and lisping. There is a small, intensely sore area high on his right leg between his thigh and scrotum, but nothing can be seen. His tongue is coated with creamy white fur.

The battle in the femoral lymph nodes is only beginning. The macrophages in the nodes, and neutrophils and blood proteins from the surrounding blood vessels, all join in the struggle. For the defending cells there can be no limited tactical goals, no strategic withdrawals, no oil weapon, nor peace conference at which they can hope to attain by cunning what they failed to win in battle. In this war there is only absolute victory or annihilation.

By now, a few plague bacilli have reached the lungs through the blood, lodged there, and multiplied briefly before being overcome by the lungs' defensive macrophages. Fortunately for Mike Bailey he quit smoking cigarettes several years ago and his lungs' defensive systems are healthy and vigorous. For a few hours his sputum contains *Y. pestis*, but they soon disappear. His heartbeat is now irregular and much faster, up to more than 110 from its usual 72. His eyes are becoming noticeably bloodshot, and a foul-smelling brown coating is beginning to form on his lips, teeth, and tongue. Although his face is bloated, it still shows the strained expression of a man in pain. Nearly unconscious, Mike screams in agony when an orderly washing him presses lightly on the almost invisible sore spot on his thigh. By now there are several lumps there the size of peas.

The morning of his third hospital day brings no relief. His blood pressure is dangerously low. He is still getting penicillin, but his temperature remains high, and his physician considers adding a broad-spectrum antibiotic to the treatments already ordered. The laboratory tests are consistent with generalized poisoning, probably of bacterial origin. Later gram-negative bacteria are seen in the blood, but the physician will have to wait several days for them to be identified—if they ever are.

When Mildred Bailey visits her husband that day she is shocked at his condition. His speech is no better, and he is conscious less and less of the time. He leaves sentences unfinished, sometimes even words. He does not know where he is, nor how he got there. The femoral bubo, now the size of a golf ball, keeps him in agony. It has become hard in the center, which is surrounded by a gelatinous, swollen, and inflamed area.

The next morning Mike's fever drops more than three degrees and remains lower through the day. But the following day it soars again, and the bubo is now a throbbing mass the size of an orange. Additional antibiotic therapy is begun with a broad-spectrum compound, and the next day his fever drops dramatically. Yet the next day it rises, although not as high as before. And so it goes. Low temperature in the morning, high in the afternoon, with a gradual trend toward normal. The bubo is still large and terribly tender, but less painful than before.

Early in his second week in the hospital, Mike's bubo collapses into an open abscess in the center where the lymph nodes had liquefied during the battle against *Y. pestis*. His fever disappears and the abscess heals slowly. By the middle of the third week he is sent home with instructions to continue taking antibiotics and to return twice a week to have the dressing on his thigh changed. The bubo heals slowly without incident, although plague bacilli remain in it weeks later.

Mike Bailey was lucky. With inadequate treatment—and his was barely adequate—buboes can form chronic ulcers, usually because of secondary infections with organisms other than *Y. pestis*. These ulcers may lay bare muscles, nerves, and blood vessels. They are especially dangerous in the groin because they can lead to fatal hemorrhage from the pelvic arteries.

Mike Bailey survived an attack of bubonic plague, although not recognized as such, but he was never to be quite the same again. He stayed at home six weeks before he could return to work, and he could no longer do his accustomed heavy labor. But he was alive, and glad of it.

It might seem as if wily *Y. pestis* had frustrated and baffled Mike Bailey's defenses, so that his recovery was due only to the miraculous powers of the antibiotic drugs. This is not true. People survived bubonic plague millenia before the "antimicrobial age," and in Mike Bailey's case, he received the drugs too late and in amounts too small to have much effect on the outcome. Mike Bailey survived, as about half the victims of bubonic plague always have, because of his immune response to the foreign substances within him.

The response to a gram-negative bacterium like the plague bacillus consists largely of the stimulation of certain cells in the body to produce antibodies—relatively specific proteins that attach to the surface of *Y. pestis* cells, thereby labeling the invaders as foreign and undesirable.

Since the body has frequent experience with gram-negative bacteria, it contains some antibodies against all such organisms. When such antibodies attach themselves to *Y. pestis* the rate at which the defensive cells engulf the plague organism may be greatly increased, although not necessarily the rate of destruction of the bacillus. The attachment of anti-gram-negative antibodies may also facilitate the attachment of other serum proteins that, without the ingestion of the bacteria by defensive cells, can cause destruction of the plague organism.

These reactions slow the attack of *Y. pestis;* in very light infections they may be decisive, but recovery following the bite of a highly infective flea requires much more.

The initial invasion of *Y. pestis* sets off an intricate system of defensive responses within the body, compared to which a computer-directed network of missiles, bombers, and nuclear submarines is as primitive as a stone axe. An important part of this defensive reaction is the production of quite specific antibodies against the plague bacillus. But it is only important if the plague-infected victim lives long enough (a week or ten days) to benefit from it.

Within Mike Bailey's body there were cells capable of producing antibodies against *Y. pestis* and closely related organisms. The bacterial invasion stimulates their multiplication and transformation into antibody-producing cells. Some days after the initial attack, some of these cells are in full antibody production, and numerous others are being made ready.

The individual cells producing antibody against the plague bacillus live only a few days, but they have a busy life. During this time each cell may produce as many as two thousand anti–*Y. pestis* antibodies every second, or some two hundred million antibodies a day, and each antibody molecule is a large and complex structure containing tens of thousands of atoms.

These antibody molecules, after attaching to the plague bacillus, greatly enhance the rate at which *Y. pestis* are both engulfed and destroyed by the defensive cells—neutrophils and macrophages—regardless of the presence of the F-1, V, and W antigens on the bacterial surface.

Within a week or so of the initial flea bite, antibody production is in full swing. If this sector of the body's defenses responds vigorously enough and if *Y. pestis* has not lodged in a protected environment like the covering of the brain (the meninges), the victim survives a bubonic plague infection without treatment and will for some months be immune to further attack. Mike Bailey's immune response was vigorous enough to save his life.

Not everyone was as lucky. A warehouseman working a few blocks away developed septicemic plague in which the bacillus multiplied rapidly in the blood and in the liver and spleen. The site of entry was never identified, and he was found to have plague only after his death. Whether the plague bacilli were injected by a flea bite directly into the blood or whether they were simply poorly filtered by the lymph nodes is unknown. Initially the liver and spleen quickly removed *Y. pestis* from the blood; many of the organisms were killed. Then they began to multiply in these organs and in the bone marrow.

The first symptoms appeared on a Saturday morning. Severe headache, mild fever, and overwhelming fatigue were the only early signs. But, by Sunday night, the man was unconscious much of the time, and his family called an ambulance to rush him to the hospital. By then, his spleen and liver had swelled so much that they protruded from under his ribs. Like Mike Bailey's, the warehouseman's pulse became rapid and irregular; unlike Mike he had only a moderate fever. In the hospital doctors began antibiotic therapy at once. During the night he had frequent nosebleeds, and blood seeped from the lining of his mouth. His blood-clotting rate slowed to one-fourth of normal. Blood—and *Y. pestis*—appeared in his urine and stools, and he began to have superficial hemorrhages under his skin. Shortly after midnight Sunday, he developed a corneal ulcer in his left eye. A few hours later he was dead. There were no swollen lymph nodes.

On autopsy, plague bacilli were found in his blood, in all of his organs including his lungs, and in his ulcerated eye. He had been ill less than forty-eight hours.

The third case of rat-borne plague involved a truck driver who transported loads from the docks to warehouses scattered around the city. In his case, the bacillus lodged in his lungs. There was little involvement of the lymph nodes, and the liver and spleen filtered out and destroyed the bacteria remaining in the blood. But on the outer surface of the lung they grew steadily. Finally, they did enough damage to the previously healthy tissue to break through into the lung's inner surface (the surface in contact with the respired air) in several places. This drastically changed the nature of the disease. *Yersinia pestis* now had access to a nutrient medium nearly two square yards in area, moist and warm. Even more significant, this surface communicated directly to the outside world through the throat and mouth of the young driver. In Mike Bailey and the warehouseman the disease occurred in the essentially closed lymphatic and circulatory systems, respectively. In those cases, *Y. pestis* had few opportunities to escape. But the vast surface of the lungs in contact with the outside air gave the bacilli such an opportunity.

The victim developed a high fever. His mother nursed him at home until he became delirious; then she and her husband drove their son to the hospital. In his lucid moments he complained of severe pain in his upper right abdomen.

The physician who examined him considered that his general condition, the abdominal pain, and the laboratory tests indicated acute appendicitis or an already-ruptured appendix. The doctor ordered preoperative medication, but his patient died on his way to the surgical suite. He had been in the hospital less than half a day.

Death was acribed to bacterial pneumonia. By the time a sputum culture revealed the presence of *Y. pestis,* the young man's mother was dying of pneumonic plague and his father was severely ill. Shortly after, two nurses, a nurse's aide, and a staff physician also became sick. All received large quantities of antibiotics and they, like the boy's father, survived the infection.

Health authorities sought out contacts of the young truck driver to examine them and give treatment to abort any plague infection they might have acquired. One was found to have plague bacilli in his throat even though he had no symptoms of the disease. Another friend collapsed and died in the street before the investigating team could locate him. He never had any symptoms and might have been missed as a plague victim except for his known association with the first case and the fact that his face after death appeared so unusually dark.

Pneumonic plague is potentially the world's most infectious and deadly disease. It can spread easily person-to-person in the same way as influenza, measles, and the common cold. Unlike them, it is nearly uniformly fatal if not treated vigorously within hours of the appearance of symptoms.

Nearly all bubonic plague victims, whether fatal cases or not, have some plague organisms in their lungs. Fortunately, it is unusual for even 20 percent of bubonic plague victims to develop the pneumonic form, and the usual rate is less than half that.

When *Y. pestis* does reach the lung, more than 95 percent of them may be killed in the first six hours of infection; the remaining 5 percent are contained within macrophages. If they are destroyed and there is not reinfection, that is the end of the pneumonic threat. If not, they begin to multiply swiftly, the number of plague bacilli doubling about every six hours until the victim succumbs. This happens long before more than a small fraction of the vast surface of the lung is infected.

A person exposed to pneumonic plague may show no symptoms for, rarely, as long as ten days. Equally rarely, he or she may be ill within hours. Most often, two or three days elapse before the initial symptoms of fever, headache, and aching back and limbs appear. For the first twenty-four hours the victim is incapable of spreading the disease. Lung symptoms do not appear immediately, and the victim has the signs of a severe generalized infection.

By the second day of illness it is usually clear that the lungs are involved. Stethoscopic examination reveals signs of congestion that a chest X ray may also detect, although not always. Coughing begins or becomes more frequent, and the sputum, clear at first, becomes increasingly dotted or streaked with blood. Often the pneumonic plague victim suffers little pain, although he or she may be delirious and weakened to the point of collapse. Death usually comes for the victim between the second and the fourth day. Even the most sophisticated treatment, unless given very early in the disease (when it is extremely difficult to diagnose correctly), may not change the outcome, and everyone in contact with the victim is in serious danger of contracting the disease and subsequently transferring it to others.

Even in epidemics of pneumonic plague, comparatively few of the victims die in hospitals. Sometimes they develop few symptoms until they are overcome by massive amounts of the plague toxins and collapse, lose consciousness, and die. In this form of the disease, in which there is little coughing of plague-infected sputum, the advancing armies of *Y. pestis* multiply beneath the surface layers of the lung. So long as they do not penetrate into the inner surface of the lung, the disease remains in a "closed" form, which, like the other closed forms of the disease, is relatively noninfectious.

One-quarter to one-half the human victims of simple bubonic plague recover even without treatment. In contrast to the relatively benign bubonic plague, recovery of untreated septicemic or pneumonic plague is extremely rare.

Death from plague of whatever sort is the result of poisoning by the toxins of Y. *pestis*. Whether the organism multiplies in a lymph node, in the blood, or in the lungs, large amounts of toxins are liberated from dead plague bacilli into the circulatory system of the victim. The results are, among other things, a steeply falling blood pressure, coma, and death.

Basically, death from plague is a special case of death from that class of diseases known as gram-negative bacteremias—that is, the presence in the blood of large numbers of gram-negative bacteria of whatever kind. Anyone in the terminal stages of plague will have Y. *pestis* swarming in their blood. The endotoxin of plague is similar to the endotoxin of other gram-negative bacteria, and the most important general symptoms of plague closely resemble those of other diseases in this category.

Whether caused by Y. *pestis* or not, gram-negative bacteremia is a serious medical problem, although the dimensions of the problem are controversial. Total U.S. deaths from gram-negative bacteremias this year will be not less than ten thousand, even in the absence of epidemics. Thus, in spite of a sophisticated armamentarium of antibiotic drugs, our defenses against this class of infections are less than impregnable. It is widely believed that lowering the fatality rate among victims of gram-negative bacteremia by the development of new drugs is unlikely. It is a disconcerting conclusion. The organisms usually involved in the common gram-negative bacteremias are far less capable of invading and multiplying in the human body than is the ferocious bacillus of plague.

11

The First Quarter-Century

In the first quarter of the present century the Third Pandemic spread across the oceans to new lands, where the disease had either never been seen or had been long absent. Nor did it neglect old lands for new. Hong Kong, the city where Yersin and Kitasato labored to discover the causative agent of the disease, had plague every year for thirty years. In nine of these years there were moderately severe epidemics, the last in 1914. India suffered horribly. By 1918 the Third Pandemic had claimed at least ten million lives on the subcontinent.

The Third Pandemic brought plague to Vietnam early in the century. The disease was always more severe in the south, but even in the worst year, 1910, the incidence was far below that which accompanied the large-scale American military buildup in 1965. Thailand was infected shortly after Vietnam. There were 586 plague cases reported in Thailand in 1917; 580 were fatal. Indonesia was infected with ships carrying rice in November 1910. From 1920 to 1927 there were between eight thousand and ten thousand fatal cases each year.

The vicious little outbreak in Maryborough, Australia, in 1905 was neither the earliest nor the worst attack of plague on that continent. Plague-infected rats were first found on a wharf in Sydney in February 1900, and the disease soon spread to humans, causing more than 300 cases. Fifteen months later the disease struck again and caused another 139 cases. In 1921–22 plague returned to Sydney on the S.S. *Wyrema*. The result was 10 fatal cases from a total of 35.

In the thirty years following reinfection in 1899, Egypt had more than nineteen thousand cases and ten thousand deaths. In upper Egypt about 13 percent of the cases were pneumonic plague.

Plague arrived by ship in Morocco in 1909. Two years later there was a violent epidemic with eight to ten thousand deaths. A ship from Casablanca carried the disease to Dakar, in what is now Senegal, in April 1914. First there was pneumonic plague, and then bubonic. Some nine thousand persons perished. In 1920 another eight thousand died.

Plague is an ancient affliction of central Africa. The disease may have originated there spontaneously, or it may be a very old colony of the central Asia focus. Ancient Hindu writing suggests trade, probably in slaves and ivory, between India and the "Men of the Moon," before the Christian era. The Men of the Moon were presumably the natives living near the Ruwenzori Mountains, "The Mountains of the Moon," on what is now the border between Zaire and Uganda. Plague may have reached South India as a result of this commerce.

Even earlier there was a vigorous traffic in slaves and ivory between the Arab countries and central Africa, via Abyssinia (now Ethiopia) and the Rift Valley. The Arab traders rested on the shores of Lake Baringa and then went south into Uganda or labored east over the mountains, into Kenya. The Plague of Justinian probably followed those ancient caravan routes from central Africa into Egypt.

The disease erupted again in central Africa in the early years of the Third Pandemic. Nairobi, capital of Kenya, had an epidemic in 1902; in 1912 the disease broke out on the eastern slope of Mount Kilimanjaro, the ice-sheathed sentinel standing guard on the Kenya-Tanzania border, in what was then German East Africa.[1]

The outbreak lasted only a month during the spring rainy

season. There were three cases of bubonic plague, followed by fifty-five cases of the pneumonic form. All ended in death. Several natives of the village of Gasseni, where the epidemic began, were apparently infected by flea bites. One, possibly more, developed pneumonic plague, and the epidemic ignited. As a Dr. Wünn, a German medical officer reported, "The sick had not been previously isolated. On the contrary, 20 or 30 people sat around each patient, howling and consoling with him. Some might throw their arms around him or bed his head on their laps."

A native woman trained as a nurse came to Gasseni to help in the first week of the epidemic, then returned to her home in a neighboring village. She became violently ill; a day later she was dead. Unwittingly she had brought pneumonic plague to her village. There soon followed sixteen more cases, and sixteen more deaths.

Dr. Richard Lurz, a medical officer of the Imperial German Colonial Army, was ordered to the area to institute control measures, and he did so with great vigor. He also made the important observation that the disease was carried by house and tree rats native to the area; the black rat had not yet invaded central Africa. Unfortunately, his report was published the year before World War I began, and it was generally ignored. Until 1952 it was dogma that there was no wild-rodent plague in central Africa. Then plague was discovered in the Rift Valley in both the black rat and the native rodents, and Dr. Lurz's paper came to light after forty years of obscurity.

Kenya had plague consistently from 1902 on, and in Uganda there was human plague every year for forty years after 1906.

After 1907, South African health authorities agreed that the disease had been eradicated from the rodent population there. Then in 1914 they received a rude shock. A malevolent epidemic of pneumonic plague broke out on an isolated inland farm. The experts soon learned that from an almost wholly urban disease of rats, plague in South Africa had become an almost exclusively rural disease. Plague was transmitted from urban rats to the native rodents, largely gerbils, where it has remained ever since, slowly spreading across the Union of South Africa and beyond.

Plague erupted in the Orange Free State in South Africa in December 1923, in both rodents and man. The epizootic was intense. In some regions more than 90 percent of the gerbils and one species of mice were annihilated, along with nearly half the carnivores that preyed on them. In a four-month period the epizootic had covered over fifty thousand square miles (thirteen million hectares), an area the size of Alabama or Bangladesh, and caused 329 human cases and over 200 deaths.

Following initial infection in 1898, plague was reintroduced into the port city of Tamatave on Madagascar in March 1921. An epizootic resulted that virtually wiped out the rodent population and caused 107 human cases; 71 were fatal. In June pneumonic plague appeared in the city of Tananarive on the island's high plateau. The disease then spread to the rodent population on the plateau, where it has remained ever since.

As befits an ancient plague focus, the Soviet Union also had plague epidemics in the early years of the Third Pandemic. Between the beginning of the pandemic and the first All-Russian Antiplague Conference in 1927, there were nearly forty-five hundred plague cases reported in Russia, in some seventy-three separate epidemics. About 70 percent of the reported cases were pneumonic.

The hosts of plague in Soviet and Chinese Asia and Mongolia are the marmots called tarbagans by the Russians. These are large animals weighing up to nine pounds (four kilograms), whose relatives live in mountainous areas in both Europe and the United states. In Asia they are hunted for food and fur.

Mongolian folklore warned tarbagan hunters to leave sick animals alone. But when the hides fetched high prices, as in 1910 and again a decade later, unskilled hunters from China came in search of the animals. Many, with their families and friends, sickened and died. The first of these epidemics of what was sometimes called tarbagan sickness and was actually pneumonic plague took sixty thousand lives; the second, in 1920, killed ten thousand.

The natives of Mongolia were more careful. An ancient legend taught the nomads of the Gobi Desert that each tarbagan hunter was condemned to spend his next existence as a tarbagan. The parts of the animal that must never be eaten, said the legend, were the lumps of fatty tissue under the shoulders, for these were the remains of the dead hunter. The fatty lumps contained the axillary lymph nodes, which, in a plague-infected animal, might teem with plague bacilli. It was a useful bit of folklore. Still, accidents happened. A tarbagan could be taken that did not yet appear ill, yet its flesh and fur might swarm with plague bacteria or infected fleas, respectively. Epidemics arose both from tarbagan fleas and from eating inadequately cooked meat.

The Third Pandemic also struck the British Isles, although not on the scale of earlier epidemics. Plague appeared in Glasgow after an absence of 235 years, causing sixteen fatalities in the fall of 1900. A year later, another group of five cases appeared in a rag shop near the site of the previous outbreak. Rats infected with plague had not been found at the time of the first incident, but the second outbreak brought closer scrutiny. When a group of five cases was discovered in a single hotel, a search disclosed infected rats in the basement and a rat epizootic in progress in the neighborhood. In August 1907 there were two more cases in Glasgow, again in a rag store.

Rodent and human plague was discovered in other British seaports during the early years of the Third Pandemic. Cardiff, in Wales, Bristol, Hull, and London were struck by one form or the other. Liverpool also had the disease. Between the end of September and the end of October 1901, there were eleven cases in Liverpool, all in four families living in the same locale: eight of the victims died. Then, in July 1914, the pestilence again afflicted a single household leading to ten cases and four deaths. Again no infected rats could be found.

In this period plague also returned to rural England in a series of local outbreaks that are still the subject of controversy.[2]

Suffolk County, England, lies about sixty miles (one hundred kilometers) northeast of London. Ipswich, the largest city, is a grain-milling center. Early in this century, grain ships from all over the world sailed into the bay formed by the rivers Stours and Orwell and then moved a little way up the Orwell to Butterman's Bay. There grain was loaded into lighters for the trip upriver to Ipswich.

Charity Farm Cottages commands an excellent view of Butterman's Bay on the River Orwell, but on December 9, 1906, Mrs. Church was not enjoying it. She was seriously ill and her chest hurt. Her younger daughter cared for her as best she could, but as the mother's condition worsened, the girl became frightened. She called Dr. Carey and then ran quickly to another cottage near Charity Farm where her older sister lived with her husband. The two daughters and Dr. Carey did what they could, but it was no use. Three days after the beginning of her illness, Mrs. Church died.

Five days later, Mrs. Church's older daughter became ill. In two more days she was dead. The next day, Thursday, December 20, the younger daughter sickened as well. The neighbors in that sparsely inhabited region tried to help. Mrs. Goodchild lived half a mile from Charity Farm Cottages and looked after both of Mrs. Church's daughters during their illnesses. Mrs. Goodchild herself became desperately sick on Christmas Eve; she died the day after Christmas. On December 27 one of her sons became sick; her husband fell ill the next day, and her second son on New Year's Eve. Both her husband and her younger son were dead in four days; the other son, now an orphan, recovered.

Mrs. Goodchild's mother, Mrs. Woods, left her home (fifty miles away) at once when she heard of her daughter's illness, arriving in time to bury her and to care for her son-in-law and two grandsons. Then, Mrs. Woods was stricken. Three days later she was dead.

The unfortunate Mrs. Church of Charity Farm Cottages had passed her disease to seven other persons, five of whom died. Her younger daughter recovered, as did one of Mrs. Goodchild's sons. All the deaths were registered as caused by acute pneumonia. In retrospect they were probably plague, although it was never confirmed.

Almost exactly three years later, the disease reappeared. It was in a small and overcrowded cottage near the mouth of the River Orwell inhabited by the family Rouse—mother, father, five children—and a multitude of fleas.

On Sunday, December 19, 1909, Mrs. Rouse awoke with a headache. Christmas was less than a week off and there was much to do, but she felt so bad that she remained in bed until ten o'clock. She vomited on arising. Over the next few days she became steadily sicker. She suffered from diarrhea and frequent vomiting, but she continued to work around the house as long as she could. On Wednesday, December 22, her oldest child, a daughter, Honora, eighteen, helped her mother upstairs and into bed. It was 4:30 in the afternoon. At 5:00 Honora went upstairs again. Her mother was dead.

A physician was called when Carrie Rouse, fourteen, and her nine-year-old sister, Alice, were stricken. Carrie was dead three days later, and Alice died two days after her first sign of illness. Dr. Hart wondered if they had been poisoned, so quickly did they die.

Then the oldest son, William, fell ill and died in forty-eight hours. The youngest son, John, Honora, and their father all became ill, but recovered. The disease was probably plague, both bubonic and some secondary pneumonic, but it was diagnosed only retrospectively (and tentatively) some nine months later when the disease struck Latimer Cottages (on the opposite side of the River Orwell from the Rouse home, and several miles upriver) and claimed four victims.

Dr. Carey, the same doctor who had attended Mrs. Church of Charity Farm Cottages four years earlier, was called on Tuesday, September 13. Although there was little he could do, he did note that all four victims showed signs of lung involvement. Dr. Carey had invited Dr. Herbert Brown of Ipswich to consult on one case and had also enlisted the help of Dr. Llewellyn Heath, a bacteriologist. Dr. Brown took blood and fluid samples, and from both these specimens Dr. Heath grew cultures that he identified as *Y. pestis.* Plague had unquestionably returned to rural England.

A sick rat was caught near Latimer Cottages. It died. A hare was shot in the same vicinity. By October 12 both were found to be infected with *Y. pestis.*

Two experts who had been with the Plague Commission in India came to Suffolk to investigate the outbreak. They initially trapped and examined 568 rats and, later, 40 rabbits. Seventeen rats (3 percent) and two rabbits were infected with plague. An intensive campaign was carried out to rid the area of rats, and thousands were killed.

More than a year after the deaths at Latimer Cottages a young sailor turned into sick bay at the Shotley Royal Navy Barracks near the mouth of the Orwell. He had cut himself while cleaning a rabbit. Seriously ill, he later developed pneumonia and was isolated. He entered sick bay on Tuesday, October 10, 1911, and was not free of infection until January 14, 1912, more than three months later. The organism had attacked the iris of both eyes, and although he survived the disease and lived to the age of seventy-six, he was almost completely blind.

Plague struck again in June 1918 and killed two persons in Warren Lane Cottages, about a mile from Shotley Barracks and midway between the rivers Stour and Orwell. An army bacteriologist confirmed the presence of *Y. pestis.*

During 1912 nearly 250,000 rats were killed on both sides of the Orwell, but no sign of plague was found. Then, in the next two years, the plague bacillus was found in a few rats, seven ferrets, and a rabbit. No infected rats were found after 1914, but it is not clear that anyone looked for them. A suggestion was made in 1950 that it might be profitable to reexamine the area, but the officials of Suffolk County violently rejected the suggestion.

It seems certain that Suffolk was infected by ships from such plague-ridden ports as Alexandria, Egypt; Valparaiso, Chile; and San Francisco, all of which shipped grain to Ipswich in the first decade of this century. From one or more of these ships infected rats escaped into the Suffolk countryside and in turn infected both rabbits and ferrets, presumably by flea transfer.

Argentina was infected early in the Third Pandemic and, in

the first thirty years of this century, had over six thousand cases of plague. Peru received the disease in 1903 and had human cases every year for more than half a century, with nearly seventeen hundred victims in 1908 alone. Peru has had more human plague than any other country in the Americas.

Formosa was stricken in 1896 and suffered some twenty-four thousand fatal cases of the disease up to 1917. Portugal, the Philippines, Shanghai, and various cities around the world were afflicted early in the Third Pandemic.

By the end of the first decade of the twentieth century, plague was firmly established in both North and South America and was slowly extending its reach in several countries. During this period both the San Francisco epidemics and the outbreak in Seattle took place.

Paris also suffered a recrudescence of plague during the Third Pandemic that was apparently triggered by the arrival of an infected cargo from India in 1917. The first human case was reported in December, and there was rat plague in the two years following. In 1920 there were ninety-one confirmed cases of human plague in Paris, mostly among ragpickers, and there continued to be both rat and human cases up to 1935. Fifty-six victims of the disease died. Black rats infested with *X. cheopis* have been found in Paris at least as recently as 1946.

In the summer of 1912 plague struck Cuba and Puerto Rico. The U.S. surgeon general suggested that the larger U.S. ports should check whether the disease had spread to them. The Louisiana State Health Department promptly began a rat-trapping program in New Orleans. Almost immediately, plague was found. On Monday, June 17, 1912, an infected rat was trapped on Stuyvesant Docks. It was a lucky accident. Six months and seven thousand rats later, the total of plague-infected animals found remained at one.

For two years there was no further sign of plague in New Orleans.[3] Then, in mid-June 1914, a young man died in Charity Hospital with symptoms highly suggestive of plague. The disease was never confirmed.

Two days later, on Friday, June 19, the first official case was recognized on the Gulf coast when a forty-nine-year-old man was admitted to Charity Hospital. He died after nine days.

Dr. Rupert Blue was now surgeon general, and he went immediately to New Orleans to manage a plague-control program. Headquarters was a small structure at 163 Dryades Street. The building was hardly wide enough to accommodate the proud legend emblazoned above the door in eight-inch-high gold letters: *U.S. Public Health Service.*

New Orleans was then a city almost two hundred years old. The population, nearly four hundred thousand, was spread over a large area, mostly in one- or two-story wood-frame houses built close to the ground. The wharves along the Mississippi River were another problem. They were state-owned, and there were jurisdictional problems in securing funds for ratproofing them.

From the beginning, the authorities and the press were completely frank about the nature of the problem. The result was that there was cooperation from all levels of society. And foreign countries, convinced that no effort was being made to conceal the true situation, responded by not embargoing goods from New Orleans.

From mid-June through the end of December, there were thirty human plague cases in New Orleans and ten deaths. Plague-control measures were begun, and extensive rodent surveys for evidence of plague were instituted at the same time.

A year after the first case, more than 378,000 animals had been received for inspection. These included some 200,000 rats and nearly as many mice, in addition to muskrats, guinea pigs, mink, rabbits, opossums, squirrels, and a puppy. Only rats and mice were plague-infected. The first infected rat found since 1912 was taken on Saturday, July 11, 1914, in a shed behind a coffee shop at 1904 Magazine Street. Some 250 more were found by year's end.

Procedures similar to those used in San Francisco were used to fumigate buildings, but they were hopelessly ineffective. Two buildings were fumigated with sulfur as thoroughly as possible, and the flooring of the buildings was removed as soon as fumigation was completed. The area under the floors swarmed with live rats, apparently unharmed. The only dead animals were those that were plague-infected; they had presumably succumbed to the disease.

Rat trappers were paid on a straight salary basis. By the third month the number of rats caught declined sharply. Perhaps the rat ppoulation was depleted by the trapping campaign. But some asute student of human nature in the upper echelon of the antiplague campaign thought otherwise. He reduced the daily pay of the rat trappers slightly and then substituted a bounty for each rat and added a bonus for each plague-infected rat nearly equivalent to three days' regular pay. The total rat catch increased immediately. When next it decined it was because rats were becoming very difficult to trap, not because of boredom on the part of the trappers.

There was a single human plague case in New Orleans the following year, 1915, and one in 1916. Also in April 1916, a British vessel, the S.S. *Trevelyan*, arrived in New Orleans from Karachi. She harbored thirty-eight rats, one of which was infected with *Y. pestis*. It was only the second plague-infected rat found on board ship in the United States. The S.S. *Eggsford* arrived on September 20. She had had no contact with any known plague ports for over a year. Nevertheless, her complement of sixty-nine rats included one that carried the disease.

Meanwhile, in California, eradication programs directed against the ground squirrel had been going on for a decade: the program in the Bay Area had been especially vigorous. There were only occasional human plague victims, and there was growing optimism in public-health circles that plague would now be limited to isolated individual cases. The threat of epidemic plague was a well-laid ghost of the distant past. Then, in August 1919, the situation changed dramatically.[4]

On Monday, August 11, and again two days later, a thirty-two-year-old Oakland man, hereafter called Victor Boone, hunted squirrels in nearby Alameda County and brought them home to eat. On August 15 he was taken ill, with a fever, pain in his right side, and congestion in the lower part of his right lung. Two days later Boone developed a tender swelling in the armpit (axilla). The axillary swelling was lanced that day and the next. The afternoon of the following day, Wednesday, August 20, Victor Boone died.

While Boone was in the hospital, he was visited by two friends, a couple his own age. Five days after Boone's death the man became ill. Three days later he was dead. His wife was stricken the day her husband died but recovered. She was the only victim of the epidemic to live.

On Friday, August 29, Boone's landlord was sick; two days later a nurse who had attended Boone also came down with the disease. The landlord died on September 3, the nurse the next day. By September 7 three more persons had died; all were contacts of the nurse and the couple who had visited Boone during his illness. All these deaths were certified as the result of influenza with pneumonia. The great influenza pandemic of 1918 had only recently passed.

After the seventh death, the city health officer became suspicious. Four more persons died in the next two days, including two physicians who had treated some of the previous victims. Only then was it confirmed that the deaths were caused not by influenza but by pneumonic plague. The last two victims of the epidemic at least had the comfort of knowing what was killing them.

In three weeks Victor Boone's squirrel-hunting expeditions had led to fourteen cases of pneumonic plague in Oakland, of which there was only one survivor. The disease had already struck its last victims before it was diagnosed.

The New Orleans newspapers carried accounts of the Oakland epidemic. Some delicious shivers ran down Creole spines at their reading; their own experience with plague epidemics was only three years past; fortunately plague had been eradicated in New Orleans.[5]

Then, two days before Halloween 1919, a thirty-three-year-old man died in Charity Hospital—of plague. In the next few months there were eleven more cases in New Orleans and four more deaths. In the same period, two ships carrying rodent plague came alongside the piers on the Mississippi. On Christmas Eve 1919, the S.S. *Managua* arrived with a cargo of bananas and rats from Nicaragua; one of the rats had plague. Early the next year, the S.S. *Historian* brought, among other things, forty-eight rats and a mouse. Again, one of the rats had plague.

New Orleans had seven cases of human plague in 1920; three were fatal. It had its last reported human case, to the present, in June 1923. Altogether, the city had fifty-one cases and eighteen deaths, and imported cases continued to arrive by ship for several years after the last indigenous case.

The year 1920 saw the spread of the disease to other Gulf coast ports.[6] In Pensacola, Florida, a sixteen-year-old boy died on June 2, after a two-day illness. From the middle of June to the end of August there were nine more cases. Of the ten plague victims in Pensacola, seven died.

Plague was first reported in Galveston, Texas, on Wednesday, June 16, 1920. The victim died the next day. By early November, eighteen cases had originated in Galveston. Two of the persons infected left the city during the incubation period or early in the course of the disease. One, a twenty-year-old dock worker, went to Port Arthur and died there. The other infected patient went to Houston, where he recovered. Two-thirds of the Galveston cases were fatal.

June 1920 was a busy month for the forces of plague control along the Gulf coast. Human plague was reported almost simultaneously in Pensacola and in Galveston and Beaumont, Texas. Beaumont is some 75 miles (120 kilometers) east of Galveston, and inland on the Neches River. Beaumont had fourteen plague cases in the space of two months. Six of the cases were fatal.

Because of the death of the young dock worker from Galveston in Port Arthur, rodent surveys were begun in the latter city. One infected rat was found. It is unlikely that the rat was infected by the young man from Galveston. Probably rodent infection had been present in Port Arthur for some time before the spring of 1920. Infected rodents were found in Pensacola and in all the Texas cities that had plague in 1920. They were not found elsewhere. It was forty years, however, before a really sensitive test for animal plague was developed. Rodent plague was, and is, probably much more widely distributed than was indicated by the earlier surveys.

In 1924 the most vicious pneumonic plague epidemic ever to occur in the United States broke out in Los Angeles.[7] A fifty-year-old Mexican national, whom I will call Jose Lucero, fell ill on Wednesday, October 1. He had a femoral bubo that was diagnosed as venereal disease. He recovered. Jose's four-year-old daughter became ill at the same time and died four days later. Following an autopsy, her death was acribed to lobar pneumonia. It was, in fact, bubonic plague with pneumonic complications.

Most of the Mexican community in Los Angeles, including the Luceros, lived on the eastern edge of the city in the Macy Street district. It was here the epidemic occurred. The Lucero home was half a block from a rooming and boardinghouse at 742 Clara Street, run by Luceno Samarano, who lived there with her second husband and family. Nine days after the death of Jose Lucero's daughter, Lucena Samarano became ill and died five days later. She was thirty-nine. Autopsy did not reveal the cause of her death. Lucena's husband was stricken on October 22, three days after she died. A practical nurse who had cared for Mrs. Samarano also developed the symptoms of her former patient. The nurse died in three days, and Mr. Samarano in four.

The preliminary phase of the epidemic was over. Two days later plague attacked in force. On Tuesday, October 28, fifteen persons became sick. One was the older sister of the practical nurse. A friend of Lucena Samarano, her mother, her son, an uncle, and four cousins were among the victims, as were her husband's mother and one of his sons by a previous marriage. Two boarders in the house were attacked, as was the priest who administered the last rites to Mr. Samarano. Every person stricken on October 28 died, most within three days.

October 29 brought seven more cases. Two were sons of Mr. Samarano; one was a woman who had nursed him, and two were his friends. A sixth victim was another boarder in the Samarano house, and the seventh was Lucena Samarano's older sister. From this group, two recovered, the youngest (Raul Samarano, age six) and Mr. Samarano's nurse.

On Wednesday, October 29, a resident physician of the Los Angeles County General Hospital answered a call from the Mexican community just across the city line in Los Angeles County. After visiting the home, he requested an ambulance to take two of the sick persons to the hospital. He could not definitely diagnose the disease, but he thought it was highly contagious, since several families in the neighborhood seemed to be suffering from it.

On Thursday another thirteen patients were taken to General Hospital. The following day, October 31, an autopsy was performed on Lucena's twenty-five-year-old cousin, and the plague organism was discovered. Lung sections from Mr. Samarano confirmed the diagnosis. By then there were thirty cases. Eleven victims were dead, and sixteen were dying. Twenty-six days had passed since the death of Jose Lucero's daughter.

Meanwhile, the young driver of the ambulance that had taken Mr. Samarano to the hospital had fallen sick the day before, as had Mr. Samarano's cousin, an eighteen-year-old girl. Also stricken on that day was a forty-year-old man of no discernible relation to the other victims.

The news of the epidemic spread from Los Angeles on that Halloween 1924 in rather strange ways. First, the assistant superintendent of the L.A. County General Hospital wired federal and state authorities and medical supply houses to learn where plague serum and vaccine could be obtained but did not say why he wanted them. A Public Health Service official in Los Angeles heard about the telegram, made inquiries, and the next day sent his own telegram to the surgeon general in a prearranged code. It began, "Eighteen cases ekkil," and ended, "Ethos. Recommend federal aid." The telegram meant that there were eighteen cases of pneumonic plague and that the situation was serious.

On November 1 a nurse who had cared for the young ambulance driver was ill. The next day two more boarders from

742 Clara Street also became sick. All six cases after October 30 were fatal.

At 1:00 A.M. on Sunday, November 2, officials cordoned off the plague-infected areas and forbade the residents to leave their homes or to congregate. A seven-day food ration based on the occupancy of each house was supplied; house-to-house searches for other victims were made; and a Spanish-speaking priest and a social worker were brought in to explain the situation to the frightened and bewildered residents.

Another boarder of the Samarano's became sick on November 4. Two children in a home found to have plague-infected rats living under it were struck by the disease, one on the third and one on the seventh. An older woman, a friend of the ambulance driver's nurse, fell ill on the eleventh. There were three subsequent cases with no known contacts between November 22 and January 10. Six of the last seven cases were bubonic, rather than pneumonic, plague.

Residents of areas outside Los Angeles read details of the plague epidemic's progress in their local newspapers. San Francisco newspapers gave it thorough coverage as did the *New York Times* and the *Washington Post.* The Los Angeles newspapers, however, referred to the disease as the "strange malady" and "pneumonia," sometimes accompanied by the adjectives "virulent" or "malignant." The newspapers were not entirely to blame, since this was the story reporters received from the city health officers. On November 16, when the epidemic was essentially over, the Los Angeles newspapers referred to the disease as pneumonic plague but added that this was a "technical term" for "malignant pneumonia." The truth was exactly the opposite. "Malignant pneumonia" was an euphemism for pneumonic plague.

The call of the superintendent of the Los Angeles County Hospital for plague serum had not gone unanswered. As a commercial laboratory in Philadelphia later reported in its house organ,

Science has discovered . . . a serum that will stop the Swath of Death and save the lives of thousand. Los Angeles calls for help and in less than thirty-six hours the vials of serum were brought to the front lines where the battle is on against the Terror. . . .

The serum was in stock, waiting for the day when a stricken world might need it. Within an hour the life-saving remedies were packed for a three-thousand-mile journey. In a few minutes a high-powered motor car was making a record run to the flying field at Mineola, L.I. Speed laws were forgotten. The messenger of mercy had right of way.

And then, the mail plane—the shipment stored aboard, the roar of engines, and the flight to save lives was begun.

Despite the hyperbole, the serum was used in only one case, and there is no reason to think that it affected the outcome even then.

The result of the epidemic was an intensive, although belated, campaign against rats in Los Angeles, beginning on November 6. Authorities first paid special attention to the port area, rather than the Macy Street section where people were dying. There was fear that Los Angeles Harbor would be quarantined, and that it would be bad for business.

The year was almost over when the first infected rat was found in the harbor area, near a hog farm, and four miles from the harbor itself. The hog farm was demolished, but the surgeon general had already quarantined the port the week before, to the distress of the chairman of the Los Angeles Chamber of Commerce, who promptly wrote his congressman to protest. In fairness, it must be admitted that it is not clear whether the surgeon general based his decision on the presence of human plague twenty-two miles away from the harbor or on the need to force cooperation of the city health department with their state counterpart and with the U.S. Public Health Service.

By early in 1925 the epidemic was over. There had been thirty-three cases of pneumonic plague, thirty-one of them fatal, and eight bubonic cases, with five fatalities. It was, to this day, the last great urban outbreak of plague in America, and the most spectacular attack of the pneumonic form in U.S. history.

12

Man Fights Back

Each member of the plague trinity is tough, adaptable, and prolific. Together, they constitute a formidable force, unde- terred in the past by man's puny efforts to turn it aside. Plague has worn seven-league boots, a cloak of invincibility, and an air of disdain. Nothing man has done against it ever mattered very much. Humanity's lot was to weep with rage, frustration, and fear as plague swept to and fro, unheeding. Bonfires in the streets, pogroms, amulets, magic potion or solemn mass, together or separately, had no effect. Plague struck with de- mented fury, turned away, then struck again, as if mocking man's impotence.

Humankind did not remain forever defenseless. As it learned to know its enemies better, so it learned, sometimes at least, to defeat them.

Once the role of commensal rats in the transmission of plague was accepted, they became the first target of plague- control efforts. For centuries, rats had been shot or bludgeoned, trapped or poisoned. They were set upon by cats, dogs, ferrets, mongooses, snakes, and other animals. But the effect on the rodent population of all this attention was negligible.

Because of the rat's generally retiring nature and nocturnal

habits, only a few of the local population ever present themselves for direct attack by gun or club. Even when they do,
such an attack holds some hazards for the attacker, for he may
acquire disease from his small victims. Any domestic cat in
full possession of its faculties will streak for the nearest tree
if confronted by a full-grown Norway rat, and although dogs,
ferrets, and mongooses successfully attack rats, they are also
apt to acquire plague in the process.

Trapping is only modestly effective. Its principal utility is
in keeping down an already small rodent population. Even
that may fail. Rats avoid traps, newly placed in their environment, just as they avoid anything unfamiliar, and when accustomed to traps they frequently learn how to steal the bait
without harm to themselves.

The traditional poisons—strychnine, cyanide, arsenic, and
thallium—are all effective to varying degrees, but hazardous
to humans and domestic animals. Thallium is not banned in
the United States; the remaining compounds are the subject
of hearings by the United States Environmental Protection
Agency (EPA) on whether their continued use is in the public
interest.

Red squill, a plant product used as a rat poison for at least
seven hundred years, is reasonably safe and moderately effective, but only against the Norway rat, generally the easier of
the two major species to control. Zinc phosphide is equally
effective against both the black and the Norway rats. It is also
dangerous to humans, although as a black powder with a gar-
licky odor it is unlikely to be eaten by accident. It is often
incorporated into bait containing tartar emetic so that it will
be expelled by vomiting in children or domestic animals who
eat it accidently. Since neither rats nor mice can vomit, they
retain this and other poisons.

In 1943 the first synthetic rodenticide was discovered, a
compound more toxic to rats than the most potent of those
used before. Its development was followed closely by a second
substance and then by a third, and very different, agent, which
had a remarkable impact on the age-old problem of rodent
control.

The first of these three poisons, the compound known as sodium monofluoroacetate, was called 1080, the catalog number of the first sample tested. The study leading to the synthesis of 1080 was done in Poland and was a basic research investigation of the important metabolic pathway known as the Krebs tricarboxylic acid cycle. The compound proved to be a very effective rodenticide, however, twice as poisonous as strychnine, by far the most effective of the older poisons against rats. Since the tricarboxylic acid cycle that is inhibited by 1080 is vital to all animals, sodium monofluoroacetate is also effective against cats, dogs, and children.

This latter property was reemphasized in March 1976, when three small chldren (two to four years of age) died in Durant, Oklahoma, after eating wafers containing 1080 that had been carelessly left on the seat of the exterminator's pickup truck.

Animals poisoned with 1080 die within a few hours, often in the open, where the poisoned carcasses may be gnawed on by cats, dogs, or pigs. Generally, rats surviving treatment with 1080 subsequently avoid it in the future even when it is presented in a different form. Nonetheless, it is a very effective compound when it can be kept away from domestic animals and children. It is very useful in deratting ships, in place of the more cumbersome fumigation. Properly applied, it kills 85 to 90 percent of ship-borne rats. Because of its extreme danger to humans and domestic animals—there is no specific antidote to 1080 poisoning—the EPA is considering banning its use.

Two years after the discovery of the rodenticidal properties of 1080, a second synthetic compound was found. This substance, called ANTU, for the initials of its chemical name (alphanapthylthiourea), was discovered during studies on diet selection by rats. Rodent control was not under investigation. It was found, however, that Norway rats, particularly adults, were highly susceptible to ANTU poisoning, while black rats, mice, and young Norway rats were not. Dogs, cats, and pigs readily succumbed to ANTU. Rats not killed when poisoned with ANTU avoid it for as long as a year.

Animals poisoned with ANTU often die in the open within

a few hours of consuming poisoned bait. There is no specific antidote for ANTU poisoning, but it is not highly toxic to humans.

A persistent problem with most rodent poisons is the death and decomposition of an animal in inaccessible locations, a distressing event when the rotting corpse is in the walls or ceiling of a residence. Thus, much was made, for advertising purposes, of rodenticides that allegedly induced the animals to die in the open. This mythical property was commemorated in a little poem that has become part of American folklore:

> Johnny and the other brats,
> Ate up all the "Tuff-on-Rats,"
> Father said, as mother cried,
> "Never mind they'll die outside."

The most important single advance in rodent control was the discovery of a new kind of compound (warfarin) at the Wisconsin Alumni Research Foundation (WARF) in 1948. This remarkable substance has dominated rodent control ever since.

The beginning was a search for the cause of massive hemorrhages fatal to farm animals that ate spoiled sweet clover hay. After years of work, the active agent was finally isolated in the predawn darkness of Wednesday, June 28, 1939. Structurally related to Vitamin K, a naturally occurring substance involved in blood-clotting, whose action it effectively blocked, this compound, known to chemists as dicumarol, was used in clinical medicine as an anticoagulant little more than a year later.[1]

Dr. Karl Paul Link, the discoverer of dicumarol, had had tuberculosis as a student in Switzerland. Near the end of World War II, when he was exhausted by long hours in the laboratory, the old malady flared up again, and Link was forced to spend two months in a hospital and another six months in a sanatorium. There he passed the time by reading extensively on the history of rodent control.

When he returned to the laboratory, studies on the rodenticidal properties of compounds related to dicumarol began in earnest. Early in 1948, the compound now known as warfarin

was selected as the most effective. It was a derivative of dicumarol. Coumarin, the substance responsible for the characteristic sweet smell of new-mown hay, was transformed into
dicumarol when the hay spoiled. The name of the rodenticide
commemorated the initials of the institute where it was discovered, plus *-arin*, from *coumarin*.

If repeatedly eaten by rats, warfarin is a very effective rodenticide, although several times more effective against the
Norway rat than against black rats. Unlike most poisons, it
in itself is attractive to rats; another bait is not required. Rats
will nibble a small amount and then often wait to see if it
makes them ill before eating more. They quickly learn to avoid
rapidly acting compounds like 1080 and ANTU as well as the
baits in which they are used. Since warfarin and related compounds are slow-acting, however, this aversion reaction does
not occur.

Warfarin has the further advantage that an antidote (vitamin
K) is available to treat accidental poisoning in domestic animals and humans. Rats, always cunning, have learned this as
well. In the East Anglia district of England, rats exposed to
warfarin seek out marram grass growing on sand dunes, because this grass has a high content of vitamin K.

A major disadvantage of warfarin and other rodenticidal anticoagulants, besides their expense, is that rodents must have
access to such baits for two to three weeks for a lethal effect.
This is not practical in emergencies.

Despite these problems, an impartial observer surveying the
various new and strikingly effective rodent-control agents made
available in only three years in the late 1940s might reasonably
have concluded that man's centuries-old war against the commensal rodents was about to end in victory. The fleas were in
for it, too.

In 1939, the same year in which both 1080 and dicumarol
were discovered, Paul Müller, a chemist for the Swiss firm of
J. R. Geigy, synthesized a chlorinated hydrocarbon now known
by the initials of its common chemical name as DDT
(dichlorodiphenyltrichloroethane). Müller tested DDT's in-
secticidal action against houseflies and beetles. It was im-

mensely effective. He went on to develop a variety of media in which the insecticide could be dispersed and made extensive further studies of its properties. In terms of public health it was one of the most significant discoveries ever made. Müller received the Nobel Prize in chemistry in 1948 for his careful investigation of the compound, first synthesized seventy-four years earlier.

The insecticide was devastating to a wide variety of insects of both economic and medical importance. Cheaply made in large quantities, it had the very desirable property (for insect control) of persistence. Since it did not dissolve readily in water, a solution of DDT sprayed on the walls of a native hut would kill every mosquito that alighted on that wall for months after.[2]

The early results obtained with DDT were spectacular. In the fall of 1943, a typhus epidemic broke out in Naples, brought in by thousands of Italians returning from prisoner-of-war camps in Yugoslavia. The Allied troops entered the ruined city on Friday, October 1. The usual control measures against the disease were applied, but they failed. The military commanders were well aware that typhus, a disease transmitted by lice and historically almost as devastating as plague, had killed more soldiers than even the most notable military blunders.

The historically minded among them may have recalled that typhus had once before dashed the hopes of a conquerer of Naples just at the moment when he beheld the city helpless before him. In 1528 the mighty army of Francis I of France was about to administer the coup de grace to the city's defenders. Then typhus broke out in the French ranks. In three weeks, nearly half the soldiers of Francis I were dead of the disease, and the siege of Naples was over.

No Allied officer wished to see that episode repeated. Finally, almost into the new year of 1944, DDT was used for the first time. The clothing, possessions, and persons of 1.3 million Neopolitans and their neighbors were dusted with the insecticide. Three weeks later the epidemic began abruptly to decline and then ceased altogether. For the first time in the history of man an epidemic of the dread disease was stopped in its tracks. The miracle was repeated on April 15, 1945, when the British liberated the concentration camp at Belsen and found 20,000 typhus cases among 45,000 inmates.

The effect of DDT on malarial mosquitoes was even more dramatic. Before World War II, malaria routinely killed a million persons a year in India alone, and made several million virtual invalids, able to work only in the intervals between attacks of the disease. In a nation overwhelmingly composed of small farmers, the effect of malaria on food production was catastrophic. Even by 1952 there were some seventy-five million cases of malaria. Twelve years later there were only one hundred thousand. In Ceylon the death toll from malaria dropped from nearly thirteen thousand a year to zero following DDT application. In the Soviet Union, in 1946, there were thirty-five million victims of malaria. Ten years later there were thirteen thousand—only one case for every three thousand a decade earlier.

Even now, more than forty years after the discovery of the insecticide, the goal of malaria eradication from the world is based largely on careful indoor application of DDT. The one-third of the world's people who live in malarial zones owe their lives and their livelihoods to DDT. The next most effective compound is eight times more expensive and far more dangerous to humans.

Plague-carrying fleas are also highly susceptible to the insecticide. Dusting rat burrows with DDT powder killed substantial numbers of fleas. The DDT's effectiveness was multiplied when the rats carried it deep into their nests on their feet and fur.

A plague outbreak in Tumbes, Peru, 1945, was stopped dramatically four days after DDT application began. Concurrently, the number of fleas dropped over 80 percent, and the number of free-living fleas in rat burrows fell even lower after the first insecticide dusting. Rat plague was reduced 75 percent by the first DDT application and obliterated by the second.

Besides all this, the miracle compound was virtually nontoxic to other forms of life, unlike many rodenticides and compounds used then and now for insect control. Although DDT did cause eggshell thinning in some species of birds, a child who ate a handful of DDT might be uncomfortable as a result, but he apparently would suffer no lasting harm. Even workers with thirty years daily exposure to DDT in the course of its manufacture showed no ill effects from the insecticide.

As the second half of the twentieth century began, there were frequent predictions of an insect-free future after mosquitoes, lice, fleas, and other obnoxious (and dangerous) varieties were exterminated. An occasional graybeard pointed out that insects had been on earth millions of years before humans and that, in spite of much effort, man had never eliminated even a single insect species, let alone several. But such warnings were little heeded in the effulgent dawn of a new era when man would obliterate still other forms of life.

The 1940s were the beginning of spectacular successes in the control of both rodents and fleas. Two points quickly emerged. A widespread campaign against rats was dangerous nonsense when plague threatened, unless preceded by extensive treatment to kill plague-bearing fleas before they could transfer to other hosts—humans, for example. And antiflea and antirat efforts were useless unless they covered a wide area. Otherwise, rats simply migrated into a treated area to take up where their predecessors had left off.

In spite of many problems, rodent and flea control was available on a scale never before possible—for those with time and the money to pay for it. Unfortunately, in some of the most severely threatened parts of the world, public health officials seldom had much of either.

In *Songs of Many Keys*, the American physician-poet Oliver Wendell Holmes (whose son was the noted Supreme Court Justice) wrote more than a century ago:

> And lo! the starry fold reveal
> The blazoned truth we hold so dear;
> To guard is better than to heal,
> The shield is nobler than the spear.

Insecticides and rodenticides play an important part in

shielding man against the approach of plague. But, despite them, the disease attacks humans as it has for centuries. There was still need for means to repel such attack when *Y. pestis* swarmed through a crack in the wall of the cellular fortress we call man. The first method of inner defense that had the slightest effect was vaccination.

Untreated plague victims who survive usually do so because their bodies begin slowly to make antibodies in response to invasion by the plague bacillus. The very first messengers signaling that such an enemy had burst the gates starts the process of antibody production in an otherwise healthy victim, but it gathers speed with agonizing, often fatal, deliberation. Once the production of antibodies begins, the process continues, leaving the victim's blood well supplied with these proteins for some time after the last traces of infection are only a painful memory.

Vaccination against plague seeks to reproduce what happens in a plague victim's body, but in a much milder way. *Yersinia pestis* either killed or, if living, greatly weakened (avirulent), is given in small amounts. The body acts as if a full-scale invasion were underway by making antibodies against the plague bacillus. If a successfully vaccinated person or animal is then injected with virulent plague bacilli, the specific antibody proteins are there, ready and waiting, without the long and dangerous period while the antibody-producing cells slowly convert to a war footing.

Vaccination, as we know it, dates from May 14, 1796, when Edward Jenner inoculated a small boy with material from the sores of a cow ill with cowpox; he later showed that the lad was immune to smallpox. (Vaccination comes from the Latin word *vacca*, meaning "cow.") Active immunization, as developed by Jenner, results when a human makes antibodies following vaccination. In principle, passive immunization with antiplague serum, where the necessary antibodies are simply injected, should do as well.

The first antiplague serum was made by Yersin in 1897. The immunity conferred is short-lived, the serum is expensive (it is prepared from rabbit or horse serum and several hundred milliliters—a large waterglass-full—may be given by injection to a plague victim), and there is obviously the risk of severe reactions. Serotherapy is now little used.

Active immunization (vaccination) against plague is almost as old as our knowledge of the causative agent. It is more than a century older if the earliest, mostly disastrous, attempts are included. In 1895 Yersin and his co-workers showed that rabbits could be immunized against the disease by repeated injection of small quantities of Y. pestis.

But Yersin, mysterious man, again turned his back on a brilliant beginning, and the man whose name is most intimately associated with plague vaccine is a young Russian from Odessa on the Black Sea—the patient, tireless, and immortal Waldemar Mordecai Wolff Haffkine. Haffkine fled Odessa to escape death at either the hands of anti-Semitic mobs or the czar's police (two groups frequently indistinguishable) and then continued his studies in Paris before going to Bombay in 1896 to attempt to develop a plague vaccine.[3]

Finally, after much experimentation, Haffkine killed Y. pestis with heat, added phenol as a preservative, and then injected the bacterial suspension, first into himself and then into anyone else who would stand still long enough.

Those Haffkine inoculated occasionally hurled curses at his head in the days following—and with good reason. The crude vaccine made some of them terribly ill. But Haffkine believed that a definite reaction against the vaccination was necessary to provide later protection. His vaccine, although often unpleasant and sometimes briefly incapacitating, improved a vaccinated person's chances of surviving a plague epidemic.

In 1896, and for nearly four decades after, there was nothing a beleaguered physician could do once a patient contracted plague. But prior vaccination often brought a drop in plague mortality of 20 to 30 percent. This was not spectacular, but the Haffkine killed vaccine was the first weapon humanity had forged in its several million years on earth that had the slightest power against plague, and it saved hundreds of thousands, perhaps millions, of lives.

Then, in the early 1930s, scientists in Java and Madagascar

found that some strains of the plague bacillus lost much of their virulence on prolonged laboratory culture. Injection of these attenuated, but living, strains also immunized animals against severe plague infection.

The live, attenuated strains were much more immunogenic than the vaccine made from killed organisms; that is, much smaller doses produced equal immunity, and they caused less severe reactions than the Haffkine vaccines of that time. The pendulum of scientific fashion, which is as subject to fad as any other, swung so far toward the use of live vaccines that most experts concluded that there was no longer reason to use killed preparations. The controversy lives on, in relation to plague as well as to other diseases.

In the summer of 1941, the clouds of war loomed menacingly on the American horizon. It was clear that if hostilities broke out, Americans would face combat in the plague-afflicted areas around the Mediterranean or in the Far East, possibly in both.

On October 22, 1941, just six weeks before Japanese bombers dropped out of the dawn onto Pearl Harbor, the Subcommittee on Tropical Diseases of the National Research Council passed a resolution: "Resolved that, even though the available knowledge does not seem to afford definite evidence of the benefits from the use of plague vaccines, it is advisable to vaccinate, with killed plague bacilli of an approved strain, all military or naval personnel under serious threat of exposure to bubonic plague." Thus, America, although with only modest faith in the product, joined the Haffkine Institute in producing killed vaccine to protect exposed personnel. The Dutch, the French, the Chinese, and the Soviet authorities relied mainly on attenuated live vaccine. Forty years later this alignment of nations remains the same.

The killed vaccine used by the United States has a reasonably good record. In World War II there were no reported deaths from plague in the U.S. Armed Forces, despite their engagement in plague-infested areas. On the other hand, in the British Middle East Force, there were twenty-six cases of bubonic plague reported; five were fatal.

A substantial disadvantage of all plague vaccines is that a series of injections must be given well in advance of exposure to the disease. Current U.S. practice is to give the vaccine and two booster shots over a nine-month period. Initial vaccination is with one milliliter of suspension containing two thousand million killed *Y. pestis;* then, at three and nine months, two-tenths of a milliliter of a similar suspension are given. The initial vaccination may be given in two equal portions several weeks apart. Far fewer unpleasant reactions are encountered with the divided first dose.

Probably little immunity exists before the second booster shot is given—if it exists then. Even after vaccination and two boosters, the proportion of humans who do not make antibody to *Y. pestis* is a bit less than one in three. Whether the nonreactors are in fact immune to plague infection is unknown.

Soviet scientists have experimented with a variety of immunization procedures against plague in addition to the traditional inoculation. They have administered plague vaccine as an aerosol suspension to roomfuls of people at a time. The obvious advantage is that as many as several hundred persons are treated in about fifteen minutes, and the results of aerosol immunization are not far different from those of inoculation. Both French and Soviet scientists have also tried oral administration of vaccine, in both liquid and lozenge form. Both methods yield encouraging results. In critical situations the time between vaccine administrations could be shortened to as little as a week, and mass oral or aerosol administration might at least partially immunize a large number of people in the shortest possible time.

In the United States the emphasis is on the use of the jet injector for treating large numbers of people quickly. Any of these techniques is a vast improvement over the classical methods of injection under the skin or rubbing the vaccine into an abraded area. Jet injection is twelve times faster than subcutaneous injection, the aerosol method with liquid vaccine is nineteen times faster, and the vaccine administered orally is twenty-two times faster. Rubbing vaccine into an abraded area of the skin is the slowest of all.

The difficulties in plague vaccination are not in the methods for preparing or administering the various types of vaccines; they are in evaluating the results. Three criteria are used: animal-protection tests, serological (blood) analysis for antibodies, and circumstantial evidence. The circumstantial evidence is the most convincing.

For example, a survey in 1948 of several thousand cases in India, where the Haffkine killed vaccine was widely administered, showed that nearly 60 percent of the untreated bubonic plague victims died. Among those vaccinated the death rate dropped to 40 percent. Similarly, in Dakar, Senegal, in 1945, nearly two hundred thousand persons were given live vaccine to head off an epidemic. Among unvaccinated victims of plague the mortality rate was 85 percent, while in those vaccinated it fell to 66 percent.

The most recent large-scale test of the current U.S.P. vaccine arose from the American military experience in Vietnam. Although plague raged among the civilian population, there were only eight reported cases of plague among Americans.

In each of these large-scale tests, other factors could have contributed to the favorable results. For instance, in Vietnam, American combat troops wore boots with trousers tucked into them. The trousers were of cloth very tightly woven and impregnated with insecticide. The troops also used insect repellent and insecticides generously and were usually well fed and healthy.

Still it is reasonable to assume that plague vaccines of both the attenuated live and the killed types offer some protection against the disease.[4]

The vaccination of thirty million civilians in Vietnam between 1960 and 1972 was by far the most impressive application of the live vaccine in history. In the last four years of this campaign, more than seventeen million vaccinations were made, and the incidence of human plague following vaccination was carefully followed province by province.

The situation was complicated by the fact that in those regions in which the vaccination campaign was most vigorously carried out, dusting with insecticides was also extensive.

Thus, any favorable effect on plague incidence would have been the result of at least two factors, the vaccine and the pesticide dusting. But the effect on plague incidence was essentially zero. Despite expenditure of over three million dollars, the program had no detectable influence on the incidence of plague. It was an expensive, heart-breaking failure.

The vaccine commonly used in this program was prepared by the Institut Pasteur in Saigon and had a useful life of fifteen days at room temperature. District headquarters received kerosene-powered refrigerators for storing the vaccine, but under wartime conditions, some of the vaccine administered was almost certainly inactivated by age. Only a single injection was given, and although a booster shot was recommended, the Vietnamese peasants were reluctant to take even the first injection. The figures on the number of persons vaccinated are those of the South Vietnamese Ministry of Health, and there may be substantial inaccuracies. Whatever the reasons, the vaccination program failed.

Another serious problem was described in May 1974. The subject was a common live vaccine strain of the plague bacillus known as E. V., from the initials of the person from whose body it was first isolated. Millions of persons had been inoculated with this strain over the preceding thirty years without experiencing serious side effects. A sample of the strain was judged completely safe by the usual laboratory tests. Yet it caused moderate to severe plague infection in three different species of monkeys! The next result was even more serious.

A major problem with live vaccines is maintaining the immunogenicity—that is, the ability to stimulate antibody production—of the strain from which they are prepared. A common procedure is to reisolate the vaccine strain periodically after injecting a large number of the attenuated plague bacilli into the animal. Such "passaged" strains show no increase in virulence. With doses of the E.V. strain very much smaller than were innocuous to guinea pigs, however, fatal plague resulted in ten of sixteen of one species of monkey and half those of a second species. Yet guinea pigs are the standard animals in which the virulence of plague strains (and the live vaccine strains) are evaluated. This illustrates the basic question that casts a dark shadow over the evaluation of plague vaccines in animals: Is man more like a monkey or a guinea pig, and, if more like a monkey, which monkey is he more like?[5]

These disturbing results emphasize the Scylla and Charybdis of plague vaccination—on the one hand the tragic results of ineffectual vaccine administration, as to civilians in Vietnam; on the other that of inoculating humans with a preparation capable of causing serious plague infection. Unfortunately there seems to be no reliable way of telling whether one is approaching one danger point or the other.

While Haffkine was sweltering in the all-enveloping heat of Bombay, halfway around the world, in the cool valley of the Danube, the Viennese chemist Paul Gelmo was attempting to synthesize a new member of the strongly colored, nitrogen-containing substances called azo dyes.

In 1908 Gelmo succeeded in making sulfanilamide, the first member of a new series of compounds called sulfonamides. Sulfanilamide succeeded as a dyestuff because it bound avidly to the proteins in silk and wool. Bacteria contain protein. Such dyes might bind to bacteria and inhibit their growth. Over the twenty years following Gelmo's synthesis of sulfanilamide, it and other azo dyes found some medical uses.

Enter Dr. Gerhard Johannes Domagk, a research director of the giant I.G. Farbenindustrie in Germany.[6] Like many others he became interested in the sulfas, first for their properties as dyestuffs, later for their antibacterial applications. He carried out his first critical experiment on a Tuesday morning in late December 1932. Mice were injected with amounts of streptococci sufficient to cause fatal infection. Some were also injected with a sulfonamide. By Christmas Eve all the animals that had received the sulfonamide were alive. All the others were dead.

Other experiments followed, but no results were published until February 1935. In this interval Domagk's daughter contracted a severe infection. Nothing helped. In desperation, her father injected her with a sulfonamide, and she made a complete recovery. Dr. Domagk kept this impromptu experiment entirely secret until a number of other physicians reported similar results. In the first paper published on his work, Domagk also proposed a biochemical explanation for the drug's antibacterial action.

Marvelous to relate, Dr. Domagk received the Nobel Prize in medicine just four years later for his discovery of the antibacterial action of the sulfa compounds and for his explanation of their inhibitory action. Critics objected that Domagk was not the first to discover the antibacterial action of the sulfonamides and that his explanation of their mode of action was entirely wrong. But the controversy could not obscure the fact that for the first time there was a class of drugs that was soon shown to be effective against bubonic plague.

As early as 1938 sulfa drugs were used against plague. In uncomplicated bubonic plague, sulfa treatment of the victims reduced the mortality from 40 to 50 percent to 10 percent. Even in septicemic plague, in which large numbers of *Y. pestis* swarm in the blood, treatment with sulfa drugs reduced the death rate from the usual 90 percent or more to between 20 and 50 percent. Unfortunately, however, it was of no value in treating the pneumonic form. Still, the age of effective plague chemotherapy had begun.

At the same time, the antibiotic age was trying hard to be born, but it was a difficult labor. The discovery of the bacteriocidal action of the mold *Penicillium* was made by physicist John Tyndall in the eighteenth century and had been part of folk medicine for centuries before that. In 1928 it was rediscovered by Alexander Fleming.

Dr. Fleming was a hardy Scotsman who kept the window of his laboratory in Saint Mary's Hospital open except in the most inclement of London weather. He also chanced to have his laboratory directly under one in which researchers were extensively studying the properties of the mold *Penicillium notatum*. Fleming completed a long series of experiments just before he was to go on holiday. His laboratory was awash in uncovered Petri dishes filled with agar on which grew colonies of the staphylococcus he was investigating. Pressed for time, he did not wash the Petri dishes but rushed home, no doubt some hours after he had promised his wife he would arrive.

When he returned from vacation, he noticed that little greenish tufts of *Penicillium* dotted his culture plates. Around each tuft the bacteria had died, although elsewhere they had grown until they covered the agar surface. As Pasteur had said, "Chance favors only the prepared mind." Inquisitive Fleming pursued the matter of the zone of dead bacteria around each puff of *Penicillium*. He finally isolated a small quantity of the responsible compound, the first antibiotic, and named it penicillin.

Fleming's preparation of penicillin was not pure, and he concluded that it was too unstable to purify without destroying it. Impure penicillin, like the moldy bread or leather or soybean curd of centuries before, could be used only for surface infections, where the accompanying impurities were less important than they would be if the material were injected into the body.

World War II brought DDT, warfarin, and 1080 to the fore. The war that made sulfa a household word was to do the same for penicillin. In the black days of the Battle of Britain, Walter Florey, a Cambridge Ph.D. in pathology, sought work that might benefit the war effort. He finally elected to attempt to improve the production and purification of penicillin. With the help of the chemist E. B. Chain, he succeeded. For this achievement, the microbiologist Fleming of Scotland, the pathologist Florey of Australia, and the chemist Chain, previously of Berlin, jointly received the Nobel Prize for medicine in 1945.

Antibiotics are complex compounds made by microorganisms to defend themselves against other microorganisms (the sulfas are not antibiotics although they are sometimes so designated).

Naturally, penicillin was tested in the laboratory against the wily bacillus of plague. In high concentrations it killed the organisms. Hopes rose. But when the plague bacillus lodged safely inside the body of a mouse or a man, penicillin became useless, and the dreams of a great victory over the scourge of plague began to fade.

The development of penicillin, however, had an effect that transcended even the considerable importance of the drug itself. Its discovery stimulated the search for other antibiotic substances produced by molds, a tedious business that fortunately was undertaken by tireless investigators.

We have heard of Haffkine, who fled death in Odessa to save lives in India. Haffkine's teacher in the University of Odessa was the flamboyant Russian Élie Metchnikoff. He also fled Odessa for Paris and the Institut Pasteur, to which place Haffkine followed. It was Metchnikoff who first discovered that some cells in the body attack foreign cells or substances and engulf and destroy them, a process so vital to the defense of the body against plague.

Still another former resident of Odessa, half a century later, took seriously the injunction of Ecclesiasticus 38:4 that "the Lord hath created medicines out of the earth; and he that is wise will not abhor them." He patiently tested ten thousand soil microbes for antibiotic production. In 1944 Selman Abraham Waksman, then professor of microbiology at Rutgers University, discovered streptomycin, for which he received the Nobel Prize in medicine in 1952. It was soon tested for its action against *Y. pestis.*[7]

The results were astonishing. If ten micrograms of streptomycin were added to a culture medium containing nearly two million plague bacilli, in two hours only fifteen hundred *Y. pestis*—less than one in a thousand—still lived! In four more hours all were dead.

Naturally there were complications. When 1.25 milligrams of streptomycin were added to a medium containing 100 million virulent *Y. pestis* of the human strain called Shasta (for the California county where it was first isolated), all the plague bacilli died in fifteen minutes. If a quarter as much streptomycin was added, the time needed to eradicate *Y. pestis* was increased not four times, but sixteen times. When tests were made at the concentrations of streptomycin attainable in the human body, the time required to kill the Shasta strain increased from minutes or hours to between two and five days. Various strains of the plague bacillus differed in their sensitivity to the drug. Human-strain Shasta was nearly ten times more resistant to streptomycin when first tested than human-strain Modoc.

These results were discouraging. The question naturally arose whether streptomycin, like penicillin before it, would be active against *Y. pestis* in culture but useless in lower animals and humans.

The next step was obvious. Virulent *Y. pestis* were injected into mice in concentrations that would make them seriously ill with plague in thirty-six to forty-eight hours. When sulfa drugs or highly potent antiplague serum was administered at this point, two mice of every three infected still died.

Large doses of streptomycin were injected into the stricken animals whose blood, spleens, and livers already swarmed with plague bacilli. The treatment was repeated every three hours for three days. Every mouse treated with the drug survived, even though each animal, before treatment was begun, had been sliding rapidly toward death.

But more than the mindless administration of the compound was required if infected mice were to live. If the amount of streptomycin was reduced one-fourth, only the plague bacilli in the blood, spleen, and liver were killed; viable and vigorous plague bacilli survived in the lymph nodes. Forty percent of the mice treated with the smaller dose of streptomycin relapsed and later died of plague. Further experiments showed that *Y. pestis* remained in the lymph nodes of mice for at least ten days after the animals had apparently recovered from plague.

In mice with septicemic plague, in which the concentration of *Y. pestis* in the blood was many times higher than in the first experiments described, all infected animals died between thirty-four and seventy-two hours after infection. When large doses of streptomycin were administered nine hours after infection, the death toll was only one or two of every ten infected animals. When smaller doses were given, death was only delayed—all animals died. If streptomycin was not given until the eighteenth to the twenty-fourth hour after infection, most of the wretched animals perished in spite of antibiotic therapy.

The lesson was clear. Prompt treatment and adequate quantities of streptomycin were essential. Delayed or insufficient treatment often did not prevent the release of fatal quantities of plague toxins.

Pneumonic plague remained untouched by vaccines and indifferent to sulfas. Early experiments with streptomycin tested whether this potent compound could cure pneumonic plague infection in animals following their inhalation of an infective cloud of *Y. pestis*. The lungs of such animals, treated and untreated, were removed, and the total number of plague bacilli counted. The explosive course of pneumonic plague infection was clearly charted.

The lungs of an infected mouse might contain initially only two hundred plague organisms. Twelve hours later the number was no higher. *Yersinia pestis* made some initial gains, but then the alveolar macrophages, whose job it was to defend the convoluted vastness of the lung, rallied vigorously and battered the invaders down to their initial number. The first battle was won. But the war was lost. For now *Y. pestis* swept over the surface of the doomed animal's lungs like a wind-lashed prairie fire. Twelve hours later, a day after the animal had taken that fateful breath and drawn the plague bacilli into its lungs, the lungs held ten thousand *Y. pestis*—fifty bacilli after twenty-four hours for every one there had been after twelve. Two days later it was over. The lungs of the miserable little animals teemed with the vicious bacilli of plague, a thousand million of them, and the mouse was dead. Or near it. Less than three and a half days after infection with the small number of plague bacilli, all untreated animals had died.

In the early experiments, streptomycin treatment was begun thirty-six hours after infection. Six hours later, the lungs of the untreated animals contained ten million bacteria, and the lungs of the streptomycin-treated animals a mere sixty thousand. In twelve hours, the spleens of infected animals were sterile and their lungs contained only a few hundred *Y. pestis*. The day after, all untreated animals were dead. But now the lungs of the animals treated with large doses of streptomycin were free of the bacteria.[8]

These were spectacular results. They showed that Y. *pestis* was killed, in infected animals as in culture, by adequate levels of streptomycin even when the bacteria infested the lungs. The road was clear for tests on the varieties of human plague.

The first reports came from Argentina. Six persons with bubonic and septicemic plague received large doses of a sulfa drug, antiplague serum, and streptomycin. Penicillin was used if a lung infection with other bacteria was threatened. All six patients recovered.

Other results came from India. Five victims were near death from bubonic plague; two had received sulfa and antiplague serum. All were unconscious. All had temperatures of 103° to 106°F (39.6 to 41°C). Even after the administration of only small doses of streptomycin there was rapid improvement; all five patients made complete recoveries. Another fifteen victims in the late stages of the disease were treated with the antibiotics. Three died in spite of treatment; the rest lived.

There was an outbreak in a group of villages near Poona, in Bombay state. Of 286 cases of apparently uncomplicated bubonic plague, 58 percent died if untreated. When streptomycin was given such patients the fatality rate plummeted to 4 percent. In septicemic plague, 92 percent of the untreated victims died. Streptomycin reduced the death toll to only 10 percent. With the new drug one in ten died; before, fewer than one in ten lived.

In the same year as the Indian epidemic (1948), there was severe bubonic plague in Haifa, in the new state of Israel. Four victims received penicillin and sulfa drugs. The treatment had no discernible effect, in contrast to the good results obtained with sulfanilamides in India. Then three of the patients were given streptomycin. All recovered. The other victim, treated only with sulfa drugs and penicillin, died on the eighth day of his illness.

Pneumonic plague in man was the last obstacle. Could the dramatic effects in mice be repeated with a human victim?

In the early spring of 1948, pneumonic plague broke out on the island of Madagascar. The Rakotson family was cruelly hit. On Sunday, March 21, the father died of the disease; he was only thirty-eight. A few days later, the two younger sons became ill. On the twenty-sixth, the oldest son lost his twelve-year-old brother to pneumonic plague and then his seventeen-year-old brother just a few hours later.

Shortly after noon on the next day, a frightened and bewildered young man was hospitalized for observation. At 12:30 P.M. the surviving son's temperature was slightly above normal, 100°F. Two and a half hours later it had rocketed to 104°F (40°C). His physician, Dr. F. Estrade, immediately gave him half a gram of streptomycin and ordered the treatment repeated every three hours.

Young Rakotson, nineteen years old, was restless. The right side of his chest hurt. His eyes became bloodshot and his heartbeat accelerated. His throat filled with phlegm, and he spat frequently. The nurses were kept busy sterilizing the emesis basins containing the dangerous fluid and supplying him with fresh ones. Late in the afternoon of that ghastly first day, the sputum accumulating in the basin was slightly rust-colored. At seven that evening, an hour after his second streptomycin injection, Rakotson's sputum was definitely tinged with blood. Two hours later he received his third shot of streptomycin. By then he was delirious and depressed. Sleep was impossible, and his temperature continued to rise, having climbed another 1.5°F since the first streptomycin injection. Dr. Estrade spent a worried night wondering what else he could do and whether the miraculous claims he had heard for streptomycin were justified. When he visited his patient early the next morning, he was dismayed to find that the painful area had spread still further over the young man's chest.

But by 10:00 A.M. Rakotson's sputum was rusty again. By late afternoon it was whitish. Antibiotic administration continued. By April Fool's Day, his sixth day in the hospital, the boy was nearly well. Streptomycin treatment continued for two more days, and from then on, young Rakotson recovered uneventfully.

These results in human plague, especially the pneumonic form, stirred the scientific world. As one battle-scarred veteran of the war against the disease wrote, "For the first time in the nefarious history of plague, a drug which will cure the pneumonic form has been found."[8]

It was a great moment.

Additional experience showed that vigorous antibiotic therapy, if begun within fifteen hours of the first appearance of symptoms, usually saved the lives of pneumonic plague victims.

In 1948 researchers discovered two additional antibiotics that were also effective against the plague bacillus: the group known collectively as tetracyclines, and the compound chloramphenicol.

By the early 1950s a formidable arsenal of weapons stood ready against *Y. pestis.* There were vaccines, live and dead, and antiplague serum. There was a group of highly effective drugs. In addition to the sulfa drugs, there were streptomycin, chloramphenicol, and the tetracyclines. There were also DDT, 1080, and warfarin to be deployed against the living vehicles that had so effectively transported *Y. pestis* over much of the earth.

The battle of thirty centuries against one of humanity's most terrible enemies seemed to be nearing an end.

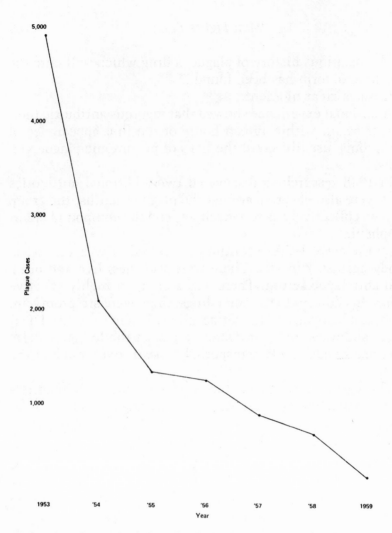

Figure 2   The End of the Third Pandemic—Human Plague,
1953–1959

13

Recent Plague
Around the World

The coming of the devil of plague,
Suddenly makes the lamp dim,
Then it is blown out,
Leaving man, ghost and corpse in the dark room.
—Shih Tao-Nan, "Death of Rats," 1792

The Third Pandemic began about 1855, but when did it end? With our limited perspective, the year 1959 is a reasonable answer. As Figure 2 shows, the number of reported cases of human plague dropped sharply from nearly five thousand in 1953 to a little more than two hundred in 1959.

This figure is based on data published each year by WHO. Plague is a notifiable disease. That is, the law requires a physician treating a case of plague (if he or she recognizes it) to notify the public health authorities of the country. In the United States, the Centers for Disease Control (CDC) in Atlanta is advised by telegram or telephone; city and state officials may be notified as well, and from the CDC the information goes to WHO headquarters in Geneva. WHO in turn publishes weekly reports and then combines them into a yearly summary. The CDC publishes its own weekly bulletin of epidemiological events in the United States. To encourage dissemination of information of public health significance, the CDC weekly report has always been freely available to professionals in the health sciences. Beginning in 1982, however, the bulletin became available primarily to paid subscribers.

WHO depends on data from the public health authorities in member countries. Individual nations elect to participate or not and decide how and what to report.

The United States reports some thirty diseases and the Soviet Union eight. India currently announces only cholera; it might report plague if it occurred. The People's Republic of China reported nothing from its founding in 1949 until 1979 when it reported the presence of plague for several years in a row.

Reporting countries may list cases and deaths from plague, or only one or the other. If they report cases, they may report bacteriologically confirmed cases and suspicious cases as well. The difficulties of evaluation are enormous. For instance, WHO reported on plague cases from 1961 to 1970 in its weekly bulletin of January 28, 1972. Fourteen months later it revised its figures for 1968 and 1969 upward nearly fourfold because of more recent information. Besides, much plague goes unreported in any form.

In areas of epidemic plague, clinical diagnosis (on the basis of symptoms and patient history) probably overestimates the total by about 10 percent, but it gives a far more realistic number than bacteriologically confirmed cases in countries where qualified laboratories are few and far between. As the Vietnam experience indicates, under such conditions only one plague case in ten is ever reported, since the diagnosis is not bacteriologically confirmed.

The number of worldwide cases declined greatly between 1953 and 1959, probably because of the combined impacts of DDT and other new insecticides and the highly effective rodenticides like 1080 and warfarin. The death rate fell also, but in spite of the availability of sulfonamides and the antibiotics for over a decade, the mortality from reported plague was nearly 40 percent in 1959 and close to 60 percent in 1960.

Then it dropped dramatically. Mortality rates must also be viewed with suspicion, but it seems that overall mortality from plague dropped from 40 percent or more at the end of the 1950s, to somewhere between 4 and 10 percent by 1974. Of course it is important to have the right kind of plague in the right place at the right time. This will become clear when we consider individual cases.

WHO's Expert Committee on Plague issued its third, and longest, report in 1959, in which it summarized its view of the world plague situation. The committee pointed out that while the fatality rate from human plague in Brazil was very low (apparently *Y. pestis* there is of low virulence in humans, something that is apparently true in Vietnam as well), the rate in much of Africa is very high. The report noted that although the incidence of plague had fallen to an extremely low level, the threat of new outbreaks was as real as ever. As a distinguished French scientist, Dr. M. Baltazard, put it in 1960, "The silence of plague today must not blind us to the fact that its present positions are stronger than they have ever been; entrenched within reach of all the strongholds of modern civilization, it may well be a disease of the future." In any case, plague is certainly not a disease of the past. Since Dr. Baltazard's statement there have been some thirty-five thousand reported cases and a total number at least several times as high.

Because plague was responsible for so much devastation in India during the Third Pandemic, it is appropriate to begin there with our discussion of recent human plague.

In the twenty years ending in 1918, at least ten million Indians died of plague. In the subsequent thirty years, nearly another three million plague deaths were reported from the subcontinent. The acute food shortages of 1946 and 1947, combined with the strife and the large movements of people accompanying partition in 1947, contributed to the total reported plague deaths in those years of nearly thirty-three thousand and forty-two thousand, respectively.

Calcutta had a mild plague epidemic in the spring of 1948. Since 1925 there had been no cases originating in permanent residents of the city, although some few cases were imported from outside. Then, on Monday, April 15, 1948, medical personnel were called to 20 Harinbari Lane. Bibi Dajafan, a forty-year-old woman, was found suffering from plague and was removed to Campbell Hospital. In the next six days there were ten more cases in the vicinity of Harinbari Lane.

Retrospectively, authorities discovered that the first case had occurred at the same address more than a month earlier, on March 6. It had not been reported. There had been eleven cases in, or close to, 20 Harinbari Lane, prior to April 15. Eight victims had died; not one was diagnosed and reported as plague.

Although nothing concerning rat deaths had been reported, it was later learned that the mother of a patient admitted to Campbell Hospital on April 17 had removed dead rats from her one-room house on the eighth, ninth, and fifteenth of that month. A plague-infected dead rat was found in the neighborhood on the nineteenth, and the inhabitants of the originally infected districts admitted that rats had largely disappeared from the area.

The second phase of the epidemic began on April 22. In the next six days 109 suspected plague cases were admitted to Campbell Hospital. Significantly, they now came from widely scattered points about the city and even from districts outside the city limits. At the peak of the outbreak a suspected plague case was admitted at an average rate of one per hour. Of the thirty-two wards and three outlying districts of Calcutta, only three reported no plague.

Then the disease declined. At the end, 147 cases were considered as plague; nearly half were very mild. Of the 74 typical cases, 17—or 23 percent—were fatal. *Yersinia pestis* was isolated from only 8 of 77 patients examined.

By 1953 the annual death rate in India was fewer than 1,400, and it continued to fall. In 1959 fewer than 200 plague deaths were reported, still fewer the next year. There were but 1,404 reported deaths from plague in all India between 1961 and 1964 and, in the latter year, only 113 reported cases.

In 1964, however, there occurred one of those inconsistencies that so frequently turn up in plague statistics. In an Indian government disease report, Mysore State lists ten plague cases, a modest proportion of the total. But, under plague deaths for Mysore in 1964, the number given is 108, nearly as many plague deaths in Mysore State as total cases reported for all

India in that year and ten times as many plague deaths in Mysore as there were reported cases!

This was not simply a typographical error. Mysore reported fewer than eight hundred cases of smallpox in the same year, but nearly twenty-six hundred deaths from smallpox. The obvious conclusion is one that persistently colors all epidemiological data: namely, that the actual number of cases of anything is often far more than the number reported.

In South India plague still existed in the 1970s in wild rodents (gerbils, the brown spiny mouse, and both common varieties of bandicoot rats), as well as in domestic mice, black rats, and the Oriental rat flea.[1] And in Calcutta and environs more than three thousand persons were vaccinated against plague in 1970–71.

In India, as in the Soviet Union, the disease has withdrawn from previously held positions. In the Soviet Union this result accompanied huge and expensive control programs. The same thing happened in India with very little effort on the part of the Indian government. A reasonable (although not necessarily correct) conclusion is that the foci that disappeared in both India and the Soviet Union were those not permanently suited to the plague bacillus and its complex ecology. This basic incompatibility led to disappearance of the disease after several decades.

Plague in India has always been predominantly bubonic in nature. The optimum conditions seem to be humidity greater than 60 percent and temperature between 69° and 77°F (20° to 25°C). The incidence of plague drops sharply in India when the temperature rises above 90°F (32°C). Pneumonic cases are generally below 1 percent of the total number of plague infections and never above 3 percent.

For malaria eradication, DDT has been sprayed in all rural dwellings in India since 1958—probably a major factor in the decline of plague on the subcontinent. In 1971, in parts of Maharashtra State, the most common flea found was *X. cheopis*. The black rat was by far the predominant animal trapped (over 99 percent) of the total, and the *X. cheopis* index, in spite of DDT, was a dangerously high 2.6 fleas per rat.

Whatever the reasons for the decline in India, there have been no cases of human plague reported there since 1967. This disease seems to have retreated, for the moment, to its stronghold in the Himalayas on the borders of Pakistan, Tibet, and Nepal.

On Wednesday, September 6, 1967, Laxmi, a sixteen-year-old girl, was tending her family's cattle near the village of Surke Mela, eighty-five hundred feet (twenty-six hundred meters) above sea level. She was ill and alone. Her family—mother, father, and three other children—were home in the village of Nawra, nearly two thousand vertical feet (about six hundred meters) below the grazing land on the terraced mountainside in far western Nepal. From where she sat leaning forlornly against a boulder it was about thirty-seven miles (sixty kilometers) west to India and about the same distance north to Tibet.[2]

The next day Laxmi felt worse and wanted to return to the village. But she had been sent to tend the cattle, and there was no one else to watch them. She could not leave. The next day she was too ill to stand. Someone from the village of Surke Mela spoke with her as she huddled in a stone stable on the mountainside. Laxmi was spitting blood by then; her abdomen hurt; she was vomiting, feverish, and coughing. Later she had diarrhea. She died that day, Friday, alone on the mountain.

Later, her family came to fetch her and wrapped her small body in shrouds. There was a graveyard a little way north of the two-story stone house in which she had lived, but her corpse was not taken there. Instead, it was carried thirty-five hundred vertical feet (eleven hundred meters) down a rough trail and cast into the foaming, icy water of the Seti River.

Seven people accompanied Laxmi's body on its journey to the riverbank. One of them, Dharam, a twenty-two-year-old cousin, fell ill some three weeks later. He had a swelling in one armpit but got well without treatment. Nevertheless, Dharam had been worried. On the day he became sick, his friend Sanke had died.

Sanke was two years older than Dharam and lived in a four-family house not far from Laxmi's family. Two weeks after the young girl's death, Sanke had gone to Surke Mela to tend the cattle. He stayed in the same hut in which Laxmi lived her last moments. On September 24, two days after he had climbed the steep path to the grazing land from his home in Nawra, Sanke too became ill. He stayed two days longer in Surke Mela and then returned to his home. He came as a messenger of death.

Like Laxmi before him, Sanke was feverish, coughed up bloodstained sputum, vomited repeatedly, and had diarrhea. Like Laxmi before him, he had no swellings or outbreaks on his skin. Sanke died on Thursday, September 28. He had been ill five days.

The month of October 1967 brought terror to Nawra and its six hundred fifty inhabitants. Seventeen people lived in the house where Sanke died. By early November, fifteen of them had been ill; twelve were dead.

One of the four families that shared the dwelling, a young couple, left the house a bit more than a week after Sanke's death to work on the rice crop. They were gone eleven days, and when they returned, they went to another house to live, hoping to avoid the sickness that had turned their former home into an abattoir.

But death had preceded them; a fifteen-year-old boy had died in their new home while they worked in the rice fields. A week after the pair arrived, the wife, twenty-year-old Jhupri, was feverish and nauseated. The next day a twenty-five-year-old woman in the same house sickened. She was dead two days later.

Jhupri recovered, after a serious illness, and her husband was unscathed by the disease.

The house next toward the mountain from Sanke's and on the other side of the steep path to Surke Mela was also stricken. It was a two-family dwelling and, like the other, made of stone plastered with lime and mud and with a stone roof. Cattle, buffalo, and goats lived on the ground floor, cooking and general living took place on the first floor, and the top floor was for sleeping. In this house a sixty-year-old man was ill on one day; next door, a fifty-year-old woman became sick five days later. Both survived. The occupants of the next house up the path to the grazing land were not so fortunate. In the space of nine days, four girls in the family, whose ages ranged from one to fifteen years, became dreadfully ill. The oldest girl died in four days and the youngest in two; the other two lived.

Nawra, in the Bajhang district of Nepal, is a two-hour walk from the district headquarters and five to seven days by foot form the nearest airstrip. It was October 30, nearly two months after Laxmi's body sank into the Seti River, before the Ministry of Health of the government of Nepal was notified of the epidemic in Nawra. Fortunately, a helicopter shortened the journey of the investigating team to half an hour.

The investigators heard tales of large numbers of dying cattle. There was no sign of dead rodents, and all of the people still sick had skin lesions. The typical skin eruptions, the stories of dying cattle, and the absence of dead rodents made it clear that the disease was anthrax. Except that it wasn't. It was plague.

A week after the first group of investigators arrived, they were joined by a CDC team. The cause of the deaths of cattle was soon shown to be rinderpest, and the human disease was correctly identified.

The outbreak had some curious features. Unfortunately, of the eighteen persons who died of plague in the village of Nawra, seventeen were already dead by the time the investigators arrived. The mortality rate was nearly 70 percent. Of the eighteen victims who died, sixteen had symptoms of lung involvement. The twenty-year-old girl, Jhupri, was the only victim with pulmonary symptoms who survived.

The remaining ten cases had uncomplicated bubonic plague. Of these, three of the victims died; the remaining seven all had skin ulcers with black scabs, which originally suggested anthrax but which were later found to be the comparatively rare plague carbuncles ordinarily associated with a mild attack of the disease (pestis minor, as it is often called).

How the disease was transmitted among the various victims is not clear. Dead rodents were said to have been seen near the stable in which both Laxmi and Sanke slept while tending cattle in Surke Mela, but none were found, dead or alive, in the village of Nawra itself. Two dogs from Nawra and two from Surke Mela were tested for plague antibodies. Three of the four were positive, indicating recent contact with plague-infected animals. As with the dogs of the Navajo—half a world away—the dogs of the Nepalese villages are not fed and must forage for themselves, so they become valuable indicators of the presence of plague in the animals that are their prey.

Both Laxmi and Sanke died of secondary pneumonic plague, presumably after having been bitten by an infected rodent flea in the stable in Surke Mela. Sanke brought the disease with him to his house in which three other families lived in separate quarters. There the disease was devastating.

Fifteen of the seventeen persons in Sanke's house contracted plague. Twelve of the fifteen victims died of it. Nearly all had swellings on the neck or trunk, along with pulmonary symptoms. They were probably victims of pharyngeal, or tonsillar, plague, which began when they inhaled large fluid droplets containing the plague bacillus. These droplets are too large to pass into the lung and cause primary pneumonic plague. Instead, they are trapped in the throat and cause swelling of the lymph nodes in the upper part of the body. Victims of pharyngeal plague, like those of primary pneumonic plague, exhale or expectorate the large *Y. pestis*–containing droplets, which may then be inhaled by someone close to them. Because the large droplets settle quickly to the ground, unlike the small droplets that cause primary pneumonic plague, pharyngeal plague is transmitted only over short distances.

The cases of uncomplicated bubonic plague are more mysterious. Neither rodents nor human fleas were found in Nawra, possibly because of vigorous DDT treatment soon after the investigating team arrived. Fleas on the villagers were the most probable vectors.

Two other points are worth mentioning. The first is that although western Nepal never before reported plague, the disease had been known in the nearby mountainous sub-Himalayan provinces since 1823 (although no cases were reported there for three-quarters of a century). Also, the properties of the plague bacillus isolated at Nawra were unlike those of *Y. pestis* in India. This suggests that Nepal is the lower fringe of the central Asian plague focus, which thus extends much farther south than was previously thought.

Another interesting aspect concerns the treatment of the villagers who were still ill with plague when the investigating team arrived. These patients were first mistakenly treated for anthrax with penicillin, which did no good at all.

Jhupri, who, with her husband, did not return to Sanke's house after the epidemic began but caught the disease anyway, was treated six days after she developed fever. She had two ulcerous areas, a swollen inguinal lymph node, an enlarged liver, and some evidence of congestion in the lower part of her left lung. By November 2 her condition was no better. Tetracycline was administered, and her temperature was back to normal two days later. However, a large bubo developed on her chest, and it remained large and tender in spite of the antibiotic treatment. A week after tetracycline therapy was begun, she also received streptomycin, and she subsequently recovered.

The day after Jhupri became ill, so did a thirteen-year-old girl from the house in which Sanke had lived. By October 31 the younger girl had no fever, but she had a pustule on the back of her neck and small but tender lymph nodes in the area of the pustule. She was given penicillin but became steadily worse over the next three days, with a temperature reaching 104°F (40°C). She received oral tetracycline on November 2, and this treatment continued for a week. After five days of tetracycline treatment she developed a rigidly stiff neck and the next day was only semiconscious.

At this point chloramphenicol was substituted for tetracycline and continued for six days, after which the girl received streptomycin for an additional ten days. Six weeks later she was well again.

She had had plague meningitis in which *Y. pestis* invaded the membranes covering the brain. There it is relatively safe from tetracycline. To bring this case to a successful conclusion required all three antibiotics used in the treatment of plague.

The point of both these experiences is that in a plague outbreak all three drugs must be available in adequate quantity. So long as plague epidemics are small enough, providing adequate amounts of drugs is not an insurmountable problem. But in an epidemic involving hundreds of cases, rather than tens, obtaining the medicines necessary to stop the outbreak might be difficult—or impossible.

There was another plague epidemic in Nepal in February 1966. Of the thirteen cases, twelve were fatal. As in Nawra, the first case came from the fields outside the village, and the disease was apparently passed person to person by the flea *P. irritans.*

In Burma, between 1905 and 1940, there were over 165,000 reported plague deaths, the largest number of any country but India. By 1949 the number of human cases attributed to plague had fallen to 650. *Xenopsyllus cheopis,* the principal flea involved, is carried by a variety of mice and the black and bandicoot rat. As in the rest of Southeast Asia, bubonic plague is the predominant form.

Human plague in Burma has shown a widely varying number of cases in recent years, but mortality has dropped steadily, thanks to the use of modern antibiotics. In 1959 there were 108 cases (34 deaths) from plague in Burmese towns (the only places in Burma from which cases are reported). In 1965 a small epidemic broke out, with nearly 300 cases reported, but the case-fatality rate was only 10 percent, and it remained low thereafter as the incidence of the disease dropped back to more nearly normal levels. For the period from 1946 to 1970, Burma had somewhat more than 9,000 plague cases.

Indonesia had almost 11,000 plague cases between 1950 and 1952. Beginning in 1950, DDT application was widespread, and in the 1960s only 115 cases were reported. Indonesia has been the scene of some of the most appalling epidemics of modern times. There were severe epidemics in the period 1932–34, reaching a maximum of 23,000 cases in the last year. The fatality rate in these epidemics was almost unbelievable; fewer than 2 of every 1,000 victims survived. These vicious epidemics were almost entirely bubonic in nature; only 6 to 8 percent were the pneumonic form.

The Texas-sized island of Madagascar has perennial plague. The disease is carried solely by the black rat and two fleas, one of which is *X. cheopis*. Pneumonic plague accounts for a third to a half of all cases. As expected, the case-fatality rate is high, and although the number of cases has greatly declined, mortality figures have improved very little.

From 1953 to 1958, Madagascar had 132 reported cases of plague. The mortality averaged 72 percent. A somewhat earlier report (1952) pointed out that only 15 percent of plague deaths on Madagascar at that time were recognized as such before the victim died. In 1959, as befits the year we have chosen for the end of the Third Pandemic, the island had only 5 cases, but three were fatal.

Between 1960 and 1970 there were an additional 143 cases, with the mortality reduced to 52 percent. This is certainly a substantial improvement over the previous mortality figures, but it is still a mournfully high number.

Plague statistics for Madagascar's great neighbor to the west, the vast continent of Africa, are spotty for recent years, in part because of the turmoil accompanying independence of the new nations and the dreary succession of military coups as one tyrant replaces another.

Late in 1951 plague broke out in Tanganyika (now Tanzania) with several hundred cases; another 162 cases followed the next year. A correlated investigation in the Rift Valley of Kenya uncovered some 70 human victims. In this focus five species of rodents maintained and transmitted the disease.

Between 1960 and 1970 the Republic of the Congo (now Zaire), Kenya, Tanzania, and South Africa reported nearly eight hundred cases of plague. Of these, Zaire accounted for nearly two hundred, of which almost half resulted from a single outburst in 1968. The mortality rate was 29 percent. This is a high figure, but it should be compared with the rates between 1953 and 1960 (when Zaire was still part of the Belgian Congo) which averaged 81 percent.

In Zaire plague exists in two foci, both in the northeast near the border with Uganda, one near Lake Albert and one near Lake Edward. Early in November 1962 the health authorities received word of an epidemic of "pneumonia" in the Lake Edward focus involving two villages. About ten days later another village, Mikondero, also reported an epidemic of unknown nature, and a WHO team set out to investigate.[3] It was no easy matter. Mikondero is a cluster of one-room circular straw huts perched on a ridge of Mitumba Mountain at an altitude of about six thousand feet (two thousand meters), twenty-four miles (forty kilometers) from the nearest road. By the time the WHO team got there, the dead were buried and the living victims convalescent. But the presence of plague was confirmed.

Several months later a five-member WHO group arrived with DDT, rodenticides, drugs, and plague vaccines. The team found, to its surprise, two current cases of pneumonic plague in the little village. Both victims received prompt treatment, their immediate contacts got sulfa drugs to prevent the disease from spreading, and the whole village population was immunized with the live E.V. vaccine. An antirat campaign began (four to six rodents were trapped per hut each night), and DDT was dusted and sprayed in and around the huts. No further cases of the disease developed. This plague focus extends into Uganda and is maintained by black and African grass rats (the black rats are the subspecies known as the Alexandrine rat) as well as the multimammate mouse and some other varieties of lesser importance. The most important flea for transmission of plague to man is the human flea, *P. irritans*. Although immunization and rat-trapping programs are under way in the focus, their effect has been minuscule. The estimated rodent population is eight million or more, while the trapping campaign accounts for some two hundred thousand per year. The little village of Mikondero had plague in 1960, 1962, and 1963, and it will probably continue to harbor the disease.

Tanzania contributed the great bulk of the plague cases in Africa in recent years, nearly six hundred between 1960 and 1970, largely in one great epidemic in 1964 that led to over five hundred cases with a fatality rate of only 2 percent. A small epidemic of pneumonic plague took place in the village of Muray in the plague focus of Mbulu. Five persons died. The outbreak was followed by vigorous control measures, and no further cases occurred.

Late in 1941, and on into the next year, Nairobi, capital of Kenya, had a vicious onslaught of plague resulting in 547 cases. Authorities set up a system of distributing cases so that patients exhibiting buboes could receive treatment at the Infectious Disease Hospital, while those without the obvious stigmata of the disease (413 of the total) were treated at the Native Civil Hospital. As expected, the mortality rates were very different. In spite of sulfonamide therapy, the death rate at the Infectious Disease Hospital was 55 percent, while that at the Native Civil Hospital was an appalling 95 percent, reflecting the usual mortality with septicemic and pneumonic cases.

In Northern Rhodesia (now Zambia) plague reappeared in 1956 after an absence of nearly forty years. The result was a localized outbreak relatively quickly controlled with DDT and warfarin in addition to treatment of the patients with sulfa drugs, streptomycin, and tetracycline. In all there were thirty-six cases; five were fatal. The rodent and flea vectors were like those of the Lake Edward focus.

The gerbil is the principal wild rodent involved in plague maintenance in South Africa. The multimammate mouse, one of the most widely distributed and abundant rodents in Africa, serves as the domestic rodent that transfers the disease to man. The reproductive potential of each rodent species is awe-inspiring; the two varieties of gerbils each can have four litters a year of three to six young each, while the multimammate mice have up to twenty offspring per litter. Thus, the losses in epizootics or control campaigns are quickly made up. The black rat still plays an important role in the plague of town and city.

There were more than nine hundred plague outbreaks in South Africa between 1919 and 1943, with over two thousand cases. On July 7, 1947, in Johannesburg, a laboratory worker who had handled both plague cultures and plague-infected tissues became ill. He had received many injections of the live attenuated vaccine, the last just two weeks before. The man acquired pneumonic plague in the course of his work and died in four days.

Two years of heavy rains in southern Africa beginning in 1966 led to a rodent population explosion in late 1967. By the middle of February 1968, human plague cases began to occur in Lesotho. There were at least 125 victims, of whom 49 died. About the same time there were 179 cases in South-West Africa.

It is unfortunately true that widespread famine and political unrest leading to war may cause a resurgence of epidemic plague, since the disease is never long absent from most of the countries of the African continent.

The Arabian peninsula, especially in the mountainous border region between Saudi Arabia and the Yemeni states, has long been considered a plague focus, although the last known outbreak, until comparatively recently, took place in 1906. Then there was an epidemic lasting from April through July of 1951, with two hundred cases and ninety deaths. Plague broke out again in the Saudi Arabian desert in June of the following year, but there were only four cases; three were fatal. This was worrisome for all the usual reasons plus an additional one.

All Muslim males are urged by their religious leaders to make, once during their lifetime, the pilgrimage to Mecca. The height of the pilgrimage (Hadj) season is during the summer. A steady stream of pilgrims journey across the Yemeni states and southern Saudi Arabia to the holy city. Plague anywhere along the line of march menaces the hundreds of thousands of devout Muslims who gather in Mecca each summer.

Naturally, public health authorities breathed a sigh of relief when the outbreak of the 1950s subsided with no more problems than the redirection of pilgrims away from the infected areas. Then plague returned to the border region in 1969, after an absence of seventeen years.[4]

The outbreak occurred in two villages at an altitude of more than forty-seven hundred feet (fifteen hundred meters) along a steep valley draining into the Red Sea. The terrain, except for narrow regions along the streams running into the valley, is high, rocky, and barren desert. The people live in houses with very thick mud walls, pyramidal in shape and two to three stories in height. Sheep and goats are kept on the ground floor.

On Tuesday, May 6, 1969, a fifteen-year-old boy, Dafer Yahya, became frightfully ill. He had a large bubo on his neck. He died on Sunday with violet spots on his body. Although it has not been proved, Dafer probably had bubonic plague with secondary pneumonic symptoms.

Dafer's mother died on the Wednesday after his burial. During the last day of her illness her sputum was bloodstained. Her husband died a few hours later. He had violet spots all over his body and had spat bloodstained sputum for some time. The home of Dafer Yahya stood empty.

Three neighbor women and a man tended Dafer's parents in their last illness. All died.

The local health inspector visited the village on the weekend during which most of the deaths occurred. He was said to have treated another suspected case with streptomycin and sprayed the area with DDT. The suspected plague victim survived.

Another epidemic soon began under uncertain circumstances in a village about a four-hour walk from the first. Within a period of five or six days at the end of May, five women (four from one house) died. All, according to their relatives, had large and painful groin buboes.

Late in June, some three weeks after the deaths of the five women, a forty-five-year-old man, Sheikh Dahbash, returned to the second village after visiting several other communities in the neighborhood. He died following two days of chills and fever. He did not have buboes but spat blood before his death. His younger brother and his sister died with the symptoms of pneumonic plague. *Yersinia pestis* was found in the woman's throat. Sheikh Ali's wife was also ill and received streptomycin from members of a WHO team. At that time she was spitting blood-flecked sputum that later showed the presence of the plague bacillus. The WHO team left the area soon after, and thus the woman's fate is unknown. The two outbreaks had led to at least fifteen cases and fourteen deaths.

The properties of the plague bacillus isolated from the two human cases indicate that the Arabian plague focus is the southernmost extension of the ancient focus in Kurdistan (the region where Iraq, Iran, Turkey, and Soviet Armenia join).

In the decade of the 1960s, Iran itself had plague only in 1961 and 1963, after which the disease submerged and has not yet reappeared.

South America has remained a vigorous center of the disease in recent years. In addition, Mexico had some four hundred plague deaths from the beginning of the Third Pandemic until 1938.

Ecuador had 115 human plague cases in 1968 and 1969, some in areas never before infected. Since 1961 the disease seems to have invaded certain urban areas on the coast, and between 1961 and 1965 there were 808 cases of plague, fortunately with low mortality. The usual commensal species of *Rattus* form the urban reservoir (along with the domestic mice), while various species of wild rat appear to be the wild reservoir. *Xenopsylla cheopis* is the principal urban flea. Hamsters also play a role in the maintenance of plague in Ecuador, as do rabbits.

Peru reported 53 cases in 1968 and 1969, but the plague incidence there varies enormously. There were 8 cases in 1969, but 128 the following year.

Brazil led the Americas in plague cases by a wide margin, with a two-year total (1968–69) of nearly 578 cases. As of 1967, the disease was present in six states, and there was a small focus near Rio de Janeiro itself.

Plague was reported infrequently in Venezuela and only once (in 1958) in Argentina.

In the Soviet Union plague ecology is as intricate as in the United States. The disease is carried by two species of marmots, three species of ground squirrels, six species of gerbils, two species of the kangaroo-like mice called jerboas, and at least two other species of mice, hamsters, rabbits, foxes, birds of prey, and even camels.

It is strange to think of the "ship of the desert" as a carrier of plague, but camels can be readily infected, either naturally or experimentally, and may transmit the disease to humans. At least forty-four cases of plague in camels have been reported in the Soviet Union; two-thirds of them were the cause of subsequent human plague.

Infection in nature is most often the result of the camel's preference for sleeping on ground made friable by the burrowing of gerbils or other rodents. The sleeping camel may cover several burrow entrances and thus accumulate fleas from the rodent population.

To the nomad family, its camels are its major possession, and they are not wasted even in death. Usually, when a camel shows signs of intractable illness, it is killed, skinned, and eaten. Plague has been transferred to man both by flea bite during skinning and by eating poorly cooked, infected meat.

In the Soviet Union, as elsewhere, one species of plague-carrying animal has been exterminated only to be replaced by another. In the Armenian Soviet Socialist Republic, plague was carried by marmots before their extinction at the end of the last century. Since that time, plague has been found in that area (between the Black and Caspian seas) in both voles and the ground squirrels called susliks, although which is the basic reservoir is a matter of hot debate among Russian experts.

The sandy soil between the Volga and the Ural rivers in southern Russia has been a longtime plague focus. In May 1958 there was a mouse epizootic on the eastern shore of the Ural River, and most mice on that side of the river died from the disease.

A ferry carried trucks loaded with hay across the river from east to west, and the following spring, plague broke out among the susliks on the western bank. By 1962 plague was common in both the midday and tamarisk gerbils in the region between the two rivers, and in the northern region the infection in mice was also passed to the big gerbils.

Between November 1963 and June 1964 at least 80 percent

of the big gerbils in the desert portion of the central Asian plague focus died of plague. On the Iranian border of this focus, the population of red-tailed gerbils exploded, beginning in 1952, and the increased population triggered migration. As a Soviet scientist reported, "All biotypes, including those ordinarily not inhabited by rodents, were found to be occupied by enormous numbers of red-tailed gerbils. At the end of the spring rains and the onset of dry weather migrations of the rodents increased."

Fulfilling its usual role as a controller of overpopulation in higher and lower animals, plague broke out in the late fall and early winter over an area of two thousand square miles (more than half a million hectares). By the end of the year the population of red-tailed gerbils was a pitiful fraction of its former level. Nevertheless, the epidemic broke out again the following spring, because of the numerous infected fleas that survived the winter in the rodent burrows.

As with most large plague foci, several of those in the Soviet Union are slowly expanding, and plague is also appearing in regions where it was previously unknown. In all likelihood, the disease was there all along but eluded less sensitive search methods.

The Soviet Union has made the most heroic efforts of any nation to obliterate plague foci, in campaigns dating back to the 1930s, employing every conceivable method of control. The results have been discouraging, in keeping with the American experience in California. The experience has been everywhere the same. Some very small foci of wild rodent plague have been eliminated (as in the western Soviet Union) or have disappeared from natural causes (as in several parts of India). No major plague focus has ever been eliminated anywhere in the world even by the most sophisticated, widespread, and long-term efforts.

Human plague in the Soviet Union is something of a mystery. There has been no official notice of human cases for many years, but the reports of Soviet plague investigators carry the strong implication that some have occurred. At the very least, the Soviet Union probably has an incidence of human plague like that of the United States. The Soviet Union has a plague research and control effort that employs some thirty thousand persons, six hundred of them physicians, divided among eleven specialized plague laboratories and thirteen mobile research teams. The United States, with a plague focus of approximately the same size, has perhaps two dozen persons involved in similar efforts. It may be that the Soviet government is much more aware of the potential threat of plague because of the severe epidemics that the country has suffered in the past. It may simply be a way of keeping a large number of technical people gainfully employed. Or it may be that human plague in the Soviet Union remains a more serious problem than one would guess from the published figures. While in the southern Soviet republics in the summer of 1983 I tried to visit some of the regional plague laboratories. I was politely told that all such arrangements would have had to have been made before my arrival in the Soviet Union, which, unfortunately, I had not thought to do.

China too, has a long history of plague. Texts alluding to "rat pest" and "malignant bubo" were published there in the seventh century A.D.

Hong Kong's history has been described—in brief, thirty years of plague. Fukien province, northeast of Hong Kong, was also infested in 1894, and the disease spread slowly throughout the province in subsequent years. In 1941 there were 626 cases reported; 63 percent were fatal, a lower mortality than generally reported in that wartime year. Elsewhere in China, though, of a little more than 400 additional cases, more than 350 were fatal. Over forty-one thousand doses of plague vaccine were administered, but the situation in Fukien rapidly worsened. From only 626 cases in 1941, there were 5,000 reported in 1943, and 7,000 two years later.

Farther north, in Manchuria, 15,000 cases of bubonic plague were reported in the region of Jehol in 1946. In the same year a small outbreak of pneumonic plague occurred in southern Manchuria with 39 cases. Only 3 of the victims of this epidemic survived.

In February 1946, a thirty-three-year-old bacteriologist working in the National Institute of Health in Nanking became seriously ill with laboratory-acquired pneumonic plague. Vigorous treatment saved his life but did not prevent him from suffering a long illness. It was more than four months before he could return to work.

The present situation in China is somewhat obscure. When the Chinese Communists took over the country in 1949, impressive advances began in the field of public health. One of the first actions of the new government was to vaccinate three hundred million persons against plague. The incidence of plague is alleged to have dropped 80 percent in the first full year after the vaccination program began. In 1952 Mao's government launched a program involving the "five kills and the four cleans," which had the killing of rats and other disease agents and the enhanced cleanliness of village, city, and home as its aims. The results, according to the government, were the destruction of 1.5 billion rats, or approximately two per person. But preventative medicine suffered a serious lapse in the next five years. Then, on Friday, June 25, 1965, Mao Tse-tung made a blistering speech to a group of medical personnel that set the stage for a return to the previous emphasis on public health measures. As Mao put it,

> Tell the Ministry of Public Health that it only works for 15 percent of the entire population. Furthermore, this 15 percent is made up mostly of the privileged. . . . The Public Health Ministry is not a people's ministry. It should be called the Urban Health Ministry, or the Public Health Ministry of the privileged, or even the Urban Public Health Ministry of the privileged.

Shortly thereafter, the "barefoot doctors" appeared, and they still play a major role in Chinese public health. Neither barefoot nor doctors, they are largely concerned with sanitation, hygiene, and family planning. There is no doubt of the impressive impact of the public health programs and family-planning efforts in China. Some medical care has been made available to rural inhabitants, often for the first time; human population growth is under control; and the number of rats has greatly declined. The incidence of plague has apparently fallen considerably, even if perhaps not to zero as claimed by the government. The barefoot doctors carry well-stocked medical kits with the antibiotics most useful in treating plague. In areas where the disease is potentially a problem, they probably receive specialized training to recognize and treat this infection, as they do to treat other specialized ailments in other parts of the country. The unanswerable question is, how well will this imposing public health effort survive the years ahead? We can only wish it well. If it fails, the resulting disease menaces us all.

14

Vietnam

The guns and the bombs, the rockets and the warships are all symbols of human failure . . . they are witnesses to human folly.
—President Lyndon B. Johnson, April 7, 1965

Plague struck again in Southeast Asia in the early 1960s, leading to more cases than occurred in Hong Kong during all the years of the Third Pandemic. Between 1965 and 1970 over twenty-five thousand plague cases were reported in South Vietnam. The total was several times that.

The eruption of plague was probably stimulated by the most widespread destruction ever inflicted on a small agricultural country. The United States had the dubious distinction of being the first nation in recent history to employ chemical warfare against the food crops and forests of another.

The alleged purpose of what might be called the "Poison for Peace" plan, in which rice fields were sprayed with an arsenic-containing compound and other crop-destroying agents, was to reduce the food supply to the Viet Cong (South Vietnamese Communist) guerillas and the regular North Vietnamese Army troops, who together controlled substantial parts of the land and population. In addition to aerial spraying, crops were burned, deliberately contaminated with noxious substances, or thrown into rivers.

The aerial poisoning campaign began in a modest way in 1961 with only five spray flights a month. By 1966 a half-million acres (two hundred thousand hectares) were sprayed, and twice that the next year. Plans to triple this effort were confounded by the inability of the U.S. suppliers to keep up with the growing demand for plant poisons. According to the Defense Department, 12 percent of the arable land in South Vietnam was "sterilized." Over half the total cropland was sprayed at least once.

As a result of the poisoning campaign and the control of sizable areas by the Viet Cong, South Vietnam, which had been a rice-exporting country (it exported forty-nine million tons even in 1964), had to import that staple by 1965.

The food-denial program had little effect on the Viet Cong or the North Vietnamese soldiers, who could commandeer what food they needed, but it made a massive contribution to the malnutrition of the Vietnamese people.

Besides the crop destruction effort, the defoliation program, which became the largest part of the spraying campaign, was designed to strip the leaves from trees along roads and border areas, thus reducing ambush sites and making aerial reconnaissance easier. This effort was of slight military consequence (according to then Defense Secretary Robert S. McNamara and to Rand Corporation studies done for the Department of Defense),[1] but it destroyed vast areas of Vietnamese forest for decades to come. Between 25 and 45 percent of the country's forests were treated with defoliant two or three times. Vast areas of hardwood forests with a limited capacity to support rodents were replaced by bamboo thickets—ideal rodent shelter and breeding grounds.

A little later, the process of winning the hearts and minds of the Vietnamese people was expanded to include extensive bombing on or near their farmlands and villages. Over 60 percent of the bombs dropped fell on South Vietnam. The total ordnance (shells and bombs) amounted to more than 1,200 pounds (545 kilograms) of high explosive for every man, woman, and child in the country (in addition to four liters of herbicide per capita). Bomb craters now occupy an area of South Vietnam larger than the state of Connecticut. The result was that Vietnamese civilians—and plague-carrying rodents—were driven from their natural habitats and concentrated into refugee camps and urban slums.

The Vietnamese government later claimed that 43 percent of food crop acreage and 44 percent of the forests in South Vietnam were destroyed.

The "people-moving" program was a great success. Vietnam had been an agrarian land with 80 percent of the people living in rural areas. By 1971, six of every ten South Vietnamese had been forced into the slums of the large cities or the refugee camps surrounding them. There were over three hundred such camps with a total population of about 1 million. Saigon, a city built to house about 300,000 persons, became a city of 3.5 million. All told, 2 to 4 million persons were made homeless.

The refugee camps have been thoroughly described. Many were scarcely fit for human habitation, but they were ideal for igniting a plague epidemic. Since food supplies were destroyed in much of the battle zone, rice was sent in from other parts of the unhappy country. This also helped spread the disease. (The progress of the epidemic is charted in Figure 3).

A handful of plague cases were reported before 1961 (about fifteen cases a year from 1956 to 1960). From 1965 to 1970 the average reported level was over four thousand cases each year. Some of this increase was certainly the result of a shift from purely bacteriological diagnosis to largely clinical diagnosis as a basis for reporting the disease. The actual upsurge of plague cases may have begun several years before 1965.[2]

Then, in 1970, American troops began to withdraw. Public outcry in the United States had put an end to the poisoning of crops—officially at least—by the end of April; the defoliation of forests was suspended, and the spasmodic bombing was increasingly directed toward North Vietnam.

By 1972 reported plague cases in Vietnam had fallen to a level of about twenty-five hundred a year—historically still a very high incidence, but well below that of previous years. This small country of some twenty million inhabitants had become the source of about 90 percent of all plague cases reported throughout the world, an embarrassing statistic to

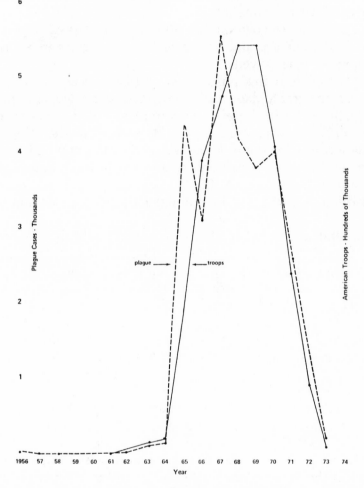

Figure 3 The Vietnam Tragedy

the Saigon government, which soon took vigorous steps. Actually reducing the incidence of plague would have been very difficult. Instead, in 1972, the South Vietnamese minister of health in Saigon made clear to his subordinates that in the future there would be no more, and preferably far less, than a thousand reported cases of plague each year, regardless of the facts. As Figure 2 shows, his instructions were obeyed.

North Vietnamese regulars and their South Vietnamese allies naturally faced exposure to the disease in the south. But plague has historically been a disease of the southern portion of the country, and so it remained. Even in the period from 1908 to 1945, when the country was under unified French rule, there were five to fifteen times as many plague cases in the south as in the north, despite approximately equal populations.

The 1970s epidemic was the first major plague epidemic to occur since the development of antibiotic treatment of the disease and of DDT, 1080, and warfarin. The results of the Vietnam experience, while heartening in some ways, clearly show that massive outbreaks can still occur under suitable conditions even in a country from which the disease has virtually disappeared.

Military policies created, or at the very least stimulated, the epidemic; it was left to the various medical corps to deal with it. They did a remarkable job. Under extremely difficult conditions, the fatality rate for treated cases was kept at 5 percent or below. In addition, a team from the Walter Reed Army Institute of Research set up a new three-story laboratory on the grounds of the Institut Pasteur in Saigon on the tree-lined Rue Pasteur and, with their Vietnamese colleagues, carefully investigated various aspects of the disease. These studies greatly broadened our understanding of plague in its modern form. Unfortunately, the knowledge was bought at the cost of much needless suffering.

All American personnel were supposed to be vaccinated against the disease; most were. All were supposed to have booster shots every six months; most did. The Vietnamese, on the other hand, whether civilian or military, were inadequately vaccinated, or not at all.

The difficulties of maintaining booster shots of vaccine, or of administering vaccine in the first place, were compounded, as already noted, by the fact that the U.S.P. vaccine first used in Vietnam had to be refrigerated and used within two weeks or its effectiveness was lost. One outgrowth of the Vietnam War was the development of a freeze-dried vaccine with much better keeping qualities.

Plague struck American and Vietnamese alike, even in the early years, although at greatly disparate rates. On March 21, 1963, a young American soldier reported to a dispensary with an inguinal bubo, fever, and searing pain.[3] He had never been vaccinated. His illness was diagnosed as a venereal disease—lymphogranuloma venerum—although no tests to confirm this conclusion were carried out. He received tetracycline by mouth; but in spite of the drug, the bubo remorselessly increased in size, and the area around it became swollen and inflamed. Penicillin (useless against plague) was given to combat this development. Thus treated, the soldier developed plague meningitis. Fortunately, someone recalled that he had just come from a plague-stricken area, and so he was given streptomycin. Soon after, a guinea pig injected with some of his spinal fluid died of plague. After three weeks in the hospital the young man was released.

Plague meningitis is a frequent result of inadequate treatment. When tetracycline is used as the only treatment of suspected plague, this complication is particularly likely, since it is difficult to achieve adequate levels of this drug in the cerebrospinal fluid.

A second American case occurred on June 22, 1966, when an immunized civilian technician developed pneumonic plague. He had had three injections of U.S.P. vaccine, the most recent about three months before. In addition, he had been given live vaccine (the E.V. strain commonly used in Vietnam) some four months earlier.[4]

On his own initiative he took about two grams of tetracycline six days after he became ill. Two days after beginning the self-treatment he was hospitalized. Some of his bloodstained sputum was inoculated into rats, and a presumptive diagnosis of pneumonic plague was made. (He had just returned from a plague-infected area.) He was isolated and given streptomycin and tetracycline immediately, and he continued to receive this treatment for eight days. In all he was given over twenty-six grams of tetracycline and nine grams of streptomycin. He recovered uneventfully.

This was a remarkable case. It suggested that an extensively vaccinated individual might live long enough even with pneumonic plague to permit its diagnosis and treatment, although untreated he would almost surely have died. Both rats injected with his sputum died of plague in four to five days.

Pneumonic plague was infrequent in Vietnam—had it not been, the epidemic would have been far worse. But when it occurred the outcome was usually not that of the fortunate technician. This form of the disease has a long history in Vietnam; cases date back to the great epidemic of 1911. A small but spectacular outbreak occurred in 1941 when a medicine man spread the disease to six families during the forty-eight hours before he developed definite symptoms of his own. Every member of all six families was dead two days after they developed symptoms.

In the late evening of Friday, September 10, 1965, a fifty-three-year-old man in a hamlet in Long Khanh province (northwest of Saigon) turned up at the hamlet health worker's home for treatment.[5] He had a fever, difficulty breathing, and blood-stained sputum. Two hours later he died. Investigation revealed that he was the fifth of his family to be claimed by pneumonic plague. His thirteen-year-old daughter had died four days earlier, his six-year-old son the day before. That morning, a man, seventy, and a woman, fifty, both members of the family, also died.

An even more extensive eruption took place a month earlier in the An Khe district of Binh Dinh province, a coastal region in the northern half of the country. On August 8 a fifty-nine-year-old man died after a brief illness. Because of his age no one was concerned over his death. But he was the initiator of an epidemic affecting forty-three persons. There were thirty-seven pneumonic and five bubonic plague cases, plus one mixed infection. Of the fifteen pneumonic cases that occurred in the first sixteen days, only two of the victims survived. Of the twenty-two pneumonic plague patients who became ill after August 24, only two died, because the disease was recognized by then. One bubonic case was fatal. Six surrounding villages were exposed, but fortunately, no further cases broke out.

This nasty little attack led to an important observation. *Yersinia pestis* was isolated from the throats (either from sputum or throat swabs) of more than 7 percent of the bubonic plague victims and from 3 percent of otherwise completely healthy persons in contact with them. Some bubonic plague patients had *Y. pestis* in their throats even though antibiotic therapy had rendered their bubos sterile. The drug concentration in the throat was apparently not lethal to the organism. Therefore, such patients were potentially infective even after antibiotic therapy had apparently cured the disease.

The throat organisms diappeared in time, with or without treatment. What is uncertain is whether such persons are potential carriers who, like the infamous Typhoid Mary, could transmit the disease to others while not suffering from it themselves.

Plague spread inexorably over South Vietnam. In 1961 only the island province of Long Khanh was involved. The following year plague broke out in three more provinces. All these were on the South China Sea; none was contiguous with Long Khanh. In 1963 the number of plague-stricken provinces doubled; all newly infected areas were neighbors of those provinces where plague had occurred the previous year. Two more provinces joined the plague list in 1964. In 1965 the plague toll soared along with the American military involvement. The number of afflicted provinces rose to twenty-four of the country's forty-four. Later the distribution changed somewhat from year to year, but the total area affected remained much the same. From Quang Tri province in the north to well south of Saigon, plague stretched across the devastated country in an unbroken chain.

Quang Nam was the third most northerly province of South Vietnam; its principal city is Da Nang. No plague had been reported there for fifteen years before 1965. Then, in September of that year, a shipment of rice arrived from Saigon. A few days later, rats began to die in the central market area; a few days after that the first human case appeared. By late May of the next year, the disease had spread to the refugee camps near the city. The overall result in Da Nang was some 270 plague cases.

The city of Hue, in the province of Thau Thein just north of Quang Nam, also had not reported plague since 1950. Then, on December 23, 1965, a worker from the central market area of the city reported to the hospital. He had bubonic plague and died three days later in spite of treatment. He had seen several dead rats in the marketplace, where food shipments came in from plague-stricken Da Nang.

Two weeks later a second case appeared, also from the market area; it was followed by 31 more in the remaining three weeks of January. In February, Hue had 115 cases, and as in the preceding month, cases began to come in from outside the city itself. March brought 4 or 5 new cases every day, and victims continued to appear, although in greatly reduced numbers, through June. Over a quarter of a million people were vaccinated in January and February. DDT was spread around the residence of each plague case, and an effort was made to locate and treat new cases quickly. The latter program was highly successful. Of over 400 cases there were only 3 deaths.

Observations made in Vietnam have important implications for plague control elsewhere. In Nha Trang, bandicoots, the burrowing rodents that are now dominant in Bombay and Calcutta, were trapped and they and their fleas examined for plague. Although they were not present in Nha Trang in the overwhelming proportions they attain in Indian cities, the bandicoot rats were heavily infested with *X. cheopis* (an average of five per animal). Some of the animals were plague-infected, as were their fleas; nearly half of the bandicoots showed plague antibodies in their sera. Flea interchange had clearly taken place between the bandicoots and the Norway and Polynesian rats and the shrews that infested Nha Trang. The recent predominance of bandicoots in Calcutta and Bombay has been advanced as a reason for the decline of plague in these cities. The results from Nha Trang make this explanation less convincing, since the bandicoots themselves seem capable of supporting an epidemic.

Early in the war, the U.S. forces constructed an army base, supply depot, and air base on Cam Ranh Bay, some twenty-five miles (forty kilometers) east of Nha Trang. There grew up around these bases a complex of fifteen villages and hamlets known as Cam Ranh City, with a total population of about fifty thousand Vietnamese. In January and February of 1966, an epidemic in one hamlet led to forty-four cases of human plague; over 80 percent were fatal. Almost none of the civilian population were vaccinated.

The U.S. military authorities had conducted intensive antirodent campaigns, but rats were still seen in daylight in dormitories and barracks, indicating a very heavy infestation. Dusting with insecticide was frequent but often ineffectual, because of the high winds and torrential rains of the monsoon season.

An epidemic began in Cam Ranh City on Thursday, February 23, 1967.[6] A patient was treated for simple bubonic plague, which was diagnosed on clinical grounds, since there were no facilities to take smears or cultures from the inguinal bubo. The Vietnamese male received streptomycin and tetracycline as an outpatient and recovered completely.

The day after the first case appeared, a wooden building was demolished in the workers' compound. As the flooring was torn up, hundreds of rats scurried for new hiding places, and the Vietnamese laborers began killing them with sticks. Four days later, seven Vietnamese from the compound came to the Twelfth U.S. Air Force Hospital with fever, nausea, and painfully tender buboes. Over the next nine days, thirty-five more patients were admitted from the compound.

In all, there were fifty-eight cases. Fifty-four were simple bubonic plague, and all the patients recovered after prompt treatment. Two cases, one an American soldier, were diagnosed as pneumonic plague. One case of certain pneumonic plague was fatal, as were two suspected cases. All military personnel in Cam Ranh Bay who had not received a recent plague booster injection were given one, and many of the civilian population were vaccinated as well. Insecticide dusting began, and the plague areas were isolated. By early March it was decided to treat all inhabitants of the workers' compound with a streptomycin injection and two grams of oral tetracycline each day for four days.

A young American private was admitted to the hospital on the evening of March 2 with fever, nausea, and a very sensitive inguinal bubo. His lungs were clear, but six hours later he showed evidence of pulmonary involvement and began coughing the following day. After two days of treatment his lungs were again clear. The bubo remained an open, draining wound for forty-five days, but the young man recovered. His case of bubonic plague progressed to secondary pneumonic plague even though he was receiving intravenous antibiotics and skilled treatment.

The other confirmed pneumonic case was not so fortunate. The day after the sick private entered the hospital, a Vietnamese civilian woman employee of the army went to a military dispensary near the supply base. She had a very red sore throat, fever, swelling around one tonsil, and tender lymph nodes in her neck. She was treated with penicillin and released. Three hours later she was back—by then near death. Twenty minutes later she died. Postmortem examination revealed pneumonic plague.

It was a dramatic demonstration of the speed with which even secondary pneumonic plague can kill a person with only mild symptoms. Probably no treatment could have saved the unfortunate woman by the time she appeared at the dispensary.

Plague ecology in southern Vietnam has some interesting and unusual aspects, some related to weather conditions, some not. The Mekong Delta is the home of about one-third of the people of South Vietnam and one of the largest rice-growing regions. Plague has been comparatively infrequent in the area, amounting to about two hundred cases between 1965 and 1972, and it will probably remain low. In the delta, rat harborages are flooded each year during the summer monsoon when much of the land is under water. The rodent population is effectively controlled by this periodic inundation of the countryside, which also yields the bountiful rice harvest.

Elsewhere in southern Vietnam the situation is different. Either under or alongside of most houses ditches or tunnels have been dug. These served as shelters during attacks by the U.S. and South Vietnamese air forces, as well as during ground fighting, and they did double duty as storage places for rice and other foods. They obviously offered food and shelter to rodents as well, and many of the rodent passages led directly into the houses above.

Interspersed with efforts to control human plague, the army medical research team continued studies of the plague-infected animals in South Vietnam. Plague organisms could be isolated from only slightly more than four rodents of every thousand examined, and from fewer than three of every thousand fleas, far below the levels thought necessary to sustain an epidemic.

Unusual human cases of plague continued to appear.[7] On November 30, 1966, a forty-nine-year-old man of Chinese ancestry was admitted to a provincial hospital near Nha Trang. He had had chills and fever for six days. Shortly after admission he lost consciousness. Two days later he was transferred to the U.S. Army Eighth Field Hospital. He was comatose and coughing up bloody sputum, but his pulse, temperature, and blood pressure were not severely abnormal. There were no swollen lymph nodes. Chest X rays revealed lung involvement, and his sputum contained organisms that could have been *Y. pestis*. The man promptly received high doses of both streptomycin and chloramphenicol, but he died in twenty-four hours, after showing only a brief period of improvement. His blood also contained the plague bacillus.

This man survived for an incredible period of ten days, at

least six of them without treatment, with either primary pneumonic or primary septicemic plague. Since he had both when he entered the field hospital, it is impossible to say which came first. In any case he showed remarkable resistance to the disease and might have survived had he been adequately treated sooner.

The Eighth Field Hospital had another unusual case three months later. The patient was a thirty-four-year-old Filipino man. He had a headache, chills, fever, and a dry cough for a day before he sought medical attention. His eyes were bloodshot and he showed general symptoms of toxicity; but neither bubos nor any other remarkable findings were present. Chest X ray was normal. Then, during his second night on the ward, he developed a large and agonizingly tender inguinal lymph node. Removal of fluid from the node showed organisms like *Y. pestis*. Immediately treatment with both streptomycin and tetracycline began. It was in vain. Six hours later the man was dead. He had symptoms clearly suggesting plague for much less than half a day before his death. Both his blood and lungs showed evidence of plague infection. Probably this was a case of pneumonic plague in which the lymph nodes initially failed to remove *Y. pestis* from the lymph fluid, so an explosive septicemia built up. Only in his last hours did the lymph node defenses begin to function. It was too late.

In the late fall of 1966, another Vietnamese man of Chinese origin was admitted to the same hospital. He had suffered for three days from fever, abdominal pain, vomiting, and diarrhea. Shortly after admission he became irrational. He had the typical small skin hemorrhages of plague on his abdomen and a large, hot, tender mass of femoral and inguinal lymph nodes. He was given streptomycin and chloramphenicol intravenously. He remained irrational for three days after treatment began, and on the third day the bubo in his groin was noticeably larger. Tetracycline was substituted for chloramphenicol and over the next two days the groin swelling subsided. Finally, after eight days, streptomycin treatment was stopped because the man no longer had fever. But the battle was not over yet.

Three days later the swelling began again, and streptomycin treatment had to be restarted. The patient then recovered. The stormy course of this man's disease illustrates the potential complexities of the treatment of plague despite potent antibiotic agents given by experienced physicians. It also emphasizes the importance of not discontinuing treatment too soon. The recommended period of antibiotic treatment is at least two weeks.

Early in 1967 plague broke out among Montagnard tribesmen in an area not previously touched by the epidemic, the Kontum province in the central highlands.[8] Between the last week in February and the first week in April, twenty-one cases occurred. The location was a fortified hamlet occupied by soldiers of the Civilian Irregular Defense Group and their dependents. They lived in deep, nearly continuous trenches covered with split bamboo and sandbags. The epidemic was in two parts; the first began on February 20. On the twenty-third, spraying with a nonpersistent insecticide (diazinon) began and continued for four days. The last case of the first group appeared about a week later (March 6). There was a three-week break until new cases began to appear on March 26, and the area was again sprayed with diazinon.

This outbreak dramatizes a problem in the use of nonpersistent insecticides in plague control. Spraying must be repeated frequently to ensure continued protection. In this incident, plague erupted again four weeks after the end of the first spraying campaign. Had a persistent insecticide been used, the second outbreak might not have occurred.

For most of the day the men of the Civilian Defense Group were outside the bunkers that served as living quarters. Their dependents, on the other hand, spent much of their time in these rather uninspiring quarters. The result was to be expected: 80 percent of the plague cases, and all the fatalities, occurred in women and children. None of the Vietnamese, civilian or otherwise, had received plague vaccine prior to the onset of the disease. Some, but not all, were given U.S.P. vaccine on February 23, three days after the first four cases were detected.

Yersinia pestis, lethal to mice, could be isolated from buboes of those patients days after treatment with vast amounts of potent antibiotics—for example, twenty-seven grams of streptomycin and eleven of chloramphenicol. In one case, *Y. pestis* was isolated both from the bubo and, more important, from the throat of a bubonic plague patient who had received eighteen grams of streptomycin and twelve grams of chloramphenicol.[9] Plague bacilli were also found in the throat of the immunized U.S. Army physician who treated these cases. Virulent plague bacilli had been isolated previously from buboes of convalescent patients as much as a year and a half after the infection had passed, but that was long before the antibiotic era.

In this outbreak in the Montagnards, as in the epidemic in the Nepalese village of Nawra later that year, many of the patients had large (1- to 1 1/2-inch diameter) ulcers, the so-called plague carbuncles, which appeared on various parts of the body—the back of the neck for example, or the buttocks. As in Nepal, these lesions, which sometimes accmpanied severe plague, bore a striking resemblance to those of anthrax.

Also in this epidemic, a quarter or more of those persons in close contact with plague patients before the patients' admission to the hospital showed substantial amounts of plague antibody in their serum during the outbreak. These close contacts of the plague victims must also have been infected with the disease, but they did not develop plague symptoms. Perhaps this was caused by natural resistance to plague, but more likely it was the result of being bitten by only lightly infected fleas, perhaps repeatedly. Such fleas may act as vaccinating agents, injecting too small an amount of *Y. pestis* to give rise to clinical plague but enough to stimulate an immune response to the organism. If this were true, it might partly explain the very low rate of plague infection among American servicemen. They were bitten by fleas, since they came down with other flea-borne disease against which they were not immunized. But these same fleas carried plague, which was a very minor problem with the American forces. Perhaps part of the effect of the U.S.P. vaccine was to establish partial immunity and thus raise the threshold for plague infection, so that a flea bite that might cause clinical plague in a nonimmunized individual only reinforced the immunity of the already vaccinated ones.

Several facts are important about this greatest of plague epidemics in the second half of the twentieth century. One is that the number of cases was much higher than the number recorded. The actual number of plague victims in Vietnam in the decade after 1964 is probably between one hundred thousand and a quarter of a million. It is also significant that 90 percent of the plague cases occurred in only thirteen of Vietnam's forty-four provinces, fortunately in thinly inhabited areas. The most densely populated regions were only lightly stricken; otherwise, the toll might have been many times higher.

The usual response of physicians about plague is that it can be easily cured by modern drugs—then they add, "*if* it is diagnosed in time." Physicians of wide experience with the disease are less certain that the cure is "easy" and are painfully aware of the difficulties of early diagnosis, especially of the septicemic or pneumonic forms.

15

Seventy Years of
Plague in America

From 1900 to 1925 plague in America had two elements: rat-borne plague, which ignited at least three of the five great urban outbreaks of the period, and wild-animal plague, which appeared soon after the first San Francisco epidemic. In the first quarter-century of American plague nearly five hundred cases of the disease were reported. About two-thirds were fatal.

The end of the Los Angeles epidemic in 1925 was the end of an era in American plague, since it was the last epidemic, to the present, in which rats were involved.

In the second quarter-century, human plague was discovered outside the seaports in which it had originally appeared. In 1934 a sheepherder died in southern Oregon; there was a human plague case in Utah in 1936, in Nevada in 1937, in Idaho in 1940. Between 1941 and 1948 there were only six cases of human plague reported in America, all in California. But the mortality figures were no better than in the first twenty-five years; four of the six victims died. The record was somewhat better for the period between 1925 and 1950. Only twenty-seven human cases were reported, but 52 percent were fatal.

Why was the incidence of plague in America so low during this time? It was certainly not because of DDT, 1080, or warfarin, since the plague incidence had fallen before any of these compounds were in use. It was probably not because of the disappearance of infected rats from ships, since ratproofing did not become really effective before about 1936. Part of the drop was probably the result of an increased emphasis on sanitation and ratproofing, but it is unlikely that this is the whole explanation. Like many other aspects of the coming and going of plague, this decline retains a disquieting air of mystery.

In 1949 there was a new development. New Mexico challenged California for the plague championship of America. And New Mexico won hands (or bodies) down. The center of human plague activity in the United States had moved substantially eastward where it was to remain. Although no human plague was reported in New Mexico until eleven years after wild-rodent plague was discovered there, and in Arizona it was yet another year before the human disease appeared, New Mexico had all three of the human cases reported in 1949 and two of three the following year; Arizona had the third.

Wild-rodent plague was a very modest contributor to human misery in the United States even up to 1964. On the average only slightly more than one case occurred each year. The level of three cases a year was apparently exceeded only three times— in 1910, 1936, and 1959. Also, between 1900 and 1964, there were frequent intervals of one to four years in which no cases were reported at all. Then, after 1964, the situation took a sharp turn for the worse.

The year 1965 saw the worst outbreak of human plague in America in four decades. It was also a landmark year for two other reasons. In every year since then, the disease has occurred. In addition, the number of cases in the "bad" year of 1965 was equalled or exceeded in five of the next twelve years. The average for the interval 1965–77 is more than nine times the yearly average since the Los Angeles epidemic ended in 1925. Some of the cases in recent years are worth examining in detail for clues to the nature of contemporary American plague.

On Tuesday, September 10, 1957, a girl whom I shall call Linda Blake had a fever. Linda was four years old and lived in

Wichita Falls, Texas, close to the Oklahoma border, about a hundred miles northeast of Dallas. Six days later she was hospitalized. By then her blood took four times longer than normal to clot and she had subcutaneous hemorrhages all over her body. On the second day in the hospital she died of plague.

Investigation revealed no plague-infected animals near Wichita Falls, but Linda and her family had recently returned from a visit to Boulder County, Colorado, a region of enzootic plague in which infected ground squirrels were found soon after. Although it is not certain, it is likely that the little girl handled sick or dead squirrels in Colorado and then carried the infection to her home in Texas. The transport of human plague from one part of America to another was to become a regular feature of the disease.

In June 1959 and eleven-year-old boy contracted plague from the nearly tame chipmunks in Yosemite National Park. The next month a slightly older girl caught the disease from a rabbit brought to her home in Bernalillo County, New Mexico, by her pet dog. The boy recovered. The girl died. In 1959 four cases in three states (two in California, one in Colorado, one in New Mexico) involved three different species of animals.

Another case in 1959 had nothing to do with wild animals, but it had some interesting and frightening aspects. A young man, here called Robert Price, worked as a chemist at the Army Laboratory at Fort Detrick, Maryland, where the principal interest was biological warfare. Robert was twenty-two years old and single. His work involved chemical analysis of *Y. pestis*; he had received the U.S.P. plague vaccine in March and a booster shot on August 10, 1959.[1]

On Thursday, September 1, Robert awakened at seven A.M. as usual. Although he had been completely well the night before, now he had chills, fever, and general weakness. In spite of these symptoms, he went to breakfast and to the laboratory. But, as the morning wore on, Robert got progressively sicker, and before lunch he returned to the barracks to lie down. At five that afternoon he entered the hospital. He was alert and cooperative, but he was a very sick young man. There were indications both of meningitis and pneumonia.

He was put in isolation and three hours later was given oral tetracycline. Although his condition had worsened in every way, he remained awake and helpful. By midnight he was coughing bloody sputum. It contained organisms resembling *Y. pestis.*

Robert had vomited most of his eight o'clock dose of the antibiotic and all of the midnight one, so intravenous administration was begun instead.

By three A.M. Robert's face had darkened, his temperature was 105°F, his pulse rate had accelerated from the normal level of 70 or less to 120, his blood pressure had fallen further (to 90/60), and his breathing rate had increased to 40 from the normal 25. He had been sick for twenty hours. His doctors doubled the rate of tetracycline administration and began streptomycin injections every six hours.

The vigorous and timely treatment finally took effect, and eleven days later Robert Price was discharged from the hospital, although indications of damage to his liver by the plague bacillus persisted for nearly two months. His blood showed antibody to *Y. pestis* on the ninth day of his illness, but fewer than five months later it had disappeared. This case raises a number of questions.

What if Robert's illness had started on Saturday morning instead of Thursday, and he had decided to spend the weekend in nearby Baltimore or Washington, as he often did, rather than in his barracks? What if he had not recently received the U.S.P. vaccine—did it make any difference? What if he had not been known to have worked with *Y. pestis,* so that he was suspected of pneumonic plague almost from the moment of his hospital admission and was treated by physicians aware of the most effective treatment of the disease? All things considered, Bob Price was a lucky man. Besides losing his own life he could have easily started an epidemic of pneumonic plague in an urban hospital or a crowded eastern city.

Three years later there was another laboratory infection with pneumonic plague at the Microbiological Research Establishment at Porton, England; the interests of this organization were much the same as Fort Detrick's. The victim was an experienced professional microbiologist. His infection was fatal, but perhaps he intended it so. He died on August 1, 1962, in the Oldstock Hospital, Salisbury.

In 1960 and 1961 plague in America was plague in New Mexico. This was not cause for parochial indifference by those living elsewhere. In both years the potential for spread of the disease far beyond the borders of the Land of Enchantment was apparent; in one case it was real.

In February 1960 two men were hunting cottontail rabbits on the New Mexico prairie in the southeastern corner of the state. The hunting was good—too good. A few days later both men were hospitalized with bubonic plague (first diagnosed as tularemia) contracted from fleas on the rabbits they had shot. The men were well treated and both recovered. The important aspect of these infections was that both young men were U.S. Air Force officers whose job it was to ferry jet aircraft to South America and to England. Fortunately, both were off duty at the time their symptoms became apparent. It might have been otherwise.

In that area rabbits live in close association with field and grasshopper mice as well a with cotton, kangaroo, and wood rats. The latter had been nearly wiped out by an epizootic. The other rodents were highly plague-resistant, but the disease spread first to the very susceptible rabbits and then to the equally susceptible men of the U.S. Air Force.

In 1961 there were three cases of plague in New Mexico. The first victim will be called Sam Duran. Sam, thirty-eight, worked in a sawmill in the village of Pecos, southeast of Santa Fe. He had hunted in wooded areas near his home in late June. On Friday, June 22, he herded sheep near the ruins of an ancient pueblo. On Saturday he was very sick. The following Wednesday afternoon, Sam Duran was admitted to the hospital in Santa Fe. His face was bluish, both lungs were inflamed, and his breathing was shallow. At three o'clock the next morning Sam Duran went into severe shock; a short time later he was dead. Autopsy revealed that he had died of pneumonic plague. He had neither swollen lymph nodes nor *Y. pestis* in his blood. Plague was never suspected, and he was not isolated, although he was put in an oxygen tent. Happily, no one else was infected.

Sam Duran was a simple man. He had never flown in a jet to South America or to England. He was probably unsure as to where Cambridge was—either of them. But the next victim of plague in New Mexico knew where both these academic citadels were; he worked in one, as a geologist at Harvard University.

This thirty-eight-year-old man had spent several days wandering through the arroyos west of Santa Fe analyzing evidence for ground movements in the area. It was Saturday, July 22, when he noticed a small sore at the base of his left thumb; he gave it little thought. Four days after his flight back to Boston, he felt tired, sick, and feverish, with pain in his left armpit, a headache, and intermittent nausea. That evening his family physician stopped by his home and noted that the young geologist had a moderately high temperature and several slightly sore lymph nodes under his left arm. But he did not appear seriously ill.

The next morning he went to his physician's office. He felt better then, but by afternoon his temperature had risen and he vomited after eating. The swollen lymph nodes were larger and much more painful. The family's physician decided to put him in the hospital early the next day. It was too late.

During the night the victim became restless, his breathing became steadily more difficult and painful, and he began coughing up blood. He was rushed to the hospital but turned increasingly blue and collapsed in shock in the X-ray room. No pulse was obtainable and external heart massage, artificial respiration, and drug stimulation all failed to revive him. His death was diagnosed, several days postmortem, and with the assistance of the New Mexico health authorities, as caused by plague, bubonic initially, progressing to septicemic and pneumonic. He had been seriously ill for only a few hours.

Two of the three plague cases of 1961 developed into the pneumonic form; both were fatal. Even in the antibiotic era the odds of a pneumonic plague victim surviving are not good primarily because of the problem of diagnosing the condition.

It is difficult at best; it is made more so since many physicians think the disease no longer exists.

The third plague victim of 1961 had simple bubonic plague, was diagnosed promptly, and recovered uneventfully.

In 1962, and again in 1964, no human plague was reported in the United States. In the intervening year, there was a single case in which the patient, a young Navajo sheepherder, died hours after admission to the hospital. It was December, food was scarce, and he had killed a rabbit to feed his dogs. The rabbit bore plague-infected fleas.

The year 1964 was the proverbial calm before the storm. It was the last year up to the present (1985) in which no plague was reported in the United States. This peaceful interlude was followed by the New Mexico plague epidemic of 1965, the circumstances of which might easily have led to the dissemination of the disease throughout the country.[2]

It began (it was later recognized) on Monday, June 21, when a three-year-old Navajo girl was treated in the outpatient clinic of the Public Health Service Indian Hospital in Gallup. She had a sore throat, a high fever, and evidence of an upper respiratory infection. She was given penicillin, and her mother was instructed to continue treatment at home in the hogan near the town of Red Rock, some eight miles north of Gallup.

Prairie dogs had warned of the epidemic. They have a unique place in Navajo culture. The Indian children make pets of the young animals, and the older Navajo delight in the antics of the gregarious creatures who share their often bleak surroundings. Besides, prairie dog, either cooked on a spit, or roasted in the fire in a blanket of moist earth, is a delicacy and an important source of protein.

But in the spring of 1965, the Indians knew something was wrong. Before lambing time in May, prairie dogs were, as usual, everywhere. With the leisure that came with the end of lambing season, the Navajo noticed that the prairie dogs were gone. Around the burrows were clouds of blue-bottle flies and the scent of the passage of death. Here and there forlorn heaps of the little animals lay huddled in groups of two or three, sociable even in death.

In Red Rock, meanwhile, the little girl first felt somewhat better and then very much worse. On Thursday, July 1, she entered the hospital with a high fever, a pulse rate nearly twice normal, and symptoms of meningitis but no lymph node swelling. She improved after appropriate treatment and was discharged after twenty-four days in the hospital. Her chart read, "Gram-negative meningitis." A few weeks later it was changed to "Plague" when plague antibodies appeared in her blood.

A week after the little girl from Red Rock was hospitalized, a two-year-old boy who lived in an abandoned railroad car between Gallup and Red Rock also entered the hospital. By August 1 it was clear that he had plague. That the disease had erupted on the vast reservation was bad news at any season: in 1965 the timing was horrible.

In mid-August was the Gallup Intertribal Ceremonial, which draws Indians and tourists from far away, ordinarily some thirty thousand persons in all. Two weeks later came the Navajo Tribal Fair, with crowds twice as large. There was another complication. Each year in August, about seven thousand Navajo children travel to schools in the West and Midwest to further their education and to escape the searing summer heat of the desert. The possibilities for catastrophe stretched off into the distance like the sere hills of the reservation.

There were many obstacles to effective action. The area involved spanned two states and included federal, private, and Indian lands. Vaccination was out of the question—its effect was far too slow to contain an epidemic. The immensity of the reservation, the poor-to-nonexistent roads, and the fact that so many of the Navajo spoke neither English nor Spanish further hindered efforts to contain the disease. The army was asked to help; so were the Fish and Wildlife Service and the CDC.

Plague did not wait for the various organizations to agree how best to attack it. Late in July a nine-year-old boy came down with plague after helping his father skin prairie dogs; the boy had a cut on his finger that opened the way for the plague bacillus.

By early August the bilingual radio station was broadcasting warnings in Navajo to avoid prairie dogs, a disconcerting notice for a family of eight who had just set up camp in a remote part of the reservation. The site was surrounded by a colony of prairie dogs that the family had intended to hunt for food. They stopped hunting when they heard the message on their portable radio, but it was too late. The four-year-old girl in the family and her three-year-old cousin developed the disease and were rushed to the hospital in Crown Point. Both recovered.

By mid-August America was experiencing the most massive emergency control measures against plague in forty years. Local physicians and the population were alerted to the presence of the disease. The symptoms and the role of wild animals were described in the newspapers and on radio and television. A first-aid booth was set up on the fairgrounds for both the Intertribal Ceremonial and the Navajo Tribal Fair. Public health nurses toured the grounds and camping areas looking for sick people and providing information on plague. The Navajo Tribal Council endorsed efforts to control prairie dogs and their fleas.

Insecticides were applied first to the fair grounds and the encampment areas and then to more remote regions; prairie dog burrows near homes were fumigated, and in more isolated districts the animals were poisoned with 1080-treated grain. Domestic dogs and homes were dusted with insecticide.

On Thursday, August 26, a public health nurse and a Navajo assistant were returning to Gallup from a clinic they had conducted. It was late in the afternoon when they caught sight of a horse and wagon drawn up in the shade of a cottonwood and a woman and two boys signaling for help. In the wagon was a perilously sick fourteen-year-old boy. It had taken the family an hour to drive the wagon to the highway from their hogan near Red Rock, whence the first plague case had come nearly two months before.

Taken immediately to the hospital, the boy already had a high temperature but no swellings and no signs of lung infection. He was nearly unconscious. His condition remained stable for the first day. Then, on Friday evening, his temperature rose to 105.4°F (nearly 41°C), his breathing became labored, and he began coughing up bloody sputum. A chest X ray revealed extensive lung infection. The boy died at 10:20 that night. He had been ill three days. The physician who tried to revive him by breathing into his throat through a plastic tube had some anxious days after the diagnosis of pneumonic plague was confirmed, but there were no further cases among the boy's family or the medical staff. As in the cases of the disease four years earlier, pneumonic plague was so rapidly lethal that the victim was dangerous to others only for a comparatively short time before he died. It is not always so.

There were two other cases that were probably plague in the 1965 epidemic but were never confirmed. Then, with the early arrival of cold weather in the fall, the epidemic came to a halt. Epizootics had extended over an area nearly twenty-three thousand square miles, almost the size of Rhode Island, Delaware, New Jersey, Connecticut, and Massachusetts combined. The prairie dog colony at Long Lake, where the next-to-last case occurred, was completely wiped out. But an average of forty-two fleas could still be collected in each abandoned burrow more than six months after the epizootic had passed.

The plague-control program ended its emergency phase in October. More than one hundred thousand prairie dogs had been poisoned, in addition to the untold numbers that perished in the epizootic. Late in September the *Navajo Times* again ran one of its notices on the dangers of contact with prairie dogs, and added the editorial comment, "We are sorry that it is necessary to issue this warning about the plague. We are sorry that the prairie dogs, rabbits, and other small animals are sick with the plague, but we are even more sorry for ourselves because we sure like roasted prairie dogs."

It would be a while before anyone on the Navajo reservation ate roasted prairie dogs without a qualm.

The 1965 plague season continued elsewhere. In September a five-year-old boy caught the disease from a ground squirrel in California's Shasta County, near Mount Shasta, a popular tourist attraction.

The eight confirmed (and two possible) cases of 1965 made it the worst year for plague in America since 1924, although, unlike the Los Angeles epidemic, there was only one confirmed and one probable death from the disease in 1965. The 1965 epidemic was accompanied by epizootics in Colorado, Utah, Arizona, Nevada, and California, in addition to New Mexico.

The following year widespread epizootics continued. Late in May 1966 a five-year-old Navajo boy died of plague in the Monument Valley Hospital in Mexican Hat, Utah. The disease was not identified until three weeks after his death. Plague soon struck Arizona and New Mexico again. Before the year was out, six cases had accumulated. One was a thirty-nine-year-old housewife living in Santa Fe, New Mexico; another was a seventy-two-year-old man from the New Mexico mountain community of Servilleta.

He first consulted a physician on Tuesday, June 7, two days after the beginning of pain in his right groin. He was given medication and spent most of the next three days in bed. Finally, because of the inguinal swelling, burning thirst, nervousness, and inability to eat or sleep normally, he again sought medical help. The physician suspected diabetes. The man was hospitalized in Albuquerque, but by the time he got there, he was confused and barely able to walk.

On admission his right inguinal lymph nodes were swollen to two to three inches (five to eight centimeters) in diameter and surrounded by an inflamed area of another four or five inches. The tentative diagnosis was no diagnosis at all—it simply stated the symptoms—and the old man was given erythromycin, penicillin, and a low level of tetracycline.

Four days later he was, not surprisingly, sicker than ever. The area of inflammation was spreading, and his blood pressure was dangerously low (80/0). Prior treatment was suspended, and chloramphenicol was ordered. The next day, Monday, June 13, he had chest pain and was spitting blood. Three days later, material from one of the swollen lymph nodes was positive for *Y. pestis,* and retrospectively, so was the blood culture taken during the hospital admission tests eight days before.

His physicians next lowered the chloramphenicol level and

added tetracycline and streptomycin. Marvelous to relate, the tough old gentleman survived the long period of misguided treatment, recovered and, in due time, returned to his mountain home. Numerous rodents were found close to his house, and in July *Y. pestis* was isolated from a chipmunk and from a cottontail rabbit in the surrounding country. The old man raised rabbits, one of which died late in May, but it could not be checked for plague.

This case was strange enough but an even more bizarre one was to follow.

A twenty-one-year-old soldier had returned to Fort Worth, Texas, from duty in Vietnam.[3] During his last days there he had torn down rat-infested buildings near Saigon. As usual, the elementary precaution of treating buildings with insecticide a few days before their demolition had been neglected. As the rats scurried for shelter, the soldiers in the unit vied to see who could kill the most rats by stomping on them. Later, the man who was soon to leave for Texas carried the dead animals to a disposal area.

It was Monday, August 15, 1966, when he noticed a small swelling in his left groin. Over the next week it grew larger, hotter, and more painful. In a few more days he entered the hospital with chills, fever, and headache. He had received the U.S.P. vaccine twice in the year prior to his illness.

The soldier was admitted to the veterans hospital in Dallas on August 29 with a diagnosis of incarcerated hernia. He was scheduled for surgery, but fortunately, that diagnosis was ruled out by a surgical consultant. Another consultant later suggested lymphoma, and part of the lymph node was removed on September 7. Two weeks later yet another consultant suggested the possibility of plague. The lymph node, which had been examined before with no result, now showed the probable presence of *Y. pestis*. Further tests on the organism at Walter Reed Army Institute of Research confirmed the diagnosis, although *Y. pestis* was never cultured. Two weeks later the young man was transferred to Brooke General Hospital at Fort Sam Houston. He was finally discharged on November 28 after a total of 104 days of illness, of which 90 were spent in the hospital. It was the first case of plague imported into the United States since the S.S. *Manila Maru* docked in New Orleans forty years before.

Also in 1966, plague-infected fleas were found in six different locations in California, spanning almost the entire state, and infected rodents were found in eight regions. An emergency control program began, and there were no human cases.

In 1967 and 1968 New Mexico had no human plague for the first time in nearly a decade. In 1967, however, there were three American cases, one in Arizona, two in Colorado; one of the Colorado cases was fatal. The next year Arizona and Colorado each had one case; the fatal case that year occurred in Idaho in October. The victim was a thirty-two-year-old man and the source of the infection was probably a snowshoe hare (usually called rabbits).

From the epidemiological standpoint, the most remarkable case was that of a six-year-old girl (she would have said she was six and a half) in Denver, Colorado.[4]

I will call her Janice. She lived in a two-family brick house on a street lined with ancient elms, maples, and cottonwoods. It was only four blocks to City Park, and the park and the houses for some distance around it were home to a substantial squirrel population.

It was a summer evening, June 9, 1968. Jan began vomiting about eight o'clock, and her mother noticed she had a fever. The vomiting went on. It went on all night. It went on all day Monday, and all of Monday night. By Tuesday morning Janice was still feverish, her throat was inflamed, and her right ear hurt. There was one thing more. She had a tender spot under her left arm. Her mother felt gently—there was a lump, hard and tender, the size of a golf ball. She promptly called a taxi to take her daughter to the hospital. By then, Jan's lips and the skin under her fingernails were blue; she had a high temperature and a racing pulse.

Doctors examined Jan in the emergency room, admitted her to the hospital, and started penicillin and sulfa treatment and extensive testing. The child's condition improved, but by the next day the swollen nodes under her arm had grown grotesquely; the golf ball was now a tennis ball, or something more. By the end of the first week in the hospital the great lump had subsided somewhat, Janice's temperature was down—although still above normal—and although her first blood culture had grown gram-negative rods, a second had not. At the end of the second week she was sent home. It was Tuesday morning.

Alas, on her first morning at home on the tree-flanked street, little Janice awoke with the familiar ache in her armpit. The swelling had returned, more painful than ever. Her mother was baffled. After all, her daughter had just come home from the hospital, she had no fever, and she was hungry. Jan's mother decided to wait and see. By the next afternoon she knew she had waited long enough. It was not that there were any new developments—Janice still had no fever and her appetite was good. But she was in pain. Jan and her mother returned to Children's Hospital.

The physician who examined her in the emergency room noted that the swelling in the axillary nodes had increased and that swollen lymph nodes were appearing on the little girl's neck. He suggested that she come back the following week.

Fortunately, Janice came back and was admitted to the hospital the next day and put in an infectious-disease ward. The intern assigned to her was fresh from medical school; Janice was his first patient since he had received his M.D. It was a case he would remember. In consultation with the pediatric resident, he decided to wait until the results of the most recent blood cultures came through before ordering any further antibiotics. The blood cultures had been sent to the CDC in Atlanta. Sixty miles away, at the CDC laboratory in Fort Collins, Colorado, was one of the most sophisticated group of plague experts to be found anywhere in the world, but they had only just arrived there after moving from San Francisco. Besides, no one even suspected plague, so the blood cultures went to Atlanta.

June ended. July began. Little Jan was taken to surgery and the swollen lymph nodes opened and drained. Then, at two o'clock on Wednesday afternoon, July 3, the telephone rang in the pediatric nursing station. It was the CDC reporting that the organism from Janice's blood was probably *Y. pestis.* Other calls from Atlanta reached the CDC laboratory in Fort Collins and the Colorado State Department of Health. Bubonic plague had struck in the geometric center of a major western city.

In less than a year there had been three cases of human plague in Colorado; both the others were misdiagnosed. One was called a streptococcal sore throat and the other tularemia. The error was fatal in one case; the other victim was left with permanent damage to his central nervous system. Every effort was made to prevent such a tragic outcome in Jan's case. The efforts were successful.

There remained the question of where she had gotten the disease. That seemed simple enough. Colorado abounds with plague-infected animals, and Janice had probably encountered one on a trip to the nearby mountains. But Jan had not been out of the city. She had visited an aunt on the other side of town, and she had played around her home and in City Park. That was all.

It was obviously enough. It was soon discovered that people had been finding dead tree squirrels around her neighborhood all spring. An intensive search began that ended in the detailed examination of 768 animals. More than one in ten of Denver's Eastern fox squirrels were plague-infected. The city health department had received reports of dead squirrels for several months but had taken no action to determine the cause. There was plenty of action now.

In July and August hundreds of sick or dead animals were examined for plague. These included two dozen Norway rats, none of which had the disease. All the infected animals were Eastern fox squirrels rather than the ground squirrels native to Colorado. Over three hundred stray domestic dogs were also tested; all were negative. Plague-infected squirrels were found close to Stapleton International Airport and to Lowry Air Force Base, faintly ominous findings themselves, but not relevant to Janice's case.

In spite of the presence of dozens of plague-infected squirrels in Denver, no evidence was found of dogs having been in contact with plague-stricken animals. This suggests that even stray urban dogs are of little value as sentinels of plague.

Besides the search for infected animals, steps were immediately taken to kill the fleas on the squirrels in the various parks of the city, especially in the areas where large numbers of plague-infected animals were located. Authorities set up as many as eight hundred bait boxes to dust the animals with insecticide when they came to get the bait. Finding a suitable bait was little problem. Eastern fox squirrels were wild about peanut butter. But there was a problem of traffic management. The squirrels were supposed to enter the bait box, be dusted with insecticide, take a mouthful of peanut butter, and leave to make room for the next squirrel. Unfortunately, no one had explained this to the squirrels. The first squirrel to find a newly stocked bait box stayed there gorging itself on all the peanut butter. Only then did it waddle contentedly homeward for a postprandial nap.

The solution was to coat small pinecones with peanut butter. In this convenient form—the squirrely equivalent of a Big Mac—the squirrels took one piece of bait to their nests and let other squirrels have a turn at the remaining feast.

The Denver epizootic—the first ever reported in city-dwelling tree squirrels—meant that flea exchange with wild rodents was taking place even in an urban center of nearly a million and a half population. An alternative explanation was that someone had brought an infected squirrel into the city from elsewhere in the state. This explanation would have received strong support if a Colorado ground squirrel or other native animals had been found in the city and infected with the disease, but no such animal was ever discovered.

Fortunately, Denver's rat population is small so the probability of transmission of plague from a fox squirrel to a domestic rat to a human is extremely low. What if a similar event occurred in the approximately four hundred squirrels in New York's Central Park, with its proximity to the city's huge rat population?

In 1969 the number of plague cases in the United States was

double that of the preceding year. In 1970 the number more than doubled again. All the cases in 1969 were in New Mexico. None of the cases was fatal, in spite of the fact that in only one of the six was plague considered in the initial diagnosis (although only one case was atypical).

On Saturday, May 31, 1969, a twenty-year-old girl living in a commune near Placitas, New Mexico, became ill.[5] She took tetracycline tablets every six hours for the next two days. She developed a tender, painful swelling in the right armpit, however, and an inflamed breast and shoulder on the same side. She was later admitted to the Bernalillo County Medical Center in Albuquerque. The diagnosis was gastroenteritis! Her condition steadily improved, and she was discharged after nine days and given oral tetracycline to take at home.

A young man in the commune came down with plague two days later. His case was diagnosed as venereal disease. His life may have been saved because his neighbor, the girl who had just returned from the hospital, shared her supply of tetracycline with him. Later he was hospitalized and treated with streptomycin and tetracycline after the organism in his blood was identified as *Y. pestis.* The source of both infections may have been a pet kitten.

A few weeks later a three-year-old boy from the rural community of Jemez Springs was hospitalized in Albuquerque. The admission diagnosis was viral meningitis or rickettsial infection. He was given penicillin, although the drug has no effect on either viruses or rickettsia. Finally, *Y. pestis* was identified, and the boy was discharged a month after his illness began with a still detectable bubo under his left shoulder blade. His recovery was complicated by congestive heart failure.

The next-to-last plague case of 1969 occurred in October. On Wednesday, October 1, a thirteen-year-old girl was admitted to the Los Alamos Medical Center in the small community of Los Alamos, site of a then Atomic Energy Commission laboratory operated by the University of California. The girl had picked piñon nuts in the forested areas around the town on the previous Sunday. That evening she noted a red area, like an insect bite, on her upper left arm. She soon developed a fever, pain in her left armpit, and a sore neck. When she entered the hospital she had an axillary bubo three inches (eight centimeters) in diameter, and a swollen spleen and liver. The attending physician considered cat-scratch fever, tularemia, and, for a change, plague, in the initial diagnosis, and the girl was treated with tetracycline. She made a rapid recovery. It was the first case of plague reported in Los Alamos County in the twenty-six years of its existence. The actual source of the infection was never precisely identified.

On the basis of surveys made before and since, however, we know that plague exists in the abundant vole and deer mouse populations as well as in rock squirrels, chipmunks, and rabbits in Los Alamos County and in contiguous areas including Bandelier National Monument.

The infection is maintained in mice living in nearly inaccessible locations on the precipitous canyon walls. When the rodent population overflows its normal habitat, plague appears on the mesa tops and in the valleys between them.

In the first seventy years of known plague in America, it gradually was discovered over a much wider area than originally expected and found to be present in an almost bewildering variety of animals.

The extensive distribution of the Eastern fox squirrel has been mentioned, as well as its role in plague. An even more ubiquitous creature is the deer mouse that certainly plays a major role as a host of the disease. This little animal's range covers North America, with the possible exception of the Deep South. The Eastern fox squirrel is found (as of 1964) from the Canadian border south to Mexico and the gulf, and from Colorado east to central Pennsylvania. Both of these species, and probably others, provide a small furry corridor over which wild rodent plague could pass to extend its domain toward the rising sun.

16

Plague in the 1970s: Worldwide

In the first years of the 1970s, plague refused to behave as befits an obsolete disease, although there was an early period of marked improvement. The worldwide incidence of plague reached a fourteen-year low in 1973, nearly as low as that in 1959, at the "end" of the Third Pandemic. Then, alas, in 1974, there were more than three cases for each one the year before. In 1975 the number of reported cases dropped, but this was in part the result of incomplete reporting from South Vietnam. Even so, there was an average of four new cases of human plague reported every day in 1975.

Throughout the first half of the 1970s, Asia contributed about 80 percent of the world's total plague, with Vietnam the major source. Indonesia, however, after reporting only 11 cases in 1970, and none in the next two years, had a sudden flare-up of the disease in 1973, with 130 victims and suspected victims. The overall mortality rate for the 218,000 cases of plague between 1911 and 1939 in Indonesia was 99 percent!—probably due to ignoring clinically mild cases. A later estimate was 70–80 percent for bubonic and 100 percent for pneumonic. Subsequently, the overall mortality was reduced to 46 percent by the use of antibiotics.[1] Burma had an even more dramatic record. From only 17 cases in 1973, plague claimed 680 Burmese victims in 1974, 275 in 1975, nearly 500 in 1976, and almost 200 more in the first half of 1977.

After an absence of fourteen years, plague returned to Cambodia (now Democratic Kampuchea).[2] Its arrival was expected. It was first reported on February 17, 1972, from the hospital in Prey Veng some thirty miles (fifty kilometers) east of the capital, Pnompenh, on Route 1 to Saigon. There were ten cases with three deaths. Early in May plague broke out farther east on Route 1, in the town of Svay Rieng in the "parrot's beak" region where Cambodia juts into Vietnam. For over a month several new cases in Svay Rieng developed each day, 109 in all. The population of the town had more than tripled when the outbreak began. Most of the newcomers were women and children driven from their homes by the fierce fighting going on around them. By the end of August the population of Svay Rieng was five times its normal level, and the refugees living in temporary shelters were the principal victims of the disease.

During the worst of the epidemic in Svay Rieng, the town was encircled by hostile troops, so the medical team and the necessary supplies—dusters, DDT, and antibiotic drugs—were flown in by helicopter. Pnompenh, its population likewise swollen more than three-fold by refugees, also had plague, but it was kept at a very low level, perhaps because the city had been for years one of the cleanest in Asia. Of 130 cases of plague in Cambodia only 5 were reported to WHO.

During the first half of the 1970s, the Americas were in second place after Asia as suppliers of plague victims, accounting for 9 percent of the total up to 1974 and over one-third in 1975.

Peru had substantial plague in 1970 and 1972 (128 and 118 cases, respectively) but very little in other years. Brazil reported over 1,300 human victims in the same six-year period; more than a third of the cases occurred in 1975. Bolivia had 87 cases, more than half of them in 1970, and none at all in 1972 and 1973, while the United States had 46 cases, some each year, but with nearly half the total in 1975. In Ecuador only 69 persons were stricken with the disease in the first half of the 1970s; the disease returned in 1976 after a two-year absence. The United States had substantially more reported human plague in 1975 than did Zaire and more than Lesotho, Bolivia, and Peru combined.

The continent of Africa was in its usual third place in the plague sweepstakes during this time, supplying less than 7 percent of the total between 1970 and 1974. In 1975 Africa reported fewer than one-third the number of plague cases reported in the Americas.

Namibia (formerly South-West Africa) made the largest contribution to plague in Africa with a single outbreak in 1974. This apparently resulted after a brush fire caused a mass migration of wild rodents into close contact with human inhabitants. Also in 1974, plague was reported for the first time ever in Rhodesia (Zimbabwe), and it increased in 1975. Then it had more of the disease than any other continental African country, perhaps because of spilling of the rodent migration from its southern neighbor, Namibia. Madagascar and Zaire reported plague each year (1970–77) and Tanzania, Guinea, and Lesotho had intermittent outbreaks; the most important in Tanzania was an eruption of pneumonic plague on the western side of Kilimanjaro. In 1972 South Africa's only case was that of a farmer who contracted the disease from the bite of a plague-infected kitten.[3]

Libya also joined the ranks of the plague-stricken in 1972. The disease had never before been reported there. Then, early in the year, sixteen cases occurred around the village of Nofilia, near the Mediterranean Sea, about halfway between Tripoli and Benghazi. Plague has apparently continued there, but no details are available.

In most countries the majority of cases resulted from epidemics concentrated in small regions. A third of the cases in Vietnam in 1974 came from Quang Nam province in the northern part of the country. Ninety-six percent of Burma's cases in the same year came from the Taunggyi district of Shan state, southeast of Mandalay. Ceará and Bahia on the Atlantic coast of northeastern Brazil north of Rio de Janeiro accounted for 93 percent of the cases reported in Brazil in 1974.

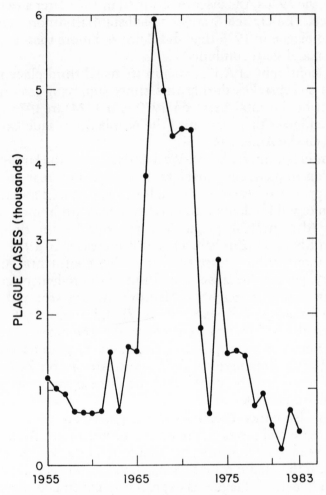

Figure 4   Human Plague Worldwide, 1955–1983

In 1978 only 766 cases and 31 deaths from plague were reported to WHO, down from 1,447 cases and 67 deaths the year before. But plague increased in both Africa and the Americas. In Africa the increase was largely due to an outbreak in Kenya. There were 68 cases in Bolivia and 6 in Peru, with only 3 deaths. Burma had 171 cases and 6 deaths while Vietnam reported 314 cases and 8 deaths.

The next year was better still. Only 505 cases and 56 deaths were reported around the world in 1980. Africa had 80 cases and 20 deaths, divided among Angola, Kenya, Madagascar, and Tanzania. The Americas had 147 cases and 7 deaths (sharply up from 1979). Brazil reported 98, and Bolivia 26 cases of plague and 2 deaths. Most of the plague in Brazil occurred on two inland plateaux in Ceará State in people with known contact with rats, mostly in people under sixteen. Clustered cases were common; nine in one house, two in a neighboring house, for example.[4]

Figure 2 showed the "end" of the Third Pandemic. Figure 4 extends the results on plague incidence to 1983. The steady decine of the 1950s may have signaled the end of the Third Pandemic, but it did not signal the end of plague epidemics of imposing size.

17

Plague in the 1970s: U.S.A.

The plague situation in the United States continued to deteriorate after the 1960s. In 1970 there were nearly twice as many cases in New Mexico as in the year before, nearly evenly divided between males and females from two to thirty-nine years of age. One case was associated with plague in a pet kitten. There were three cases in California. The only fatality was a forty-nine-year-old man in Oregon who died six hours after entering the hospital. He became confused and ill four days after dressing a wild rabbit he had shot. It was the first case of human plague in Oregon in thirty-six years.

A pet dog, generously supplied with fleas, was implicated in another case, that of a twenty-year-old woman in Santa Fe, New Mexico, but the association was not proved. This woman's case was diagnosed as incarcerated hernia—one of the favorite misdiagnoses of bubonic plague—but the error was corrected by taking a sample from the bubo before she was subjected to unnecessary surgery.

Perhaps the strangest of the 1970 cases in New Mexico involved a collaboration of sorts between pueblo medicine

men and physicians in an Albuquerque hospital before the
disease was cured to the satisfaction of all parties.[1]

The most concerned party was, of course, the victim. He
was a thirty-nine-year-old Pueblo Indian, a college graduate
and the governor of a pueblo north of Albuquerque. In May
he suddenly developed severe headache, nausea, vomiting, and
fever. The next day he became confused and afflicted with
teeth-chattering chills. He had no known contact with rodents, there were no lymphatic swellings, and his spinal fluid
was clear. He was acutely ill. He spoke and thought slowly,
but there was nothing definite about his symptoms.

He was treated in an Albuquerque hospital with penicillin,
which naturally had no effect. On his third day in the hospital,
physicians carefully reexamined him for the presence of enlarged or tender lymph nodes. None was found. Convinced,
reasonably enough, that he was receiving no benefit from the
treatment, the governor returned to his pueblo, where the
medicine men (with one exception) conducted an elaborate
curing ceremony. As part of it the governor went alone to a
sacred cave some miles from the pueblo.

On his way there, the governor was first mystified when
the woods seemed to part before him as if the branches were
swept aside by some unseen hand and then astonished when
the usually gloomy cave brimmed with light. Entering, he saw
a procession of the ghosts of men he had known from the
pueblo—among them his own father. His father talked to him
at length, telling him that he was too young and too important
to the pueblo to die. Another elderly ghost then turned him
around and directed him to return to his people. It was several
hours later when he reached the pueblo. He felt much better.

Meanwhile, the two blood cultures previously obtained were
found positive for Y. pestis, and the governor was asked to
return to the hospital. He did so, although he considered himself to be well. He was readmitted with a temperature of 101°F
(38°C) and a small left inguinal bubo. He still appeared somewhat confused. After treatment with streptomycin and tetracycline for a week, he was discharged in good condition.

The outcome pleased nearly everyone. The governor was

happy to be cured and credited the pueblo medicine men with his recovery. The physicians who treated him in Albuquerque were pleased to have such a puzzling case correctly diagnosed and effectively treated. And the medicine men—all but one— were pleased as well, for the same reason.

Early in the spring of 1970, the governor, as the tribal officer responsible for maintaining order, had fined a young medicine man for drunkenness and disorderly conduct. Only a few weeks later the young man was again the center of a disturbance, and the governor had him jailed. The tribal council met and favored a much stiffer fine, the usual punishment for a second offense, but the governor insisted on a jail term, and his opinion finally prevailed. The young miscreant knew who was responsible for his sentence and, livid with rage, he publicly threatened the governor with death.

The day after the young man was released from the tribal jail, the governor was stricken with his violent illness. The other medicine men were not surprised when he returned from the white man's hospital little better than when he went— what did Anglo doctors know of spells and witchcraft? They then took measures appropriate to the source of the governor's illness, as they saw it. When he returned from the cave they, and he, were satisfied that he was cured.

But a spell broken rebounds against the person casting it. Consequently, no one in the pueblo was surprised that the first cousin of the young and unruly medicine man died the following week. And they nodded knowingly when, six months later, the young man himself was killed in an automobile accident.

Widespread epizootic activity continued in 1971, and plague-infected rat fleas were found in Tacoma, Washington, for the first time in seventeen years. Norway rats, an occasional black rat, and three species of mice intermingled in the affected area of south Tacoma, which is a mixture of small, old houses, commercial sites, and vacant lots. Rodents frequented empty buildings, trash piles, and blackberry thickets.

In spite of the epizootic activity, it was a mild year for human plague. One victim was a young Navajo woman who had cleaned and eaten two prairie dogs some days before. And plague struck Oregon again; the victim was a ten-year-old boy from Pendleton. He apparently acquired the disease while staying in a lakeside cabin in the northeastern part of the state. Both patients recovered.

The next year was even better. There was only a single plague case, a young student of Northern Arizona University at Flagstaff, who had helped two friends skin a bobcat. The young man was a nail-biter with numerous hangnails that apparently provided entry for the plague bacillus. As usual, he initially received penicillin, the modern panacea for all infections. Later, *Y. pestis* was identified from his swollen lymph node, and more appropriate treatment was begun. He recovered without incident. It was the first confirmed case in America of plague transmission from a wild carnivore to a human.

The year 1973 marked the beginning of a sharp upturn in human plague in the United States. There were widespread epizootics in California and Arizona. In California, Lava Beds National Monument was closed until control measures could be completed. Nearly five thousand acres (two thousand hectares) of Navajo reservation land near the Colorado border of New Mexico were treated with insecticide, and emergency control measures also had been applied in two southern Colorado counties the previous year. The prairie dog population continued to increase until, in the town of Cortez, Colorado, prairie dogs within the city outnumbered human residents.

Two human cases accompanied the epizootics. One was a sixty-four-year-old resident of El Paso, Texas, who had apparently acquired the disease during a month-long stay on a New Mexico ranch. The other victim was a nine-year-old girl who lived not far from where the plague-infected bobcat had been shot the year before. She developed a plague infection in her right eye as well as in her armpit. Belatedly her illness was identified as plague and specific treatment was begun. Her condition improved rapidly, although the pupil in her infected eye remained dilated for some time thereafter. Both 1973 victims of plague survived.

In 1974 there were four times as many cases as in the preceding year, and for the first time since 1970, one case was fatal.

Epizootics continued. At 9 A.M. on Saturday, June 22, campers already settled in the popular Moraine Campground in Colorado's Rocky Mountain National Park were moved out, and officials closed the campground following the discovery of plague in deer-mice fleas in the area.

In 1974 plague started in earnest just four days after the closing of Moraine Campground. On that Wednesday evening, Louise Williams, a twelve-year-old Navajo girl living in Mentmore, New Mexico, began to vomit. She also had a severe headache and a general feeling of illness. The next morning she visited the pediatric clinic of the Gallup Public Health Service Hospital with a temperature of 104°F (40°C) and mild tonsilitis. There was no evidence of meningitis, lung involvement, or swollen nodes. She was sent home after the customary penicillin injection.

Louise was normally a very active, healthy girl, an enthusiastic horsewoman, and an animal lover. Perhaps the latter trait was her undoing. Whatever the cause, Louise did not feel better the next morning, and later that day she was admitted to the hospital in Gallup. Two and a half hours later, Louise Williams was dead. Plague bacilli had invaded her spinal fluid and blood. She now had widespread subcutaneous hemorrhages and a mass of enlarged lymph nodes high on her left thigh.[2] She had died without ever showing typical symptoms.

The source of her fatal infection is uncertain; she may have picked up a sick mouse or prairie dog to comfort it. On the Sunday before her illness, she had gone with her family to church at Rocky Point, five miles west of Gallup. That night Louise and some relatives went to a hogan about five miles north to tend the family's small herd of sheep. There was past evidence of plague both around the hogan and in the vicinity of Louise's home in Mentmore, but none of her companions in either location became ill.

In a Public Health Service office in Gallup there is a map. On it, marked and numbered, are the locations of 146 prairie dog colonies in the area. Each is checked once a month for signs of plague. The four "dog" towns near where Louise had been were checked, but there was no evidence of recent infection.

A five-year-old boy living in the suburban part of Salt Lake County, Utah, became ill in late August. The source of his plague infection was never traced, but he had visited a neighboring home where the children of the family had collected ground squirrels, field mice, and Norway rats to feed a pet owl. In preceding years rodent or flea plague had been reported in half of Utah's twenty-six counties.

Other cases occurred in Gallup and Santa Fe as the summer of 1974 went on. A nineteen-year-old man became ill on Tuesday, September 24, in Santa Fe. The case was diagnosed as incarcerated hernia and surgery was performed. No evidence of hernia was found, but a second incision revealed a swollen, gangrenous lymph node. The unlucky young man recovered uneventfully.

A six-year-old girl became the second victim of the disease in Los Alamos, but again, the source of the infection was unknown. The family had two dogs and three cats and there were chipmunks and field mice near their home.

In late October the disease returned to Gallup. The victim in this case was a twenty-eight-year-old physician who, on Sunday, October 26, noticed an area of painful inflammation on his left little toe and pain in his groin on the same side. He treated himself with oral penicillin for the next six days. It is somewhat comforting to find a physician treating himself as inadequately as he might treat a patient similarly afflicted. The young man doggedly continued his hospital work even though he had little appetite, a nagging headache, and a moderate fever. On the following Saturday he consulted a colleague. By then he had a stiff neck and a swelling in his groin. Material from the bubo was presumed positive for *Y. pestis* and suitable treatment was begun. The young physician made a rapid recovery.

The source of his infection is also uncertain. It may have

been acquired on a camping trip to Colorado or from his two dogs and a cat.

The disease refused to go away with the coming of cold weather. On Monday, November 11, a sixty-two-year-old woman developed symptoms that led to her hospitalization the next day. She had skinned and dressed two flea-infested cottontail rabbits while on a hunting trip in northern New Mexico the previous week. The rabbits were still in her home freezer; the bone marrow of both animals contained *Y. pestis.* Still another victim contracted the disease, possibly from a pet cat, near Albuquerque in early December. In 1974 rodent populations increased in parts of California and in Arizona, New Mexico, Colorado, and Utah, and carnivores with high levels of *Y. pestis* antibodies were found throughout Oregon and in parts of Montana. The official reaction in Montana was to stop plague surveillance for fear of finding more!

A December case of plague in New Mexico is unusual, and normally no further cases would be expected until early spring of the following year. It did not work out that way. The 1975 plague season, on its way to becoming a record year for human plague in America, got off to an early start.

The case of Danny Gallant, whose name appeared in the opening pages of this book, began what was to be the worst year for human plague in the United States since the Los Angeles epidemic ended in 1925.

Danny's experience in February 1975 had several unusual aspects. One was that he caught the disease from an infected coyote, dead for some time. There were no fleas on the animal, but Danny had a hematoma on his right middle finger, a consequence of having it smashed between the leaves of a table five years before. This hematoma apparently provided entry for the plague bacillus from the coyote's blood. Although flea bites are the usual source of infection, cuts, severe hangnails, even blood blisters can provide portals for wily *Y. pestis.*

A coyote had never before been implicated as a source of human plague infection. This was significant because coyotes may travel 100 miles (161 kilometers) a day or more, thus transmitting the disease over a considerable distance. And they are increasingly penetrating the suburbs of every large western city. The coyote population of Los Angeles in 1975 was estimated at four to five hundred. They are found from Maine to California, except for the South, and from the Arctic coast of Alaska far into Mexico.

Of course, the scientific aspects of the case were of secondary interest to Danny Gallant and his family. The boy entered the hospital on Thursday, February 13, five days after skinning the coyote. Plague was considered in the initial diagnosis, and streptomycin treatment was begun. Later, tetracycline was substituted, and Danny was sent home after six days with instructions to continue taking the drug orally. Two days later, however, he was rehospitalized with symptoms of plague meningitis. Danny eventually received chloramphenicol and was discharged a second time, about three weeks after his initial admission. He completely regained his health, but it was a long time before he felt like tossing a ball through the orange basketball hoop over his garage door. Danny was a slender, wiry boy of seventy pounds (thirty-two kilograms) when he and his friend skinned the coyote; by the time he left the hospital for good, he was sixteen pounds (nearly eight kilograms) lighter.

No one else in Danny's household developed symptoms, and his friend, Dale, with whom he had skinned the coyote, remained well, as did the rest of his family.

Following Danny's adventure, nearly four months went by before the disease appeared again. It was another unusual set of cases in an unusual year.

The victims were all Navajos living in a cluster of hogans near Tuba City, Arizona, some thirty miles east of Grand Canyon National Park. On Tuesday, May 7, the first case, a thirty-one-year-old woman, was hospitalized in Tuba City with symptoms of bubonic plague; her three-year-old daughter followed her mother to the hospital the next day. Their symptoms were nearly identical; both were later confirmed as plague victims. In the mother's case there was a serious complication. She was pregnant, near term, and the baby was showing signs of distress. As we have seen, plague toxins may cross the placental barrier and do serious damage to an unborn child.

It was a difficult decision. The mother had *Y. pestis* in her blood. Even if the infant was not being poisoned by plague toxins, it would be exposed during delivery to the organisms in its mother's blood. On the other hand, each drug used for the treatment of plague has undesirable properties in pregnancy. Streptomycin passes into the fetus and localizes in the eighth cranial nerve causing possible disturbance of hearing and balance in the newborn. Tetracycline causes liver damage to the fetus and discoloration of the baby teeth; it may also cause growth inhibition by localizing in regions of new bone growth. Chloramphenicol crosses the placenta readily (as do other drugs) and may cause aplastic anemia or the "gray baby" syndrome, most often in premature infants, with a mortality rate of about 40 percent.[3]

The attending physicians finally made their decision. They would treat the mother vigorously with streptomycin and begin artificial induction of labor, then treat the baby after delivery as if it were also plague-infected. Mother, daughter, and newborn son recovered without incident. A week later another child got plague. She was not so fortunate. Treated with synthetic penicillin three days after her illness developed, she died three hours later. Although she never exhibited clear-cut symptoms of plague, both her blood and lungs yielded *Y. pestis*, and her organs showed signs of extensive damage by the plague toxins.

The little girl had lived with her parents and a younger child in a citrus orchard in Ventura County, California, between Santa Barbara and Los Angeles. She had no insect bites; and although the family kept cats, dogs, chickens, and rabbits and there were black rats in the orchard and rat droppings in the rabbit hutch, there was no evidence of an epizootic and no one else was affected by the disease. There had been fatal human plague in Ventura County in 1956, and an epizootic in wood rats a decade later.

Another month went by before the next case appeared. The

story of Ralph Fulp's incredible battle with pneumonic plague is told in the next chapter.

Near the end of June, a girl three and a half years old contracted plague at her home in San Juan County, Utah, but recovered.

As July began, New Mexico's reputation as the prime plague state of America was beginning to suffer. Only one of the six human cases in the United States had occurred there, but the balance was about to be redressed. Of the next fourteen cases, New Mexico contributed thirteen.

All three of the plague cases in July were simple bubonic plague. They involved two boys, nine and fifteen, and a girl, twelve.

The girl lived on the Navajo reservation near Sheep Springs, some thirty-five miles north of Gallup, in the northwestern corner of the state. She was treated for probable plague, and her fever fell after administration of streptomycin for twenty-four hours. But the antibiotic level then had to be reduced because the drug was causing tissue damage. The girl's temperature immediately rose, so she was given intravenous chloramphenicol and, later, tetracycline. In a few weeks she was well again.

Six days after the Navajo girl was hospitalized, a fifteen-year-old boy in Pecos, New Mexico, at the southern end of the Sangre de Cristo Mountains and 170 miles (275 kilometers) east of Sheep Springs, sickened with plague, and in six days more, a nine-year-old boy living near Elk Mountain, some 30 miles northeast of Pecos, was also stricken. The first boy had a left-groin bubo and, later, some evidence of meningitis, but he regained his health without unusual difficulty. The nine-year-old, with similar symptoms, underwent exploratory surgery for incarcerated hernia. *Yersinia pestis* was cultured from the necrotic lymph nodes exposed in the operation. He had an uneventful convalescence. The source of the first infection was not identified, but the second boy had handled several dead rodents poisoned with anticoagulants.

So far, only one of the nine reported cases of human plague had been fatal. That relatively good record was not to last.

In August there were four more victims; three were females—two were three years old, one was sixty-four. The other sufferer was a fourteen-year-old boy. One of the girls and the teen-aged boy died, one from bubonic, the other from secondary pneumonic, plague.

Charlene Brown, the girl who died, was Navajo and lived within a few miles of Red Rock State Park. She had been treated as an outpatient two days before and appeared to be recovering. Then her condition abruptly worsened, and she died in the hospital emergency room.

On the day of her death, a rodeo began in the park, to be followed, a week later, by the Navajo Tribal Ceremonial, a situation reminiscent of that in 1965. Authorities began an intensive dusting and bait-box campaign to protect visitors to the area.

Although the source of Charlene's infection remained uncertain, her family owned several dogs and cats, and the cats had recently brought home dead field mice.

August brought developments in the animal world as well. A United Press dispatch told of foot-long Norway rats nesting in palm trees along the beach in Fort Lauderdale, Florida, and living off the debris left by swimmers and picnickers. Although the Norway rat is typically a burrowing animal, this report emphasized (were emphasis needed) the fact of rodent adaptability.

Also, early in August, many prairie dogs died in Bailey County, Texas, northwest of Lubbock on the border with New Mexico. *Yersinia pestis* was found in prairie dog fleas, and the Muleshoe National Wildlife Refuge—where the epizootic was first discovered—was closed until control measures could be completed. Aerial surveys of the county indicated that epizootics might have occurred in several other rangeland areas earlier in the spring and summer.

On August 4 Moraine Campground in the Rocky Mountain National Park was closed again when two plague-infected ground squirrels, one sick and one dead, were found in the area. Glacier Basin Campground in the same park was closed shortly after for the same reason.

The second three-year-old girl and the sixty-four-year-old woman who exhibited plague symptoms early in August lived within a few miles of each other near Cuba, New Mexico. The girl's case was uneventful. But the older woman was thought to have an incarcerated hernia. That she had plague instead was discovered only during exploratory surgery. She was the second plague victim in a month to go to the operating room instead of the isolation ward. Four plague-stricken field mice were found in the Cuba area in the north-central part of the state.

Further surveys by New Mexico's Environmental Improvement Agency also disclosed a plague-infected ground squirrel within the city limits of Santa Fe, the second such incident during the year. Thus far, Santa Fe had no human plague, but it was soon to arrive.

The last human plague victim of August was a Californian, fourteen-year-old William Handley, who, on Monday, August 25, developed symptoms. The boy had spent the summer with his maternal grandparents in the village of Carlito Spring, in Tijeras Canyon east of Albuquerque.

By Wednesday, William Handley was short of breath. He had what might have been insect bites on his left arm, and he had caught wild rodents to feed the household pets.

The next day his parents took him to a physician in Albuquerque. The doctor's presumptive diagnosis was viral hepatitis, and he urged the boy's parents to consult their family physician. The family then drove to their home in California's Marin County, north of San Francisco, where William was again seen by a physician. He was not hospitalized. Two days later his face was dark, his breathing shallow and painful, and he was coughing. Chest X ray showed fluid accumulation in both lungs, and he was put in the hospital. On Monday he was transferred to a hospital in San Francisco. He died a few hours later.

Death was caused by secondary pneumonic plague. He never had swollen lymph nodes, nor were any found on autopsy. The plague bacillus apparently gained early access to his blood and multiplied vigorously there, leading to the relatively rare septicemic form of the disease. *Yersinia pestis* then infiltrated his lungs, with fatal results.

William Handley's case was difficult to diagnose correctly, and only prompt diagnosis and vigorous treatment could have saved his life. The boy had potentially exposed 130 persons to pneumonic plague. All were given prophylactic tetracycline and were watched carefully, but no other cases developed. William's death was the first from pneumonic plague in America in a decade. And, for the second time, New Mexico had exported a pneumonic plague case to a major American city.

The year 1975 was the first in half a century when there was more than a single pneumonic plague case in America. The average had been less than one such case each decade. In 1975 there were two cases ten weeks apart; a third case was imminent.

The first plague attack of September bore an unpleasant resemblance to the last one of August: again septicemic plague, presumably from a flea bite, went directly to the pneumonic form. The victim was a thirty-year-old woman living in Ruidoso, New Mexico, in the south-central portion of the state. Her disease deveoped less explosively than in the previous pneumonic cases, and the condition was quickly and correctly diagnosed and effectively treated. A dog she owned died. Its corpse contained *Y. pestis.*

Epizootic plague had menaced the citizens of Santa Fe for some time. By mid-September the first human case appeared. The victim was a twenty-eight-year-old woman, mother of two children and five months pregnant with another. The physician who examined her recognized the disease, as did his patient. Proper treatment was begun at once, and she made a full recovery. In January 1976 she gave birth to a six-pound baby boy.

The next victims were two sisters and a cousin, three, ten, and twelve years old, who lived in the tiny village of Petaca, some fifty miles north of Santa Fe. The children convalesced uneventfully after serious illnesses. The last two cases of plague in New Mexico for the month of September were two more girls, one eight, one eleven years old. One child lived in Glo-

rieta, eight miles southeast of Santa Fe, and the other in Tesuque, a few miles north. In both cases the parents of the
children recognized the disease, probably because of the intensive publicity given the earlier cases, and they both got
swift and effective care, with good results. So far, none of the
September cases of human plague had been fatal. Then, on
Monday, September 15, an eighty-year-old woman living in
the small mountain community of Greenwood, Colorado (population sixty), developed fever, chills, headache, and abdominal pain. She entered the hospital in Colorado Springs on
Friday and died the next afternoon. Plague bacilli from her
blood were not identified until ten days later.

The little town of Greenwood, some twenty-five miles east
of Pueblo, Colorado, and about one hundred miles south of
Denver, consists of twenty to thirty homes clustered along a
small creek. Although some of the houses are in excellent
condition, others are dilapidated, some are abandoned, and
accumulated trash offers good nesting sites for rodents.

Six days before her illness, the victim and her husband had
noticed a dead animal odor from near their bathroom. The
corpse could not be reached, but the woman put mothballs
behind the partition concealing the dead animal in hopes of
suppressing the stench. After her death a dead wood rat was
removed from the wall, another was found in the basement,
and a dead rock squirrel was located in a tree near the house.
The rock squirrel contained plague antibodies, but the two
wood rat corpses were too badly decomposed to give reliable
results.

Probably, the woman's infection came from fleas from the
dead wood rat behind the bathroom partition that may have
been driven into the house by the odor of mothballs, although
fleas could also have come from the dead rat in the basement.
There was evidence of an epizootic in rock squirrels in the
area, and rock-squirrel fleas were found in large numbers in a
wood-rat nest. The fleas had transferred to wood rats after their
usual hosts died during the epizootic.

The 1975 plague season in America ended in the second half
of September. On September 20 a ten-year-old girl in Santa Fe

developed the familiar symptoms but made an uneventful recovery after suitable treatment. She was the last plague case of 1975.

The plague year ended with twenty confirmed cases and four fatalities, a case-fatality rate of 20 percent, or one in five. The modest improvement over the usual rate was probably the result of the wide publicity given the early cases in New Mexico. The generally heightened awareness of the disease increased the chances of its early diagnosis.

Two of the cases of 1975 involved the relatively rare septicemic form, and the incidence of pneumonic plague was also higher (15 percent) than usual. Of the victims, five were male and fifteen female; three of the four fatal caes were women or girls.

Plague in 1976 got off to another early start. The first case, a fifteen-year-old Navajo boy who lived in Moenave, Arizona, had premonitory symptoms on Monday, February 24 and was admitted to the Tuba City Indian Hospital (thirty miles east of Grand Canyon National Park) on Thursday. Later that day he began coughing frothy, bloodstained sputum containing organisms resembling *Y. pestis.* His blood pressure fell rapidly and his blood-clotting time rose. Fortunately, he was young and strong and received good treatment. He ultimately recovered with no serious aftereffects.

Two or three days before his illness he had found a dead (or dying) cottontail rabbit a mile or two from his home. He dismembered the animal and fed it to his dog. Fleas from field mice near his home were positive for *Y. pestis,* and three of seven serum specimens from dogs at the boy's home also showed antibodies to plague. As in the preceding year, there was a pause after plague declared its intentions before it struck again. In the interim the disease was found in prairie dogs in southeastern Colorado, along the New Mexico and Oklahoma borders, and on April 1 the New Mexico Environmental Improvement Agency began the distribution of free flea powder to any pet owners who wanted it.

Southern California was again the site of an early case in 1976. On Sunday, April 13, a forty-five-year-old man who lived twenty-five miles southeast of Bakersfield had chills, fever, and a right inguinal bubo. Later, he developed a generalized rash, jaundice, and a cough. The following Saturday he visited the emergency rooms of three Bakersfield hospitals before gaining admission to the isolation room of Kern Medical Center. By then his sputum was tinged with blood, he had a right-sided pneumonia, and bacteria resembling the vicious bacillus of plague were found in his peripheral blood (blood taken from a fingertip or earlobe), in material aspirated from his throat, and in a skin lesion on his right arm.

The tentative diagnosis was plague, and he was started on chloramphenicol. It was too late. The man died on Sunday, April 20, one week after his illness began and on his second day in the hospital. Six members of his household and sixty-seven persons at the three hospitals he had visited received prophylactic tetracycline; but no other cases appeared. Investigation revealed ground-squirrel deaths around the victim's house.

Two weeks later, Reyes Lovato, a sixty-three-year-old woman who lived in Santo Domingo Pueblo, halfway between Albuquerque and Santa Fe, New Mexico, died in an Albuquerque hospital of secondary pneumonic plague. She had skinned a rabbit and a pack rat five days before her illness began. There were signs of a possible rodent die-off in the area around the pueblo, and the plague bacillus was isolated from a dead pack rat found nearby.

By May 1, 1976, there had been as many cases (three) of secondary pneumonic plague as in the entire preceding year; two of them were fatal.

There were three more widely separate plague cases in May. All the victims were women, ranging in age from sixteen to thirty-nine. The sixteen-year-old contracted the disease in Coconino County, in north-central Arizona, but recovered. The twenty-two-year-old girl was a resident of Pueblo, Colorado (eighty miles south of Denver), who apparently encountered the disease in Phantom Canyon, forty miles northeast of the city. The older woman lived near Tijeras, twelve miles east of Albuquerque, New Mexico. On Saturday, May 12, she had the familiar symptoms accompanied by a left inguinal bubo and a small pink, healing lesion on her inner left thigh. She was twenty-two weeks pregnant. The woman made a complete recovery and her baby arrived in the world as a normal, healthy infant.

The woman had noticed fleas on her dogs and cats before she became ill. Early in June the area around her home was treated with grain containing a systemic insecticide. Such compounds combine the merits of being harmless to the host animal but lethal to the fleas that feed on them. The recent development of such agents and the means for applying them is a substantial advance in plague control.

Shortly after this case was discovered, it was followed by a second in a nearby area. A twelve-year-old girl also acquired the disease in Tijeras Canyon. Her parents recognized the symptoms, and that helped ensure rapid treatment and speedy recovery.

A seventeen-year-old boy in Dixon, New Mexico, about thirty-five miles northeast of Santa Fe, also had plague a few days later, which he had apparently caught from a flea on a pet dog.

Meanwhile, wild-animal plague began to appear in many areas of Colorado. The Devil's Kitchen picnic area in Colorado National Monument in west-central Colorado, fifteen miles from the Utah border, was closed when authorities noted that all of nearly four hundred prairie dogs had suddenly vanished. *Yersinia pestis* was isolated from one dead animal. The disease also appeared in animals in the Rocky Mountain National Park, some forty miles from the Wyoming border in north-central Colorado, as well as on the Fort Carson military reservation, seventy miles south of Denver, and in the vicinity of both Vail and Aspen, two areas separated by thirty miles of mountains. Late in June a plague-infected prairie dog was found within Denver itself.

A twelve-year-old boy in Rio Arriba County in northern New Mexico and a girl the same age in Coconino County, Arizona, also contracted the disease in June but got well without incident following treatment.

On Friday, June 20, a five-year-old girl developed a red papule on her chin while camping with her family in the Plumas-Eureka State Park in the Sierra Nevada, 140 miles (225 kilometers) northeast of San Francisco. They were in the park five days and slept at night in a floored tent. On Monday, June 23, the little girl entered the hospital in San Francisco. She later developed swollen and painful nodes on the right side of her neck but made a good recovery after suitable treatment, although the painful lymph node on her neck that had grown progressively larger had to be incised and drained.

Meanwhile, officials had closed the Plumas-Eureka State Park the day after the little girl's disease was identified as plague. Evidence was quickly found of a die-off of both chipmunks and squirrels over one-third of the campground, including the spot where the girl had camped with her family. The area was dusted with DDT.

There were other developments during this time. On Saturday, June 19, 1976, Colorado Governor Richard Lamm telegraphed Russell Train, administrator of the EPA, requesting permission to fly four thousand pounds (1,800 kilograms) of DDT from California to Colorado. The governor proposed that the insecticide would be used only to dust rodent burrows as a plague-control measure. The request was approved, but the transaction helped to focus national attention on wild-animal plague in Colorado.

By early July, the seeds from the national publicity about Colorado's plague problem were beginning to sprout, although, in terms of human plague, the problem was relatively small. The Colorado Environmental Health Service (EHS) and the Denver Chamber of Commerce reported hundreds of long-distance telephone calls from potential tourists worried about plague. One caller asked Dr. J. Douglas McCluskie, director of the EHS, if the roadblocks had been taken down. It was a difficult question to answer in a word, since there had never been any roadblocks. Other callers asked if plague had spread throughout the city of Denver. It was evident that—even in the last quarter of the twentieth century—plague retained its power to elicit rumor and fear.

There were also three more human cases in July, only one

of them in Colorado. Two of the victims were boys, one sixteen and the other five. The older boy lived in Apache County, Arizona, near the New Mexico border. The other boy lived in Albuquerque but was infected while visiting relatives in Harding County, New Mexico, in the northeast corner of the state not far from the Texas border. Human plague had never before been reported in Harding County. Like the first three cases of 1976, this boy developed the pneumonic form of the disease. He became ill on Thursday, July 10, and was hospitalized the following Monday. Both he and the boy in Arizona ultimately made complete recoveries. The third case of July 1979 was five-days-old, apparently the youngest plague patient ever studied in the U.S.[4] The child lived near Montrose, Colorado, where a plague epizootic was in progress in rodents near the child's home. She had primary septicemic plague, possibly related to a "bug bite" on her right knee, but she was well treated and recovered uneventfully.

On Wednesday, August 4, the Egyptian consul in San Francisco notified the New Mexico authorities that residents of the state could not enter Egypt unless they had been vaccinated against plague. This, besides being silly, was contrary to International Health Regulations, which do not require vaccination against plague under any circumstances. U.S. officials clarified the situation and the Egyptian order was withdrawn. The Egyptians at least knew where the action was. They did not call Colorado.

A week after the notice from the Egyptian consul, New Mexico had its seventh case of 1976—a two-year-old boy living in Las Vegas, sixty-four miles east of Santa Fe on the other side of the Sangre de Cristo Mountains. Probably infected by fleas on the family's pets, he was soon well again.

On Thursday, August 12, fifteen-year-old Jason Roybal, a junior at Albuquerque's Del Norte High School, was on an outing with his family on the crest of Sandia Mountain, which dominates the northeastern skyline of the city. Sandia Crest is a popular launching point for hang gliders, and Jason and his family, along with some fifty other persons, sat on the rocks and watched the frail craft as they swooped toward the plains below. Chipmunks were everywhere, dining happily on the scraps left by careless picnickers and shamelessly soliciting the watching crowd for more.

By Sunday Jason had a high fever. His father is a retired naval officer and, on Monday morning, Jason was taken to the emergency room of Kirtland Air Force Base Hospital in Albuquerque. A throat culture was taken, and the boy was sent home with instructions to take aspirin and cooling rubs for his fever.

On Wednesday morning Jason was listless, nauseated, and complained of pain, like that of a pulled muscle, in his left groin. Later that day, he was admitted to the base hospital and treated with oral penicillin for a streptococcal sore throat because of the results of the earlier culture. His blood pressure, pulse, and respiration were normal, and there was no sign of lung infection. He did have several severely painful and enlarged lymph nodes in his left groin. Tragically, these classical stigmata of plague were ignored. Had material from them been examined at this time the outcome might have been different.

Wednesday night Jason's condition steadily deteriorated, but the decline apparently went unnoticed. On Thursday morning Jason had pneumonia in both lungs, and his blood pressure had fallen sharply (to 80/50). Samples were now taken from the inflamed nodes in his groin—the fluid in the sample swarmed with gram-negative, bipolar staining rods. The possibility of plague occurred to someone and streptomycin treatment was begun. It was too late. At 11:30 that morning, a week after the outing on Sandia Crest, Jason Roybal died of pneumonic plague. On autopsy he had, among other things, external hemorrhages on his heart and acute pneumonia.[5] For over twenty years there had been only occasional plague cases in the vicinity of Albuquerque. Then there were six cases in twenty-two months.

The last plague victim of 1976 was a fifty-nine-year-old woman in Velarde, New Mexico, thirty-four miles north of Santa Fe. She had an atypically mild case of the disease and spent only a few days in the hospital.

There were two other events of 1976 with bearing on plague.

On Wednesday, September 17, the army announced that it intended to use anticoagulants to poison Beechey ground squirrels in the vicinity of Fort Ord, California, to reduce the danger of plague. The ground-squirrel population had risen an estimated tenfold in four years, in part because of the poisoning of coyotes that helped control the ground squirrel density.

The Humane Society protested the army's proposal. The army clearly had a point, but there is a question, based on what we know about plague ecology and the past history of squirrel control in California as an antiplague measure, of whether attention might more profitably be directed toward the field mice and deer mice in the area. A systemic insecticide that would kill the animal's fleas without harming the animal itself could be used. And fewer coyote killings might help to solve the ground squirrel problem in a less objectionable manner.

Then, on the last day of September 1976 the New Mexico Environmental Improvement Agency announced that rats were a serious problem in at least six New Mexico cities, including Albuquerque. Rat control in Albuquerque was to become a city responsibility since federal funds had run out. Considering the mounting plague problem in and around the city and the rising rat population, the loss of control funds is ominous.

Contrary to expectation, there were sixteen cases of human plague in the United States in 1976, making it the second worst year in half a century. Three of the cases were fatal; the case fatality rate was 19 percent, a bit less than one in five. There were nearly as many cases of human plague reported in 1975–76 as occurred in the Los Angeles epidemic of 1924–25. Fortunately, the incidence of pneumonic plague was far lower.

As mentioned before, the observed incidence of this highly communicable form of plague had been about one case per decade for fifty years. In the 1975–76 epidemic there were eight cases. No one knows the reason, but it is a disturbing trend. The fatality rate of pneumonic plague in the United States in this two-year period was 50 percent.

As in the preceding two years, the 1977 plague year got off

to an early start. In mid-February a thirty-eight-year-old man was exposed to the disease after skinning rabbits near the town of Craig, Colorado, in the northwest corner of the state. Originally diagnosed as tularemia, his disease progressed to pneumonic plague before it was correctly identified. The man made a satisfactory recovery in spite of the delayed recognition.

This early case, in the light of the events of 1975–76, raised the specter of another bad year for human plague in the United States. Fortunately, the effects of two years of widespread epizootics among the plague-bearing animals, coupled with the devastating drought that struck all the states (with the exception of Texas) that normally have enzootic plague, seemed likely to reduce the population of plague-infected animals and thus the risk of human contact. This hope was soon dashed.

The next victim, stricken in mid-June, was a three-year-old Navajo boy who lived near the Zuni reservation in the western part of New Mexico. He recovered, but only after surviving the serious complications of myocarditis and pericarditis (inflammation of the heart muscle and of the fibrous covering that encloses the heart), probably caused by the toxins of *Y. pestis.* Later in June a forty-three-year-old man living about twenty-five miles (forty kilometers) north of Santa Fe developed the disease but recovered uneventfully.

June's most spectacular case was that of a young wife and mother whose home was ten miles (sixteen kilometers) west of Flagstaff in Arizona's Coconino County. On Monday, June 13, this twenty-three-year-old woman very suddenly became ill. By Wednesday she had an extremely sore throat and a large, tender swelling on the right front side of her neck. She was hospitalized in Flagstaff, and cultures of her blood were started along with penicillin therapy. By the next day the swelling on her neck had become so large that it interfered with her breathing, and she had exploratory surgery to drain the expected "abscess." No abscess, but rather a single large decomposing (necrotic) lymph node was found. Other antibiotics were started, but none were relevant to her as yet undiagnosed ailment.

The day after surgery, X rays showed that both lungs were now involved with the disease. Pneumonic plague was suspected, and the young woman was treated with streptomycin, tetracycline, and steroids. On Friday her blood cultures and cultures from the lymph nodes in her neck were growing organisms identified by CDC, Fort Collins, as *Y. pestis*. The usual complications ensued. Her blood-clotting time became abnormally long, and both platelets and red blood cells began disappearing from her blood as the widespread hemorrhages under the skin, so typical of advanced plague, began to appear. But proper treatment had started in time and the woman's condition gradually stabilized. Although she recovered she required extensive plastic surgery to replace the massive amounts of tissue that had to be removed from her neck.

The young woman, her husband, and their six-year-old daughter had noticed, a week before the woman's illness, that their pet cat was uncoordinated, drooling, and coughing blood. Both adults peered into the cat's mouth in an attempt to find the cause of its illness. The sick cat disappeared the day before the young woman became ill; it was later found dead, and *Y. pestis* was isolated from its tissues.

In retrospect it is clear that the unfortunate woman acquired pharyngeal plague from her plague-stricken cat; this subsequently developed into pneumonic plague. Sixty-seven potentially exposed persons were given antibiotics and were watched carefully, but there were no more cases. The source of the cat's infection is not known.

In July there were five more cases, two in New Mexico, two in Oregon, and one in California. One New Mexico victim was a five-year-old boy, the other was a thirty-six-year-old man. Both received prompt and proper treatment and made good recoveries, although the older man had a severe illness and was still hospitalized six weeks after it began. One Oregon victim was a twenty-one-year-old man who lived near Klamath Falls not far from the California border. He also developed mild pneumonic plague but ultimately recovered, although he was originally treated for a streptococcal sore throat. The second Oregon case was a thirty-three-year-old woman living in the coastal community of Coos Bay. Her illness was originally diagnosed as Legionnaires' disease (it was secondary pneumonic plague), but she was treated with gentamycin and made a fortuitous recovery. There had been no previous evidence of plague along the Oregon coast. A three-year-old girl from San Diego, California, also contracted the disease in the Lake Tahoe region. Her case was fatal.

August brought three more cases. Late in the month, a Navajo woman in her middle forties was admitted to the Zuni Indian Health Service Hospital with an axillary bubo. She recovered, but the source of her infection remains, as usual, unknown. The case of a fifteen-year-old Navajo boy in Apache County, Arizona, was more straightforward. He had shot twenty-three prairie dogs and helped prepare them for cooking and eating. After a critical illness (his temperature once reached 106.2°F, or 41.5°C) he recovered.

The other August case remains an enigma. Dr. Joseph T. Cordell, a fifty-five-year-old veterinarian, had been working for several years at the Society for the Prevention of Cruelty to Animals clinic in the small town of Arroyo Seco between Monterey and Salinas, California. He worked very long hours and often, rather than returning to the house in which he had a room, he slept on a mattress on the floor of the clinic. On Friday, August 12, he became ill in his rooming house. His landlady was not home, and he was too sick to seek other help. On Sunday the owner of the house returned, and it was she who drove Dr. Cordell to the hospital in San Jose. He had pneumonia, pains in his chest, shaking chills, and fever. Physicians began intensive treatment but it was too late. He died the following Wednesday of massive pneumonic plague infection. He had either primary septicemic plague complicated by the pneumonic form of the disease, or else primary pneumonic plague.

All animals that died in the clinic were incinerated immediately so they could not be checked for plague. None of the living animals showed any suspicious symptoms. Arroyo Seco is on the southern boundary of Fort Ord, and, as we have seen, that area has had plague problems in the past. But an intensive search disclosed no infected animals within the military reservation, and no infected animals in the vicinity of Arroyo Seco.

Dr. Cordell lived a reclusive life with few close associates, and those associates were reluctant to shed any light on his activities in the few days before he died. At this point the events leading up to Dr. Cordell's death from pneumonic plague near the densely populated San Francisco peninsula remain shrouded in unwholesome mystery.

September brought four more cases, two in New Mexico, one in Arizona, and one in California, plus another suspected case in Arizona. None was fatal. One victim was an eight-year-old boy who lived in the uranium mining town of Grants, New Mexico. He was scratched and bitten on both arms by a plague-infected cat he was trying to retrieve from a tree. Ultimately, the boy had axillary buboes under both arms; the cat died.

The sixteen human plague cases in the United States by mid-October 1977 were followed by two more in November, a sixteen-year-old boy in Colorado and a thirty-six-year-old man in New Mexico, for a total in 1975–77 of fifty-four. Fortunately, the fatality rate in 1977 was very low, although five of the sixteen victims had pneumonic complications.

In 1978 there were twelve cases and two deaths from plague in the U.S., five cases in New Mexico, two each in Arizona and Colorado, and one each in California, Wyoming, and Nevada.

The U.S. had 18 cases and 5 deaths in 1980; 13 of these occurred in six counties of New Mexico between May and September. Asia reported 283 plague cases in 1980 with 29 deaths; Vietnam accounted for 180 of the cases and 5 of the deaths.

Plague in the United States was somewhat different. Even though 70 percent of the cases came from New Mexico, human cases occurred over an area of about two hundred thousand square miles, an area as large as France or Ohio, Pennsylvania, New York, New Jersey, Rhode Island, Connecticut, Massachusetts, Maine, Vermont, and New Hampshire combined.

By the end of the seventies more than 1,100 cases of plague

had occurred in the U.S. in this century. No further plague had appeared in Hawaii since 1949, but in the continental U.S. the disease continued to extend the area in which it was known to occur. Before 1927 there had been 32 plague cases diagnosed on arrival in the U.S. and only 1 after 1927 (the soldier who went from Vietnam to Dallas).

During the seventies all but 2 of 105 victims were infected in their state of residence. Overall mortality rates, for Indians and non-Indians alike, ran 14 percent. Rabbits were the most frequently known source of infection (it was not known at all in over half of the well-studied cases). Plague continued to be a serious infection in the elderly; 57 percent of the patients over sixty died.[6]

In New Mexico plague exists in animals in every one of the thirty-two counties, although five counties (McKinley, Bernalillo, Santa Fe, Rio Arriba, and Sandoval) contribute nearly three-fourths of the human cases. On a per-capita basis, the rates in Sandoval and Rio Arriba counties are ten times higher than in Bernalillo County, in which a third of the state's population resides. Plague is carried in New Mexico by fourteen species of fleas and twenty-eight species of mammals; nearly half the cases involved domestic dogs and cats as intermediate hosts, and 80 percent of the cases are contracted in the Upper Sonoran life zone (between 5,000 and 7,000 feet above sea level). The highest risk factors for contracting the disease were availability of food and nesting places in the immediate home environment.[7]

18

The Ralph Fulp
Story

On Wednesday afternoon, June 11, 1975, the softball team of
U.S. Electric Motors in Chino Valley, Arizona, played a double-
header at Willow Park field with two of the top teams of the
Coors Tournament League. The catcher for U.S. Motors was
Ralph Fulp, a tall, husky (six feet two inches, 198 pounds),
dark-haired young man who worked evening shift on the as-
sembly line and during the day studied engineering design at
Yavapai Community College in nearby Prescott.

Midway through the first game there were runners on second and third. In a double play Ralph Fulp reached for a ball
hurriedly thrown from third base, his cleats slipped in the
sand, and he felt a stabbing pain in his right groin. In spite of
the pain, he tagged the runner out and played the rest of that
game, which the U.S. Motors team won, and the next game,
which they didn't. Later, Ralph drove home to the double-
width trailer he shared with his friend John Zelitis, an engineer
with U.S. Motors.

After two years in the army, mostly in Germany, Ralph had
returned to Phoenix in December 1974. He was an enthusiastic outdoorsman. He loved horses and competed in rodeos as
a bull rider and calf roper. He found Phoenix swollen and

confining. Like most twenty-three-year-olds, he wanted a place of his own. After visiting Chino Valley for the summer rodeo and celebration called Frontier Days, he applied to U.S. Motors for a job and, to his surprise, was instantly hired. He was soon settled in the little town on Arizona's high northern plateau.

The day after the softball game, Ralph was much sicker. His temperature had risen, there was now a definite swelling in his right groin, he was nauseated, and he had a blinding headache. He suspected flu and possibly a hernia. Just the Monday before, he had helped a friend load old telephone poles into a trailer and then unload them at the site where they would become posts for a new corral. Ralph wondered if that very heavy lifting had led to a hernia.

Whatever it was, it was ill-timed.

Ralph was still in the standby Army Reserve. The previous April he had received a letter from Lt. Col. William Kelley in Saint Louis, Missouri, ordering him to report to Yakima Firing Center in Washington State for two weeks active duty beginning Saturday afternoon, June 14. Ralph was a fire control repairman, servicing the electronic and optical systems responsible for the accurate firing of heavy artillery. He had planned to leave Chino Valley for Phoenix that evening, Thursday, and then buy his airplane ticket to Washington the next day.

Ralph Fulp packed, sold his open Bronco (he hoped to buy a four-wheel drive pickup when he returned), and waited uncomfortably for the time to leave for Phoenix. It was late Thursday evening.

Ralph spent the two-hour drive lying across the front seat of his girl friend's old blue Valiant with his head in her lap. John Zelitis and his girl, Ann, were in back. In spite of the 80° temperature, Ralph was wrapped in a heavy sheepskin coat. Once he got out of the car and vomited into a ditch. The trip seemed endless.

They drove east along Arizona 69, past Big Bug Creek, and then south along the interstate highway, U.S. 17. The area around Chino Valley is more than five thousand feet above sea level in the piñon-juniper habitat typical of that altitude in the Southwest. Phoenix is four thousand feet lower, in a largely desert area.

They passed Deadman's Wash. At Horsethief Basin the first of the giant saguaro cactus begin to dot the ever more arid landscape. The desert is beautiful in early summer, but that night Ralph Fulp took scant interest in it.

At Biscuit Flats the blue Valiant left the interstate highway and turned east again. It was nearly midnight when Ralph got out at the concrete-block house on the corner of Delcoa and Thirty-second where his parents and sister live. He walked straight from the entrance hall through the living room and then turned right into the family room, where his father and mother were watching television. He was amazed to see that the mottled green carpet had waves in it like a Goofy Golf course and great holes. "Hey, Mom," he said, almost as a greeting. "What happened to the rug?" He described for her what he saw.

Carol Fulp is a registered nurse who works evenings on the fourth floor of John C. Lincoln Hospital in Phoenix. She looked inquiringly at her son. His face was chalk white. He stood hunched over because, she soon learned, of the pain in his groin. She told Ralph to lie down on the couch and she got a thermometer. His temperature was 105°F. He explained about the flu and the possible hernia. After examining the swelling in his groin, Carol Fulp had no idea what it was, but she did not think it was a hernia.

Ralph Fulp towers over his parents. Carol is a small, pretty woman with bouffant light-brown hair. Dan, her husband, is dark-haired and slender, but wiry. When they met, Carol was in the early years of nurse's training and Dan was in the Air Force. Later, because Dan was being transferred far away, Carol decided to drop out of training and marry him. They had three children: Ralph; then, two years later, Tim; and finally Brenda Sue, now fourteen, and a freshman at Shadow Mountain High School as our story begins.

The Fulps had returned to Phoenix when Dan left the Air Force. Carol had never lost interest in nursing, and she worked for six years in a doctor's office. Then, at the age of thirty-eight, she returned to nursing school, competing with girls half her age; she graduated two years later. Ralph had the same kind of determination. He would need it.

The next day was Friday the thirteenth. Carol called Maj. John Turner of the Army Reserve in Phoenix to explain why Ralph would be unable to report for duty. She went to work that afternoon as usual.

Of that Friday Ralph remembers very little. He could not get up, and he vomited several times. When his mother returned at 11:30 P.M., she examined his groin and took his temperature. The groin swelling was now the size of two golf balls; the inflamed area around it was as big as her hand. Ralph's temperature remained high.

Carol decided to consult a physician early Saturday morning. She knew Dr. James Favata from her work in the hospital. His office was next door to Lincoln Hospital, which was not far from the Paradise Valley section of Phoenix in which the Fulps live, and Carol Fulp respected him both as a physician and as a human being.

She spent the night trying, with aspirin and cold water rubs, to lower Ralph's temperature. It was no use. The next morning she called Dr. Favata but reached his answering service instead. However, just five minutes later, Dr. Favata called to explain that he was shaving and that he would meet her in his office in a few minutes.

James V. Favata, M.D., is a youthful-looking, dark, and intense person. Born and raised in Silver Creek, New York, he received his M.D. from the University of Illinois in 1961. Following internship and a three-year residency in internal medicine, he went into practice in Phoenix in the late summer of 1965.

Ralph Fulp was lucid and cooperative, but he was obviously an extremely sick young man. After careful examination, Dr. Favata called Lincoln Hospital and asked for a wheelchair. Shortly after, Ralph Fulp was ensconced in Room 423, where the admission laboratory tests were made and X rays were taken. Later, a needle was put into the antecubital vein of his inner elbow so that he could receive a steady infusion of ampicillin, a broad-spectrum synthetic derivative of penicillin.

Dr. Favata had explained that had Ralph been on the Navajo reservation, he would say he had plague. But that seemed improbable. Although plague is firmly established on Arizona's high northeastern plateau, it had never been confirmed below the Mogollon Rim, the escarpment that separates the northeastern plateau from the more heavily settled southern portion of the state that includes Phoenix and Tucson.

Ralph Fulp's first afternoon and evening in the John C. Lincoln Hospital passed quietly. The view from his room was of the nearby mountains and the towering rocks that jut from the residential areas of Phoenix. There was a steady stream of hospital staff who wanted to see what "Carol's kid" looked like; the stream included an encouraging number of pretty girls about his own age.

Sunday morning was quiet. To pass the time, Ralph telephoned his mother before his family went to church. She kept telling him to relax and take slow, deep breaths. He tried, but he was soon panting again.

Then, at 1:30 P.M. his father and sister visited; Carol was preparing for work and would be in later.

Dan Fulp noticed that his son's arms and ears were turning black and that Ralph was gasping for breath. He almost ran to the nurse's station. Muriel Lee, an R.N. and a next-door neighbor of the Fulps, was on duty. A moment later things began to happen. Nurses and aides appeared from everywhere. The "crash cart" was rolled into Ralph's room, and an oxygen mask was put over his face. Then the sides of his bed were put up, and he, bed and all, was taken quickly down the hall to the Coronary Care Unit (CCU).

The nurse pushing the bed was a small woman. She had trouble steering the bed and keeping the oxygen bottle in place. Ralph remembers kidding her about her driving. Except for isolated incidents, he remembers nothing more of the ensuing thirty days.

Ralph's mother stayed with him that first night in the unit. He remembers telling her of the monkeys he saw on the ceiling; later he thought he was in Dr. Favata's house. At some later point he saw his sister's face pressed against the glass wall of the isolation cubicle, her eyes streaming tears. He tried to wave, but then she vanished. Ralph recalled realizing that he was bound hand and foot with heavy leather straps. It made him furious. But he was wildly delirious at times, and he is a very strong young man. The usual canvas restraints were inadequate. By then, Ralph had an array of tubes and wires inserted or attached, and they had to be kept in place.

He also remembers trying to talk. He could not. There was a hole in his throat; that discovery frightened him.

At 5:00 A.M. Monday, after spending the night with her son in the CCU, Carol Fulp went to her mother's house to sleep. She was nearer the hospital there than at home. Before eight the telephone rang. It was a nurse from the unit. Dr. Favata needed permission for a surgeon to cut a hole in Ralph's throat (a tracheostomy) so that they could better force oxygen into his tissues. Carol agreed to the operation and then threw on her clothes and rushed to the hospital.

Afterward, Dr. Favata described Ralph's appearance on that Monday. "It was the most frightening thing you've ever seen in your life. He was black from the top of his head to the tip of his toes." As a nurse put it later, "Now I know why they call it the Black Death."

In the soft night illumination of the cubicle, Ralph's color had been less apparent. Now the room was ablaze with light, since the surgeon had just finished making the incision in his throat. Ralph's mottled blackness against the white bedding was dramatic. It was accentuated by blood splattered on the bedclothes, walls, and ceiling during the operation.

Ralph Fulp, for all his usual strength and vigor, was sliding rapidly down the slippery slope toward death. The maze of monitors told the story. His blood pressure was undetectable, yet his heart raced at 120 to 140 strokes a minute (nearly twice normal) striving to force blood through his flaccid arteries. The digital thermometer registering his temperature was off scale. And the eye recorded what the instruments did not: the ominous blackness of his skin.

James Favata turned his other patients over to his associates and spent Monday either at Ralph's bedside or reading in his office to try to find out what was wrong and how best to cope with it. The day before had been Father's Day. His family planned a big party, but the guest of honor never appeared. It was Wednesday before James Favata opened the presents from his wife and children.

The disease seemed to be plague, despite what the books said about its geographical limits. But it scarcely mattered. The problem now was to keep some tiny spark of life aglow within Ralph Fulp until the antibiotics could take effect against the infection, whatever it was. Dr. Favata ordered administration of fluids, drugs to raise Ralph's blood pressure, corticosteroids, the additional antibiotics tetracycline and gentamycin, and later streptomycin. Nothing helped. Ralph sank steadily.

Had his patient been elderly, James Favata could more easily have accepted it. Life ends for us all. But to lose a brawny young man at nearly the beginning of his adult life, and to an unknown malady, was almost unbearable.

At eleven that Monday morning, Dr. Favata had to admit he was beaten. He then had the distasteful duty of asking Ralph's parents for permission to do a postmortem examination when the end came. It could be in a few hours at the most; it might be minutes. He explained that he needed the autopsy to determine what the infection was that he had fought so hard against only, in the end, to lose. The Fulps gave permission, and Dr. Favata returned to his vigil in the CCU.

Dan and Carol Fulp and the Reverend David Burrows stood in the waiting room after Dr. Favata had returned to the unit. David Burrows is pastor of the American Baptist Church in the Paradise Valley suburb. Carol Fulp is a deaconess and her husband a trustee of the church. Religious faith permeates their family.

Tears ran down the cheeks of all three adults. Then Reverend Burrows suggested that they pray. Afterward, all of them, nearly at the same instant, felt a wave of confidence and peace surge around them. They feel that, at that moment, God put his hand under Ralph's sinking body, and it sank no more.

Ralph Fulp did not die on Monday. He swung in the limbo between the living and the dead that day—and the next. By Wednesday he had a detectable, although very low, blood pressure. By then, he also had total kidney failure. But Dr. Favata concluded that Ralph would probably live, and he went home to open his Father's Day presents.

James Favata was still concerned that Ralph Fulp's massive infection might do permanent damage to his heart, lungs, kidneys, or liver. Early in the first week of Ralph's hospitalization, cultures made from secretions in his throat and from the swelling in his groin grew rod-shaped, bipolar-staining organisms with the characteristics of *Y. pestis*. The final test was the injection of the cultured organisms into mice and guinea pigs. These unfortunate animals died with the typical buboes of plague, and plague bacilli were isolated from their bodies. The diagnosis of plague, which had become steadily firmer as the evidence mounted, was now unequivocal.

The diagnosis was certain; the source of infection was not. Personnel from the CDC at Fort Collins, Colorado, were joined by a team from the Arizona State Department of Health in an effort to establish where Ralph Fulp had contracted the disease. It was a herculean job.

The investigators sought signs of a rodent die-off. They found a lower-than-usual rodent population around Prescott and Chino Valley, but it was not certain that this was caused by an epizootic.

Ralph had no evident flea bites and no history of contact with wild rodents. He had, however, been around pet dogs and cats that might have passed a plague-struck flea to him.

Ralph had a chest X ray on admission to Lincoln Hospital on Saturday. There was no sign of pneumonia. The first hint of respiratory involvement was his panting over the telephone on Sunday morning; by early afternoon he was in severe distress. Dan Fulp's alertness may have saved his son's life.

X rays were taken twice daily for three days after Ralph was transferred to the CCU. They record the relentless bacterial invasion. First the left lung, then the right. Then the spread of the plague bacilli across both. It was a race between the proliferating bacteria and the antibiotic therapy. If the spread of the infection was not halted quickly, Ralph Fulp's life was forfeit. But, as we have seen, if too much of an agent like streptomycin was used (streptomycin kills bacteria rather than only stopping their growth), then Ralph might have died from a sudden flooding of his system by toxins from the mass of dead or dying *Y. pestis.*

The proper treatment of such massive infection needs a delicate touch and some measure of good fortune. By Thursday of his first week in the CCU, Ralph's blood pressure was stable without the aid of drugs, and the area of bacterial infiltration of both lungs was diminishing.

Ralph Fulp regained consciousness in mid-July. He was still in the CCU, although now in an open room. Since pneumonic plague is potentially the most infectious fatal disease known, Ralph was kept in strict isolation in a closed, glass-walled cubicle until his lung infection cleared. Everyone entering donned sterile green gowns, bootees, masks, and gloves. When they departed, the clothing was left inside. After the disease was identified as pneumonic plague, everyone who had been in close contact with Ralph, 105 persons in Lincoln Hospital, the 3 members of his family, his girl friend in Chino Valley, and John Zelitis and his girl friend, received antibiotics to suppress infection. No other cases occurred.

When Ralph was conscious he became aware of his hands and feet. His skin had mostly returned to its normal color, but "I looked at my hands and feet and they were black. They didn't move, and if I banged them against the side of the bed they felt like rock."

Dr. Favata explained to Ralph that he would lose parts of his hands and feet, but it was too soon to tell how much.

To go to sleep in the middle of one month and not wake up until the middle of the next is a shock. To realize that portions of your hands and feet have died in the meantime is even worse.

Ralph's family had followed the spreading blackness on his extremities and knew the outcome. They waited anxiously for the day when Ralph would regain consciousness and realize what he had lost or would lose.

Dan Fulp was with his son soon after Ralph left isolation. Ralph had been conscious only a little while, and he had not entirely mastered the art of speaking. To do so he first had to cover the opening in his throat before any sound would emerge. Even then, his speech was weak and uncertain.

His father knew Ralph was trying to speak and leaned forward attentively. He only half understood the whispered word. Perhaps he didn't wish to. The second time it was clearer.

"Bullets."

Dan Fulp recoiled in horror. He expected Ralph to be depressed. What he could not believe was that his sturdy, self-reliant son thought to take his own life. Still the word was clear. And Ralph was obviously annoyed at his father's seeming incomprehension.

Later, Dan Fulp learned that what Ralph wanted was a popsicle, a particular variety of which is called "Bullet," and described on the wrapper as a "quiescently frozen confection." Dan's faith in his son's character, so suddenly shaken, was justified.

When Ralph was conscious, he was also hungry. Dr. Favata was there when a nurse asked what he wanted for his first meal in a month. Ralph replied quickly, "A six-pack of Coors and a pizza."

The nurse said no. Beer was against regulations. Then Dr. Favata spoke up. "He's been through hell. Let him have it." James Favata could have been speaking for himself.

Ralph got his beer. He got his pizza, and it smelled wonderful. Oh, for the first bite, and a swallow of beer to wash it down! But it wasn't that simple. The flood of antibiotics that saved his life had also altered the microbiological flora of his body. During the worst of his illness, blood seeped from the membranes of Ralph's nose and mouth. One result was a bad oral infection with the yeast *Candida*. His mouth was much more raw than he realized, but the first bite of the fragrant, hot pizza made it clear. He could not eat any of it. And he drank only a little beer. But the Coors did not disappoint him.

The room in which Ralph regained consciousness was his fifth in Lincoln Hospital. He had spent seventeen days in the CCU, and then he was transferred to a two-bed room nearby. There, because the groin bubo caused him so much pain (although his conscious mind was blissfully unaware of it), the swelling was incised and drained. Then potentially infectious, he had to be isolated again. Finally, on July 15, he was moved to the two-bed room where he woke up. After two weeks there he was discharged. It was Tuesday, July 29. He had been in the hospital forty-four days.

Dan Fulp had built a carpet-covered ramp leading into the cream-colored house with green wood trim. It was a great day when Ralph was wheeled through the door that he had limped painfully out of more than six weeks before. But his troubles were far from over.

That Saturday morning in June when he left for Dr. Favata's office, Ralph weighed 198 pounds. Now he weighed 143. His skin hung on him in empty folds, as if borrowed from someone else.

No one knew how much of his hands and feet he would lose. The boundary dividing living flesh and dead was still obscure. At home, Ralph could recover strength to withstand anesthesia and surgery, and the rest would give his body time to choose which tissues it could revitalize and which reject. The surgery would be a formal, final recognition of what could live and what could not.

All the skin on Ralph's hands and feet was dead. There was a definite risk of infection starting in the moist and nutritious area beneath it. Such infection could quickly extend the region of fatally damaged tissue and lead to much more extensive amputation. In Ralph's weakened condition it could even be fatal.

His hands and feet were covered with sterile bandages, which Carol Fulp had to change twice a day. Evenings, when she arrived home from work about 11:30 P.M., she spent from one to three hours cutting or peeling away dead skin. It came off Ralph's heels in pieces half an inch thick, resembling in texture and pliability the leather of his saddle in Chino Valley.

The skin contained tiny bits of cactus as mementos of the times he had run barefoot on the prairie.

Finally, the dead skin was gone, but the new skin under it was exquisitely tender. In some places bone and nerve lay exposed. A faint breeze from someone passing caused Ralph painful spasms. The plantar nerves penetrate most of the skin and muscles in the feet and the joints of the toes. These were severely damaged by the infection. If Ralph's feet were touched in the wrong way, the pain was excruciating. Inevitably it happened, and whoever was responsible felt sick with remorse. So did Ralph.

He was totally helpless. He could not feed himself. Someone had to hold the urinal for him and clean him up when he used the bedpan. When he was no longer in isolation, his father or his younger brother, Tim, took care of him. Both were only spasmodically employed, and they spent many hours a day at the hospital. They continued to help when Ralph was home, but both had to work when work was to be had.

Carol Fulp had a similar problem. She left for the hospital before 3:00 P.M. five days a week. If her husband and younger son were working, no one could care for Ralph but her daughter. Brenda returned from school in time to fill most of the gap after Carol left and before Dan or Tim was available.

Brenda Sue was self-conscious about her own changing body. Now she faced the prospect of taking total care of an adult male. Ralph, as older brothers do, had always teased her, sometimes unmercifully. Brenda's introduction to home nursing was potentially thoroughly unpleasant.

Carol Fulp talked with both Ralph and Brenda. Ralph agreed to curb his sometimes boisterous tongue, and Brenda Sue was warned of the days when Ralph, racked himself with pain, discouragement, and fear of the future, would leave her in angry tears.

Everyone in the Fulp household remarks on Brenda's metamorphosis during the time she took care of Ralph. At the beginning she was a little girl, but by the end she had become a young woman. She did what was required in a cheerful and matter-of-fact way, although some of it was not much fun, and the pain her brother felt she felt deeply as well. Brenda Sue did more than minister to Ralph's physical needs. When he was depressed, she would tease him, hit him over the head with pillows, and generally harass him until, in self-defense, he had to feel better.

Ralph was at home all of August, gaining weight, trading old skin for new, and building strength for the next phase of his ordeal.

On Thursday, September 18, Ralph Fulp was readmitted to John C. Lincoln Hospital and given a battery of tests to establish whether he was fit for surgery and, if fit, how extensive the surgery would be. His second visit to Lincoln Hospital was not a pleasant occasion. Ralph was convinced that he would die on the operating table or shortly after leaving it. He was understandably frightened.

On Saturday morning he received preoperative medication in his room. Later, a drowsy Ralph Fulp was wheeled down the fourth-floor hall to the elevators that took him to the surgical level (second floor). Normally, Ralph would have been admitted to the surgical floor, but Dr. Favata had arranged with the surgeons to put him on the medical floor where Carol Fulp worked.

Ralph's stretcher was wheeled through the double doors of the surgical suite. It made a right turn, then a left, then turned left again into the largest operating room, number four. The anesthesiologist and the surgical nurses were waiting. After Ralph was securely fastened on the table, the anesthesiologist gave him an injection and then tilted the table so that Ralph had the feeling he was standing on his head. A few minutes later, the table was returned to horizontal, and the two surgeons and four surgical nurses gathered around it.

When the surgery was completed, Ralph was wheeled across the hall of the surgical suite to the recovery room. As soon as the anesthesiologist was satisfied that Ralph was regaining consciousness, the young man was returned to his fourth-floor room, his feet and hands swathed in bandages the size of boxing gloves. When he was fully conscious and somewhat rested, his mother told him what had happened in the operating room.

The first two joints of every finger on his right hand and the first joint of every finger on his left had been amputated. Amputated is perhaps not quite the right word. The blackened portions were snapped off like so many dead, dry sticks, which is what they had become. Some of the bone ends were still jagged, and there was not enough sound flesh left around them to permit sewing a flap of skin over the ends. Grafts would have to be made later. All Ralph's toes were gone, and parts of both feet. He had worn a size 12 shoe; he would now wear a 7.

When Carol Fulp told him about his lost fingers, Ralph replied, "Well, I had the use of them for twenty-three years." The bravado faded as the impact of his losses and their effect on his future became clearer.

For Ralph Fulp it was a time of mental and physical agony. The bandages on his hands and feet were changed frequently. Often the fluid-soaked gauze stuck to the open ends of his wounds. Then his left foot became infected, and the surgeon had to reopen it. Ralph is certain that on that day they heard him on all four floors of Lincoln Hospital. The wound was cauterized repeatedly before it finally healed.

A misunderstanding led Ralph to try to walk before his feet were really healed. When his legs dangled over the side of the bed, the blood rushed to his feet; they promptly swelled and began oozing. Ralph Fulp is a very tough young man. He walked in the stainless-steel walker when he was told to, but a nurse followed, sponging up his bloody tracks. The error was corrected when one of the surgeons saw Ralph in his walker and nearly had apoplexy.

It was a bad time. Ralph had always been active. He played high school football for four years, three of them as varsity defensive end and linebacker; he was proud of his supple strength. He competed in rodeos and loved to dance, play ball, and work on machines. Now he could neither stand nor walk unaided. He could not push a button to call a nurse or change a television channel. He rang a little bell instead, since he could grasp that with his thumbs.

He had no idea of how to earn a living or what to do for

recreation. Increasingly, he found himself thinking of himself as a cripple.

There were also financial problems. It would be months before he could earn money, if he ever could. Dan Fulp and Ralph's brother, Tim, both work in construction. Dan is an electrician, Tim a dry-wall installer. But, because of the recession in the housing industry, Dan Fulp had worked about one day in three for more than a year; Tim had done little better. Besides, Tim was now married and had his own responsibilities.

Carol Fulp had a steady job that she loved, but nurses are not well paid and she often had four persons to support. That left little for medical expenses. And Ralph's bills were as spectacular as his illness.

His total hospital room bill was $5,300. He owed nearly $2,800 for drugs and medications. The bill for laboratory tests was $3,000, $1,500 for dressings and supplies, more than $1,200 for oxygen therapy and physical therapy, $1,000 for miscellaneous items (such as thirty-seven blood and platelet transfusions and the recovery room), and about $650 for X rays. The total bill from John C. Lincoln Hospital would be nearly $16,000.

There were also substantial doctors' bills. Dr. Favata had done little in the first days of Ralph's illness but to concentrate on saving his young patient's life. He continued to see Ralph two or three times a day. A surgeon did the tracheostomy on Monday, June 16; he incised and drained the bubo later on. There were bills from an anesthesiologist and a hematology consultant. One surgeon had worked on Ralph's feet, and another on his hands. Both did all possible to give him something he could use. Dr. Favata's bill was modest, considering the time and effort he expended, and Ralph Fulp begrudged no one his fees. He was alive and equipped to face the future because of his doctors' skills. But their aggregate bill of over $3,800 was, on top of everything else, overwhelming.

Ralph had medical insurance through U.S. Electric Motors in Chino Valley that supposedly included a major medical supplement. Clearly it did not. The insurance paid less than half the hospital bill, under 6 percent of his total doctors' bills, and $45 a week for twenty-six weeks as a total disability payment. The company had presumably established its assembly plant in Chino Valley in the hope of paying low wages and modest benefits. These expectations were fulfilled.

As Ralph contemplated his physical and financial situation, the end of September neared. To him it seemed more like the end of the world.

Carol Fulp and her oldest son had always been close. They talked often of what lay ahead, and she knew how deeply discouraged he was.

One day Ralph had a visitor, a pharmacist about his own age from the hospital. The young man had not worked that day; he had been out playing tennis. When he walked into Room 426 he was still carrying his tennis racket—in a shiny steel hook where his right hand should have been.

The two young men chatted a while, then the pharmacist left, and Ralph Fulp lay back on his pillows to ponder. The visit had made a deep impression. The young man earned a good living and played tennis without a right hand. Ralph still had his right hand, a thumb, and stubs of fingers. He had more to work with there than his recent visitor. Ralph began to realize that he could base his approach to the future either on what he had lost or on what he could still do with what he had.

When Ralph had returned to Phoenix after his two years in the army, he had made the discovery—shared by many young veterans—that joining the American Legion was a good way to cut drinking expenses. Ralph soon found that there were other benefits as well.

Dan Erler, an official of Post 75, visited him in the hospital. The next thing Ralph knew there was to be a benefit steak fry for him at the Legion Hall.

Barry Jipner was an old friend. They had worked together at a local restaurant, Pinnacle Peak, before Ralph had gone into the army. When Ralph was first in the CCU, Barry Jipner sat on the floor in the hallway outside for most of two days waiting for news of his friend.

Barry is an electrician. He was asked by the manager of Pinnacle Peak to do some wiring for him. Barry agreed, on the condition that he be paid in steaks. His wages, in the form of thirteen-ounce steaks, were the main course of the Legion steak fry.

The big event was Saturday, October 4. Ralph was not due to leave the hospital for at least two weeks, but he asked Dr. Favata's permission to attend. To Ralph's surprise, he got it. The conditions were that Ralph behave himself and be in by midnight. Otherwise, James Favata warned, Ralph would surely turn into a pumpkin.

Dr. Favata also wrote an official prescription. It read: "For Ralph Fulp. ℞—Ralph may get a *little* drunk tonight (if he brings a note of approval from his mother). Signed: J. Favata."

To Ralph, after months of misery, it was a fabulous party. He saw friends he had not seen since high school, and, for the first time ever, he broke down and cried for sheer happiness. When he got back to the hospital, he was beaming from ear to ear. Paula Caretto, a pretty young nurse who had watched his struggle from its beginnings, later told him she wanted to kiss him because he looked so happy. Ralph wished she had told him sooner.

Ralph's second stay in Lincoln Hospital lasted twenty-nine days. When he left it this time, life was looking better. Dan Erler, of the Legion post, had done more than arrange the benefit. He also got in touch with John Richling, an official of the Disabled American Veterans (DAV). Later, after a series of interviews and tests, the DAV awarded Ralph a monthly allowance so that he might return to school.

Others pitched in. Nancy MacKay, Lincoln Hospital's social worker, contacted Virginia Kolnick of the State Vocational Rehabilitation Department. Usually, Ms. Kolnick visited patients only after they left the hospital, but Nancy MacKay, aware of Ralph's brittle morale, persuaded her to visit him while he was still in the hospital. Virginia Kolnick's efforts resulted in a five-year grant from the department for books and tuition. Ralph had decided to become an X ray technician, and then, after he was gainfully employed in that field, to take a degree in pharmacy.

When Ralph came home from his second hospital stay, he was still in a wheelchair, but he had crutches from the American Legion to use around the house. He went to the hospital every day for whirlpool baths and exercises to strengthen his muscles and prevent his joints from stiffening.

Determined to get well and strong quickly, Ralph walked a little farther each day to build up his strength. It took eight months before he really felt he was back to normal.

On Sunday morning, October 26, 1975, Carol Fulp wrote on her kitchen calendar, "Ralph made coffee. Tied own shoes." He had tied his own shoes for nearly twenty years before he was stricken with plague. But it is harder with only thumbs and stubs of fingers.

Four Sundays later there was a barbecue benefit dance for Ralph at the Wagon Wheel Restaurant near Prescott, arranged by Sheri Tobin and two of her friends, Leona Parkinson and Chris Arntsen. Sheri teaches school in Phoenix but returns home to Prescott on weekends. She knew Ralph well; they danced together at the popular Prescott nightclub called Matt's, and she was determined to do something to help.

The entire Fulp family was present. Ralph was supposed to stay in his wheelchair for only a few hours at a time, but he remained at the Wagon Wheel from the beginning of that party to the end more than thirteen hours later.

Sponsored by the Sacred Heart Catholic Church to ensure tax-exempt status, the event was announced on billboards, posters, and radio stations all over the northern part of the state. All the food, including a steer for barbecuing and an expert to prepare it, the beer, ice cream, flowers, liquor, and advertising were donated by merchants visited by the persuasive Sheri Tobin and her friends. A Shetland pony was donated for auction, as was Indian jewelry and much more. Sheri and her friends had also persuaded half a dozen country-western bands and singers to donate their time—and pay their own expenses—to come to Prescott for the benefit.

The party was an experience that no one who attended it

would ever forget. It became a frenetic competition to see who could imagine yet another way to raise money. When the first auction ended, the new owners of the merchandise auctioned it again. The second buyers did the same. One young man auctioned half his moustache. Ralph's friend Barry Jipner is a good-looking young man with an expensively styled haircut. He auctioned his hair. It brought $200, and Barry was shaved bald right on the stage. Another young fellow did the same. The waitresses donated their tips. For the waitresses, whose earnings that day were a substantial fraction of what they might be in an ordinary week, it was a moving act of charity.

When Ralph left the Wagon Wheel, it was early in the morning of his twenty-fourth birthday. He had just attended the most memorable birthday party of his life. He was euphoric. As he said later, "I wasn't drunk. I was high on people. On all those who have given so much of themselves for me." The benefit at the Wagon Wheel raised $5,381.40.

Back in Phoenix, Nancy MacKay was busy as well. She prepared a detailed analysis of the financial position of Ralph and his family. Then she went before the governing board of John C. Lincoln Hospital. After hearing her presentation, the board voted to reduce Ralph's bill by $6,421.50.

In late December, Lincoln Hospital had its annual Christmas party. Sandy Labriola, a licensed practical nurse at Lincoln, invited Ralph to be her date for the dance. He gladly accepted. He was stronger now and walked without crutches. That night he danced; it was something he thought he might never do again. It was hard, painful, and the performance lacked the polish his dancing had before, but he loved every minute.

Meanwhile, the search for the source of his infection went on. It was October before blood samples from two coyotes in Yavapai County (which includes both Prescott and Chino Valley) revealed that the animals had had substantial exposure to *Y. pestis*. Two more coyotes with high levels of antibody to the plague bacillus were taken in the same area the next month. Also in October, a coyote with an even higher level of antibody was found in Mojave County, on Arizona's border with Nevada and Utah. It was clear that plague was no longer confined above the Mogollon Rim.

In January 1976 Ralph Fulp began going to Glendale Community College in Phoenix. He now drives himself to school in the four-wheel-drive pickup he waited so long to get. Ralph recalls the day, not long after the amputations, when Dr. Favata came into his room with a wide grin on his face. He told Ralph that it was going to be all right: Ralph would be able to drive. James Favata had driven with just his thumbs on the way from his home to his office, and it worked fine. So it does for Ralph also. We drove around northern Arizona together in his truck. He handled it expertly, and, simultaneously, a can of beer as well. I had to worry only about my own beer.

Fortunately, Ralph still has both thumbs, although the loss of skin on them was so extensive that he no longer has any thumbprints; the new skin is completely smooth and shiny.

The story is not over yet. On Thursday, August 12, 1976, Ralph again lay unconscious under the glare of the operating-room lights while surgeons worked on his right hand and foot. The jagged bone ends of his fingers were ground off smooth, and padding and skin flaps laid over them to give smoother and more comfortable fingertips. His left foot was opened to correct a new problem. In the original surgery one of the bones of the left great toe was allowed to remain in place. Now it had worked down to the bottom of Ralph's foot; walking on it had become an agony. The bone piece was removed. Unfortunately, infection developed along the incision line, and for a time Ralph had an ulcer there the size of a half-dollar and half an inch deep. Even with the special $180 shoes he requires, walking is painful.

But Ralph refuses to remain an invalid. On the second day of deer season that fall he clumped laboriously up Domingues Mountain, near Chino Valley, where this story began, and killed a deer three hundred yards away with a single shot through the head.

By midsummer 1977 Ralph was still having periodic bouts of severe swelling on his right thigh and groin. His hands and feet, however, had nearly recovered from the surgery of the preceding summer, though he could still not walk barefoot on a hard surface. Ten years after his ordeal began he still can't. His feet easily become red and raw during hot weather when he perspires, but his spirit is undampened. He limps a bit more when his feet are in that condition, but he doesn't complain. His principal complaint comes when he has to buy a new pair of shoes, since their present cost is $400 a pair. In the spring of 1984 he had just gone in debt to buy a dump truck and is working in construction and doing some welding on the side. He is married and the father of a little girl who will be three years old in May of 1985. This is Dan and Carol's first grandchild and they are enjoying her.

Ralph's sister, Brenda, was married in September 1983 and is tutoring hearing-impaired children at the high school from which she graduated. She planned to begin graduate work in summer, 1984.

James Favata, M.D., worked in Saudi Arabia as a medical administrator for two years after a heart attack made it impossible to continue private practice. He has recently returned to the Arizona State University clinic in Tucson.

Ralph had learned much in the course of his adventure. He now knows about a disease he thought no longer existed, although he still doesn't know exactly how he got it or why it was so virulent. He knows something more of pain, despair, courage, love, and friendship. He knows that people, even in this age of indifference, will still extend a helping hand.

He occasionally plays the role for others that the young pharmacist played for him. When Carol Fulp finds patients deeply depressed by their lost ability to lead the life they once led, she sometimes asks Ralph to stop and talk with them. It often seems to help. And it helps Ralph Fulp feel that his own ordeal was not completely without meaning.

19

Plague Around the World: 1980–84

Concerning plague in the U.S. at least, 1980 was the Year of the Cat, despite what the Chinese calendar said. Prior to that time only eight cases of plague in domestic cats had been reported to the Centers for Disease Control in the nearly forty years of its existence. In 1980, in New Mexico alone there were another five cases of feline plague, in addition to two others elsewhere.[1]

Some of the earlier cases of cat-borne plague we have discussed before. One was the boy near Grants, New Mexico, in 1977 who was scratched by a cat he was trying to recover from a tree. The boy's disease was diagnosed as a viral syndrome and treated with erythromycin, which has no antiviral activity. Both the cat and the boy had plague. The boy was finally adequately treated and recovered; the cat wasn't and didn't. The boy's grandfather, from whom he had acquired the cat, periodically shot rabbits around his home and fed them to his twenty to thirty cats and four dogs. The infected cat had last eaten wild rabbit six days before the boy became ill.

Another case was that of the twenty-three-year-old Arizona woman who acquired pharyngeal plague from a sick cat. Her infection subsequently developed into secondary pneumonic plague.

On Christmas Day, 1978, a seventy-six-year-old woman living near Reno, Nevada, became ill and subsequently died of secondary pneumonic plague most probably acquired from one of six free-roaming cats she fed (in addition to the two she had in her house). One of the free-roaming cats was found dead at her home of pneumonia, but the presence of Y. pestis in the cat could not be demonstrated.

The first cat-associated case in the U.S. was in a thirty-eight-year-old California veterinarian who contracted the disease in 1936 from a cat he treated for an abscess under its jaw. The cat subsequently died, the veterinarian recovered.

Of the five New Mexico cats found to be plague-infected in 1980, three were found in rural areas near Albuquerque, and two others (littermates) lived in a rural area near Santa Fe. Only one of the cats was successfully treated, the others died or were killed. Only the two kittens from near Santa Fe may have caused human cases since their six-year-old owner and her sixteen-year-old aunt also had the disease.

The sixteen-year-old left New Mexico by car for Nebraska on August 15th. Three days later she was seen by a doctor in Columbus, Nebraska, because of lethargy, and a small, tender right inguinal lymph node. Naturally he prescribed penicillin and naturally she got worse. She developed a fever with nausea and vomiting and was hospitalized and given a penicillin derivative intravenously. Despite the treatment she improved and was discharged from the hospital a week after she had left New Mexico. That day it was confirmed that her niece in New Mexico had plague. By then the older girl was on her way to Oklahoma, but she was intercepted by the Nebraska State Police, escorted back to the hospital, isolated, her bubo aspirated, and proper treatment begun. The bubo still contained Y. pestis.

This was the ninth case of "traveler's plague" in the period 1950–80. The overall fatality rate for plague-infected travelers was 33 percent, versus 18 percent for nontravelers.[2]

In the decade 1970–80 there were thirty-eight plague cases

in children sixteen and under in New Mexico; this age group accounted for 55 percent of all cases of the disease from 1950 to 1970.[3] The incidence of plague in these children was half again as high in Indian children as in Hispanics, and twice as high as among non-Hispanic children. The overall case-fatality rate was the same for all groups. In three of these thirty-eight children none of the cultures (either bubo aspirates, blood, or both) grew *Y. pestis*. These cases were confirmed by the presence of plague antibodies in the blood following the illness.

Only a minority of the children (8 percent) were initially suspected of having plague, even at the time of hospitalization, although 82 percent had the bubonic form of the disease and all had typical buboes at the time they entered the hospital. For the 18 percent that had septicemic plague the fatality rate was nearly three out of four. Of the septicemic cases 57 percent went on to develop the pneumonic form of the disease, a ten times higher incidence than in the victims of uncomplicated bubonic plague. All the septicemic cases that developed plague pneumonia died, as did one who developed plague meningitis.

The average time from onset of illness to death was slightly more than four days. Of the six fatal cases, four *never* received an effective antibiotic; the two others got adequate treatment *only* on the day of death. In all these patients there was an average delay of nearly four days from onset of illness until an effective antibiotic was prescribed although the patients sought medical attention on average one and a half days after their illness began.

These horrifying results—in a state that has accounted for more than half the human plague in the United States over the past thirty years—suggest that a tremendous amount of missionary work remains to be done among New Mexico physicians (as well as those elsewhere in the country) to raise their index of suspicion that plague may be involved when someone in, or recently from, a western state appears with a fever of unknown origin, particularly if accompanied by an enlarged, tender lymph node. Mistaken diagnosis, and its inevitable corollary, inadequate treatment, leads to the needless loss of young lives every year.

In addition to these 1980 cases in New Mexico, a forty-seven-year-old woman in Tahoe Paradise, California, died of primary pneumonic plague acquired from her pet cat. Primary pneumonic plague is that transmitted directly from a sick animal or human rather than secondarily as a complication of bubonic or septicemic plague. It was the first case of human primary pneumonic plague since the Los Angeles epidemic of 1924–25. The woman became ill on October 2 and died two days later. She was given tetracycline to take at home every six hours for a presumed urinary infection since her urine contained both pus and bacteria although she also complained of chest pains. Unfortunately, she took only half the prescribed doses over the next two days. She died four and a half hours after admission to the hospital. It was not until four days after her death that the hospital laboratory succeeded in culturing *Y. pestis.* The woman's cat had brought home a dead chipmunk eight days before the woman became ill. The cat died and was buried on September 29; it was later shown to have bilateral pneumonic plague.

The victim had a sixteen-year-old daughter living at home who slept with the sick cat on her chest, and her mother had run a twenty-four-hour day care center at South Lake Tahoe for about 150 children. She had potentially exposed 197 people to pneumonic plague; fortunately there were no secondary cases. Like 11 of the 18 California plague cases of the 1970–80 period, the woman acquired her disease in her home.[4]

Cat-associated plague continued in the following year. Dr. Robert Winters, a forty-nine-year-old veterinarian in Evergreen, Colorado, acquired the disease in March of 1981 after a cat he was treating bit him between the thumb and forefinger. The cat and the veterinarian survived, and the cat was shown to have a high level of plague antibodies. When an acquaintance learned that Winter had plague he remarked, "Gee, that's a Middle Ages disease, isn't it? Did they treat you with leeches?"[5] This from the resident of a state that routinely produces some 7 percent of human plague in America! Not that this level of ignorance is unusual. Most residents of the western states are blissfully ignorant of the presence of the disease and hence are more susceptible to accidental infection.

In March 1981 a house cat living near Cloudcroft, New Mexico, ate plague-infected rodents near its home in James Canyon and acquired the disease but was promptly and adequately treated and recovered.

The first U.S. plague case of 1981 was in a twenty-five-year-old rancher who lived in Otero County, New Mexico, about five miles from the Texas border. He had cut his left hand and then skinned a dead bobcat. The subsequent orange-sized bubo in his left armpit was aspirated and reported by the laboratory to contain gram-positive cocci. He was naturally treated for a staphlococcal or streptococcal infection. The laboratory was in error. The young man died six hours after admission to the hospital. He had been ill two days. He was not isolated while in the hospital and no isolation procedures were used in handling body fluids. Permission for an autopsy was denied, and the body was released to a mortician.

This was potentially a very dangerous situation for the mortician and his staff (as it had been for the hospital staff before the young man's death). When someone dies of plague an autopsy is mandatory. The person performing the autopsy and his or her assistant are supposed to wear surgical scrub suits, gowns, shoe covers, caps, double surgical masks, and double gloves. After autopsy the body is wiped with antibacterial solution, put into double body bags, and promptly cremated or buried without embalming, and those involved in the autopsy are given prophylactic tetracycline.[6]

When the presence of *Y. pestis* was recognized (with some difficulty) an autopsy was performed.

New Mexico had thirteen cases of plague in 1980 (one fatal), and two of the thirteen (the second and third cases of 1980) occurred in the village of Cuba, the population of which is only 1,500. As Ted Brown of the State's Environmental Improvement Division pointed out, "Most of the time in New Mexico a person is infected within a quarter mile of their home if not inside it."[7] Early the following year the citizens of Cuba banded together to clean out the trash they had been dumping for years in the arroyos leading to the Rio Puerco that provided good rodent harborage. The second case in Cuba was in a twenty-eight-year-old man who died of pneumonic plague in June. Forty-three contacts were given prophylactic treatment. The two Cuba human cases followed a prairie dog epizootic in the vicinity.

Elsewhere in the U.S. in 1980 there were five additional cases, four of which were fatal.

There were thirteen plague cases and four deaths in the U.S. in 1981. This total would have brought shrieks of horror from the public health establishment prior to 1964 when the average for forty years had been one case a year but, with an average of nearly fourteen cases a year since 1975, the 1981 total brought only yawns.

New Mexico had six cases (three fatal); Arizona, four; California, Colorado, and Oregon had one case each. The Oregon case was fatal. Five of the U.S. cases were simple bubonic plague, five were septicemic, and two were secondary pneumonic plague. From 1970 to 1981 there were plague epizootics in twelve western states: Arizona, California, Colorado, Idaho, Montana, Nevada, New Mexico, Oregon, Texas, Utah, Washington, and Wyoming. These led to 136 human cases in eight states of which 19 were pneumonic plague. Texas, Washington, Idaho, and Montana had no human cases.

The other fatal case in New Mexico in 1981 was that of a twenty-five-year-old Navajo woman who died of pneumonic plague in late July. At this point the fatality rate from pneumonic plague in New Mexico was 75 percent.

The fifth and sixth cases of plague in New Mexico were in a forty-six-year-old woman and a twenty-two-year-old man who were close neighbors in Las Huertas Canyon on the northwest side of Sandia Peak near Albuquerque. A very high incidence of rodents with plague-infected fleas was found near the Las Huertas Picnic Area.

Arizona health authorities examined twenty-seven coyotes in the area of Mormon Lake southeast of Flagstaff in the summer of 1981. Of the twenty-seven, twenty-one had antibodies to plague.

Plague also made the news in the U.S. briefly after a plague-infected wood rat was found less than a mile from President Reagan's Rancho del Cielo in the Santa Ynez Mountains some twenty miles from Santa Barbara in July 1981.

In New Mexico the state Department of Health and Environment further clarified the ecology of plague in the Land of Enchantment in the June issue of the *Communicable Disease Summary*. Animals involved in plague were divided into maintenance hosts, amplifier hosts, and accidental hosts. Those in the first category are relatively resistant to plague and include deer mice, white-footed mice, brush mice, piñon mice, voles, and kangaroo and wood rats. The second group, whose role is that of enhancing the amount of *Y. pestis* in circulation through their susceptibility to the disease, includes chipmunks, squirrels, and prairie dogs. Accidental hosts are dogs, cats, coyotes, raccoons, badgers, bobcats, and, of course, humans. The latter have no role in the ecology of plague, at least until such time as there is another epidemic of primary pneumonic plague in the U.S.

Other countries in the Americas reporting plague in 1981 were Bolivia, Brazil, Ecuador, and Peru, for a total of 128 cases and 12 deaths. The world total of 194 cases and 24 deaths was the lowest number ever reported to the WHO. The People's Republic of China had 8 cases and 6 deaths from plague in 1979, 30 cases and 20 deaths in 1980, and one nonfatal case in 1981.

Plague had been increasingly more frequent in Oregon in the 1970s with the disease reported in six (Willowa, Umatilla, Klamath, Coos, and Lake) of the state's thirty-six counties. This led to a more careful examination of the ecology of the disease in that area. The disease was found in nine species of Oregon animals (hares, three species of squirrels, marmots, and four species of mice), and the disease is enzootic in the southeastern half of the state. The yellow pine chipmunk (*Eutamias amoenus*) and the golden-mantled ground squirrel (*Spermophilus lateralis*) were plague-positive in popular recreational areas such as Crater Lake National Park. Somewhat more than 10 percent of the coyotes whose blood was sampled had been exposed to plague, but there was not a good correlation between the distribution of human and coyote plague in Oregon.[8]

A milestone in the history of U.S. plague was achieved in February 1982 when a man contracted fatal plague while hunting rabbits near Odessa in west Texas. For some reason the fatality rate of rabbit-related plague cases is nearly three times as high as for other sources of the disease. Most important, this was the first case of indigenous plague in the Lone Star State since the 1920s.

New Mexico's first case of plague in 1982 didn't occur until mid-May. The victim was a twenty-year-old woman from McKinley County whose disease was promptly recognized and properly treated at the Gallup Indian Medical Center.

The second victim from the same area was not so fortunate. In mid-July an eleven-year-old Indian boy from near Thoreau, New Mexico, died of the disease in a Gallup hospital.

Meanwhile a sixty-five-year-old woman in San Juan County had also contracted the disease in May but made a good recovery.

Jose Facundo Trujillo was not so fortunate. Trujillo, forty-two, lived alone in Vallecitos, about fifty miles north of Española. He arrived at the emergency room of the Española hospital at 11:50 P.M. on Monday, July 12, and died seventy minutes later from pneumonic plague. He had become ill the preceding Saturday. Twenty contacts were given prophylactic treatment. Just a few days earlier an eleven-year-old Navajo boy acquired plague from either a ground squirrel or a prairie dog; his case was also fatal.

A twenty-year-old Navajo woman from McKinley County was the next victim. She made a good recovery but the source of her infection was never found. About a week later a twenty-nine-year-old Santa Fe man acquired plague from a ground squirrel.

A nine-year-old boy from Nambe Pueblo was the seventh plague case of 1982 in New Mexico; he became ill in early August but recovered. Another case occurred in Santa Fe a week later in a fifteen-year-old boy.

The ninth, and final, case of 1982 in the Land of Enchantment was a man from near Raton who had bubonic plague in early October and recovered. He had killed eight squirrels in late September about twenty-seven miles west of Raton. An investigation located a plague-infected tassel-eared squirrel in the man's freezer (it was only the second time that plague was found in this species in New Mexico, and the first time that human plague had occurred in Colfax County). It is also noteworthy that the man was an employee of the New Mexico Game and Fish Department and that the tassel-eared squirrel is a protected species.

Investigations of wild rodent plague in New Mexico also revealed a rock squirrel dead of plague in the laundry room of a home in southeast Santa Fe and three epizootics in the vicinity of Albuquerque. The first was in prairie dogs on the east slope of Sandia Mountain in April, followed by an almost contiguous epizootic in rock squirrels the following month. A second rock squirrel epizootic in August occurred in the western Sandia foothills inside the Albuquerque city limits. In connection with these three epizootics control measures were taken in the environs of 201 residences.

Arizona had four cases of human plague in 1982, three of them in Navajos, and widely separated in time. The cases occurred in May, July, August, and December. Two of the victims were male and two were female. All recovered. Wild carnivore samples revealed recent exposure of these animals to plague in Graham County, Arizona, where the disease had never before been found. Graham County is northeast of Tucson.

A ten-year-old girl living southwest of the town of Warm Springs, on the Warm Springs Indian Reservation in north-central Oregon, intervened in a fight between two male cats in August and was superficially scratched on both arms for her trouble, and also received a puncture wound near her left nipple. Some days later she was ill, feverish, and had a lump in her left armpit. On August 16, 1982, she was admitted to the hospital and given penicillin. Two days later gram-negative bacilli suspected of being *Y. pestis* were cultured from her blood. She was promptly isolated and appropriate therapy begun. She was discharged from the hospital on August 23, but it was nearly a month before the bubo in her armpit had completely disappeared.

The family had five cats, four of which had current or recent plague exposure (two of the cats became ill the day after the girl). The male cat that had scratched her refused to present himself for testing but remained well. This case was unusual in that the disease had been acquired from the scratch of an apparently healthy cat. It was also noteworthy that it was the eleventh case of plague reported from Oregon since the initial case of 1934. Ten of the eleven cases have occurred since 1970; four of these cases were fatal, or 40 percent.[9]

Colorado had two plague cases in 1982, a seven-year-old male in late July, and a girl the same age in early August. Both cases were probably acquired in the same area where Huerfano and Las Animas counties meet near the town of Walsenberg in the southern part of the state. The girl had cared for a sick rock squirrel before it died.

A fourteen-year-old boy acquired bubonic plague in late July from a flea bite in Utah County, Utah, south of Salt Lake City. The boy recovered and no further investigation was made.

Wyoming had its second case of human plague when a twenty-two-year-old woman, a veterinary assistant, became ill on June 22, 1982. She developed pneumonic plague which was, a week after she became ill and five days after her hospitalization, adequately treated. She eventually recovered. The source of her illness was traced to an eight-year-old male cat, Jiggs, who was treated at the veterinary clinic on the morning of June 16. On June 17 Jiggs's condition worsened. The veterinary assistant was peering into the animal's throat when it coughed directly into her face. Jiggs died that night. The cat had been catching thirteen-lined ground squirrels near his home; 198 abandoned squirrel burrows near Jiggs's home suggested decimation by a plague epizootic.

Seven of the nineteen plague cases of 1982 were traced to squirrels, three to cats and two to rabbits, and seven were unknown. One of the cases involved either a squirrel or a prairie dog. Eleven of the victims had a flea bite, six had direct contact with an infected animal, and two cases were of unknown route of exposure.

Worldwide, the incidence of plague rose sharply after the unusual low of the preceding year. WHO recorded 713 cases and 36 deaths, up from 194 cases and 24 deaths the preceding year. Plague on the border between Uganda and Zaire claimed 153 victims (three fatalities); there were thirty-six cases and three deaths in Tanzania, the same number of cases but nineteen deaths in Madagascar, and nineteen cases and one death in South Africa. Brazil had 151 cases but only one death. The disease was also reported from Peru, Bolivia, Burma, and Vietnam.

There were no early cases in 1983 to herald the arrival of the worst year for human plague in America since the Los Angeles epidemic of 1924–25. The first three cases, all Indian males between the ages of nineteen and thirty-nine, occurred in April; all were bubonic; two occurred in New Mexico's McKinley County and one in Arizona (Coconino County). May brought five more cases, three males and two females; three were Indians, and four of the five cases occurred in Arizona (three in Coconino and one in Apache County). The New Mexico case was in Grant County. The Apache County case was an eighteen-year-old male who died of pneumonic plague on June 11. A fifty-six-year-old man died of bubonic plague in late May in Coconino County.

June was appalling. In the first two weeks eight additional cases were reported; two were fatal. Both were young males, nine and five years old. The older boy lived in Klamath County, Oregon, the younger in Apache County, Arizona. New Mexico had four June cases, Arizona, two, Oregon, one, and Utah, one. The Utah case was in Tooele County.

At this point, 25 percent of the cases had been fatal, 13 percent had been pneumonic, and 13 percent septicemic. Two of the cases had come from areas where human plague had never before occurred, one in southwestern New Mexico (San Miguel County) and one near Lake Powell in Arizona. There was animal plague in Arizona, New Mexico, Nevada, Utah,

California, Oregon, Wyoming (with a severe epizootic among ground squirrels in and near Cheyenne), Washington, and western Texas.

By the end of June, New Mexico had four more cases. Two were from the environs of Santa Fe (a woman fifty-eight and a man sixty-one), another was a forty-five-year-old Navajo woman from the Church Rock area who had pneumonic plague. Meanwhile, the pet cat of a Los Alamos family was confirmed as having the disease. It was the third cat case of 1983 and the fifteenth since 1977.

On Wednesday July 27 Bill Huey, fifty-eight, became ill at his home in Tesuque, New Mexico. He had a high temperature (101°F, about 39°C). He slept fitfully the next night, owing to chills and fever, and the next day he saw Dr. Paul Kovnat. Bill Huey was sent home with an antibiotic and aspirin to keep his temperature down. Mary Huey had to change the sheets on Bill's bed twice Friday night. Saturday was slightly better; Sunday was a lot worse and Dr. Kovnat ordered him to the hospital. Bill went reluctantly. More blood cultures were taken. By then Bill Huey was hallucinating and having conversations with people that weren't there and his temperature reached 104°F (40°C). Monday and Tuesday scarcely existed for Bill Huey; he only knew that he had a terrible headache and his chest hurt. By Wednesday morning, a week after the beginning of his illness, a gram-negative organism was isolated from his cultures but not identified. The next morning Bill Huey was told he had septicemic plague. He was discharged from the hospital after a week-long stay. There was no clue to the origin of his disease, but he has four dogs, all of which now wear flea collars. He was the twentieth case of plague in New Mexico and the thirteenth since mid-June. In the worst previous year for plague in New Mexico (1975) there had been a total of sixteen cases. That number was exceeded by mid-July in 1983.

Just before Bill Huey became ill, a plague-infected rabbit was found on the Arroyo del Oso Golf Course at 7001 Osuna, N.E., in Albuquerque, about three miles due north of two of the city's major shopping centers, Winrock and Coronado, and some five miles northeast of the University of New Mexico School of Medicine on the edge of the main university campus. This was the closest approach yet of a plague-infected animal to the city center. Usually about five infected animals are found in Albuquerque every year, but they are usually found in the foothills of the Sandia Mountains on the eastern border of the city. At the same time the state health and tourist information offices were getting calls from around the country inquiring about the safety of a trip to New Mexico.

Two days before Bill Huey became ill, thirteen-year-old Donna Marie Delattre, whose story began this book, handled and then released a wild chipmunk she found on one of her frequent, solitary excursions into the hills around St. John's College on the southeastern edge of Santa Fe. The fact that she was able to pick up the animal suggests that it was not in good health. Two days later, on the day Bill Huey became ill, Donna said goodbye to her parents and younger sister and flew to Atlanta. The next she was driven to her grandparent's home in the little mountain community of Seneca, South Carolina.

That evening she complained of a sore throat and tenderness in her right groin. She reportedly had a temperature of 104°F (40°C). The next morning (Friday) she saw Dr. J. Pruitt who noted an oral temperature of 101°F (38.3°C), an inflamed throat, tender lymph nodes in her neck, and a one-half by one inch tender right inguinal lymph node. Laboratory tests were done and oral penicillin was prescribed. On Monday, August 1, just a week after she had handled the chipmunk, she was seen again. She still had a temperature, the bubo in her right groin was growing, but her chest X ray was normal. Because of her recent arrival from New Mexico, plague was considered. She was hospitalized in the Oconee Memorial Hospital and given intravenous therapy, including streptomycin. The next morning she was breathing rapidly, she was producing bloody sputum, and she appeared moribund.

Donna was then transferred to a large, regional medical center in Greenville, South Carolina, where she was treated with intensive supportive therapy including intravenous chloramphenicol. Despite her treatment she died in Greenville hospital at 2:30 that afternoon. She had been ill less than four days. Both lungs were infiltrated by *Y. pestis* in addition to the organism in her blood and in aspirates from the groin bubo. She was the fifth case of plague east of the hundredth meridian, excluding laboratory accidents, since 1920.[10]

This was another case of "traveler's plague," that ended in the death of the traveler. Of the nine similar cases that have occurred since 1957, five have been fatal, three of them from secondary pneumonic plague. In six of the nine cases the disease was acquired in New Mexico. Colorado, Wyoming, and Oregon were the sources of the other three. Five of the victims were under sixteen years of age, and this group accounted for three of the five fatalities.[11]

Unfortunately, the appetite of the disease for human victims continued unabated. New Mexico recorded its third fatality (and twenty-fourth case) in mid-August; the victim was a thirteen-year-old boy from Eagle Nest who had bubonic plague and was promptly and properly treated. Unfortunately, the disease progressed so rapidly that the boy's defenses, even aided by potent antibiotics, were overwhelmed. Although he had been ill only a very short time before he saw a physician, he died half a day after his disease was diagnosed. Jonathan Mann, M.D., the New Mexico State Epidemiologist, called it "probably the most severe case of plague I've seen."[12] New Mexico's three fatal plague cases of 1983 were in two thirteen-year-olds and an eighteen-year-old.

On August 29, *Time* ran a two-column story on plague in the U.S., featuring a picture of Jon Mann examining a prairie dog. The story managed to crowd an incredible number of errors into a relatively short space. One was that "the human risk is limited primarily to people trekking into the wilds. . . ." As we have seen, in New Mexico and California, at least, most people are infected in or near their homes. Another error was that the exceptional number of cases did not constitute an epidemic.

That was undoubtedly what *Time's* reporters had been told, so this error, unlike most of the others in the article, can't be blamed on sloppy research. State health officials (and their politically minded superiors) don't like to use the word *epidemic* in public because of the vision it conveys of great numbers of people in a limited area becoming ill, as in the Great Plague of London, for example. In the general sense, however, any rise in the number of cases of anything that exceeds the normal "background level" constitutes an epidemic. In recent years New Mexico has had about seven cases of human plague a year. What else but an epidemic could one call a period in which twenty-seven cases occurred in seven months?

Human plague continued to appear across the West until late in the year. There was another case in Shasta County, California, late in July; otherwise the disease confined itself to Arizona and New Mexico. When it was finally over—the last case was reported from Colorado in December—there had been forty cases in all. This was a substantial jump from the previous worst year of 1975 in which there were twenty-five cases, and it continued the five-year average of the number of reported cases on the steadily rising path it had been on for the past twenty years. The 1983 total was only one less than that of the Los Angeles epidemic of 1924–25 in which forty-one cases occurred.

Elsewhere in the world the provisional totals for 1983 were 715 cases and 40 deaths, of which the U.S. contributed six. Madagascar, with 24 cases and 19 deaths, and China, with 25 cases and 15 deaths, accounted for most of the remaining fatalities. Tanzania reported 226 cases, Brazil 82, Ecuador 65, Burma 96, and Vietnam 118, while Bolivia and Peru had 21 and 17 cases, respectively. These totals may change considerably as further updates come in to the WHO.

In the December issue of *Life* magazine an article on plague appeared as further testimony to the disease's newfound fame (an article in *National Geographic* on the same subject was to appear in mid-1985). The *Life* article was written by the talented New Mexico writer, John Neery, who now lives in Tesuque where he is a neighbor of Bill Huey, the twentieth New Mexico case of 1983. The plaintive question that runs through the article, and through the interviews that preceded it, is "Why can't we simply turn to and eradicate this disease?" The answer should be reasonably clear to readers of this book. The ecology of plague is so complex that it has never been eradicated anywhere by human agency.

The incidence of human plague might be reduced in New Mexico and the other western states if more funds were available for surveillance and insecticide treatment of areas where epizootics were found to be in progress. If a "war on plague" were to be declared however, the money to fund it would probably be taken from other important health-related activities rather than from additional funds supplied for that purpose. President Nixon's "war on cancer" is a case in point. Its effect on the incidence or treatment of cancer was modest in proportion to the money spent, but it did divert much-needed funds from other vital research areas. Such fund diversions serve the political ends of "wars" on anything, but not the public interest. A "war on plague" to be even remotely effective would cost billions and might, if extraordinarily effective far beyond what experience suggests is reasonable to expect, prevent one to two dozen plague cases a year, or three to five deaths. The vast sums required could save more lives if directed elsewhere in the unlikely event that such sums were to be newly available for the improvement of human health.

Spurred by the rising incidence of human plague in the United States, as exemplified by the ghastly year just past, plague experts from Arizona, California, New Mexico, the Indian Health Service, the Centers for Disease Control, and the Pan American Health Organization met in Santa Fe, New Mexico in late February 1984 to consider how to improve prevention and control of the disease. The group agreed to design new data collection forms so that adequate information on human cases would be available in the future to guide control efforts. Insect control was held to be the key to control during epizootics, with rodent control playing a long-term role in human plague prevention. A second meeting of the ad hoc committee will take place in early 1985.

The spring of 1984, like that of 1983, was cold and wet throughout much of the West. That combination had been blamed for the large numbers of cases in 1983 since it favors both large rodent and flea populations. The 1984 plague season in New Mexico got off to an early start with a case in an eleven-year-old boy from McKinley County that was reported on March 28. The boy had acquired plague from his cat that later died. The boy recovered. Early the next month yet another plague-infected cat turned up in Jemez Springs, New Mexico. The cat was well treated and survived.

In late May the death from pneumonic plague of a twenty-four-year-old man from the mountainous Frazier Park area fifty miles (eighty kilometers) north of Los Angeles was reported. He too was believed to have gotten the disease from his cat.

There were two more plague cases in Los Angeles County in 1984, one traceable to a cat. One victim was a thirty-five-year-old veterinarian in Claremont who treated the sick animal. The other victim was the thirty-five-year-old wife of a veterinarian practicing in Bradbury in the foothills of the San Gabriel Mountains. Her husband's occupation was probably irrelevant to her case. Both recovered although the Claremont veterinarian had secondary pneumonic plague. He became ill on March 30, saw a physician for the first time on April 2, and was hospitalized after a second visit the next day. He began coughing on April 4 (ultimately exposing sixty-one people), and an antibiotic effective against plague was begun on April 7.

He had treated a cat whose symptoms were consistent with pneumonic plague, but the cat had died and its body was unavailable for autopsy. One of the veterinarian's own cats had contact with the cat that died; it also acquired plague but was promptly treated and recovered. Evidence of an epizootic was found in the area where the first cat had lived.

Since 1959, four veterinarians and one veterinary assistant have acquired plague from animals they have treated, and one infection was fatal.

In addition to these three cases in the southern half of California, there were two other California plague cases, both involving thirteen-year-old boys, one in Tulare County (for which tularemia is named), and one in Toulumne County near Yosemite National Park.

The state of Washington had one plague case in a thirty-year-old man in Yakima County, who contracted the disease in January from a bobcat he had shot, and Texas had its second indigenous plague case since the twenties when a forty-eight-year-old male contracted the disease after rabbit hunting in Winkler County. Winkler County wraps around the south-eastern tip of New Mexico.

Utah had two cases of plague by the end of August, one in a forty-six-year-old Navajo on the reservation in San Juan County, and a fatal case in an eighteen-year-old boy involved in a survival course in Garfield County in the vicinity of Bryce Canyon National Park.

Arizona had only one case by late August, in contrast to its usual record, but that case, involving a twenty-nine-year-old man in Apache County near Canyon de Chelly National Monument, was fatal.

Despite the unusual level of competition from California, New Mexico was sustaining its reputation by having ten cases of plague, or half the total of twenty reported cases in the U.S., by the end of August. There were two cases near the communities of Madrid and Mendenales (near Abiquiu), and a fourth case in the vicinity of Peña Blanca, near the Rio Grande about halfway between Albuquerque and Santa Fe, by early June. The Peña Blanca case was the septicemic form of the disease, which is difficult to diagnose, but the forty-year-old man received good treatment and recovered. In mid-June there was another septicemic case, in a forty-three-year-old man who lived just south of Santa Fe; he also recovered. He apparently acquired the disease from fleas brought home by a pet dog.

By early July there was a third septicemic case, this time in a sixty-one-year-old woman in the Rio Arriba County community of Dixon. Her case was probably acquired from fleas brought home by her pet dogs.

By August, New Mexico had still not had a fatal case of plague. This changed abruptly when a seventy-year-old man,

who lived about two miles south of Santa Fe, died of septicemic plague less than three hours after being admitted to the
hospital. Ordinarily septicemic plague, which has a 70 percent
mortality rate, occurs in only about 10 percent of plague cses.
By early August nearly 60 percent of the plague cases in New
Mexico had been the septicemic form; happily the mortality
rate was only one-third that expected.

New Mexico's eighth case of plague for 1984 was in a fourteen-year-old boy who contracted the disease in Lincoln County
but was not hospitalized until he returned to his home in
Lubbock, Texas. The next case was in a seventeen-year-old
boy who acquired the disease near his home north of Pecos,
near the popular Pecos Wilderness Area. The tenth case was
in a thirty-two-year-old man who lived in the town of Coyote,
some twenty miles west of Abiquiu.

Also in August, a fifth area in the environs of Albuquerque
yielded a plague-infected animal, in this case a dead rock squirrel in Glenwood Hills near the Sandia Mountains. Both North
and South Sandia Heights, the Frost Road Area, and a region
twelve miles south of Tijeras on NM 14 were previously found
to contain plague-infected animals.

Early in September, at the request of Representative Bill
Richardson of New Mexico, the House added $3 million to
the Health Professions Act for additional research into plague
control to be conducted by the Centers for Disease Control.

On September 3, a fourteen-month-old girl died from septicemic plague in Colorado Springs, Colorado. She was the
daughter of an Air Force officer, and her home was on the Air
Force Academy grounds. The next day a twelve-year-old girl
who lived south of the town of Tijeras, east of Albuquerque,
went to the Pediatric Clinic of the University of New Mexico
Hospital. She returned to the Clinic on Thursday, because her
condition had worsened, and Thursday night, she went to the
hospital's emergency room. She was hospitalized on Friday,
when she was diagnosed as having pneumonic plague. Her
symptoms were described as unusual. She had potentially exposed over 500 people, and these contacts were given antibiotics prophylactically. The girl is making a satisfactory

recovery. The source of her infection remains unknown although a rabbit dead of plague was found at Pine Flat picnic area, which the girl had visited. The picnic area was promptly closed.

A second Albuquerque girl, eleven years old, was also hospitalized with bubonic plague on September 10.

Of the final eight cases of human plague in 1984 New Mexico contributed half. All the victims were male, from fourteen to seventy in age, living in Bernalillo, Santa Fe, Taos, and San Miguel counties. All recovered. Of the other four cases, two were in different Colorado counties (Saguache and Jefferson), one occurred in Arizona (in a Navajo in Apache County), and one in California (in Monterey County).

The total for 1984 was an appalling thirty-one cases, the second worst year since 1924. Five of the cases were fatal (16 percent), three of the five in males between twenty and twenty-nine, of which two occurred in New Mexico and one in Utah. The two other fatal cases were an elderly man in New Mexico and an infant in Colorado.

New Mexico had sixteen of 1984's cases, with four in Santa Fe County, three each in Rio Arriba, San Miguel, and Bernalillo counties, and one each in McKinley, Taos, and Lincoln.

California had six cases of human plague in 1984; Colorado and Arizona three; Utah, two; while Texas and Washington state each contributed one case.

Another landmark in the history of plague in America was achieved in 1984 with the publication of a detailed account of the extinction of plague in the Hawaiian Islands.[13]

Although there had been 410 confirmed cases in Hawaii between 1899 and 1949—with at least 350 fatalities—and probably multiple introductions of the disease both among the various islands and with the Asian mainland in the early years of the century, the disease has apparently vanished because the complex of plague-carrying animals and fleas was not rich enough to sustain a permanent focus of plague. The black, brown, and Polynesian rats (the latter present since Polynesian times) and two varieties of the flea *Xenopsylla* (*cheopis* and *vexabilis*) maintained the infection for more than half a century, but there have been no human cases since 1949 and no animal plague found since 1957. The island of Kauai was plague-free after 1906, Oahu after 1910, and Maui after 1951. The Hamakua District on the big island of Hawaii was the last holdout. Between 1910 and 1949 there were 112 confirmed human cases of plague in the district, of which 109 were fatal, but after May 1957 neither plague-infected animals nor fleas were found.

Improved sanitation, replacement of mules by trucks and tractors after World War II, DDT application, and rat trapping and poisoning all play a role in the disappearance of the Hamakua focus. The basic proposition of the authors of this paper is, however, that the simple system of three rodents and two fleas was insufficiently diverse to insulate the focus against the effects of climatic cycles (particularly drought), when coupled with other environmental pressures.

Plague continued to be a problem in Tanzania in 1984, with 148 cases reported by the end of December, and in Madagascar (24 cases), Brazil (22), Ecuador (6), Peru (172), Vietnam (20), Burma (96), and Zimbabwe (1).

Plague struck Saudi Arabia again in 1984 leading to 37 cases. Nine resulted when an infected camel was butchered and eaten. The two butchers and seven members of a family died. At this writing (January 1985) none of these cases has been reported to WHO by the Saudi government. Libya notified WHO of eight cases of plague in 1984, for the first outbreak since 1977.

Figure 5 summarizes the history of human plague in America from 1900 to 1984. The first quarter-century was marked by the ferocious epidemics in California and the lesser ones along the Gulf coast. Human plague from wild rodents exceeded three cases a year only once (1910) during this time. This is deduced from the location of cases during the first twenty-five years and the rather arbitrary assumption that those occurring in places other than epidemic centers were caused by wild-rodent plague. If the assumption is wrong, it further reduces the level of wild-rodent infection as a cause of human plague. If the assumption is correct, the human

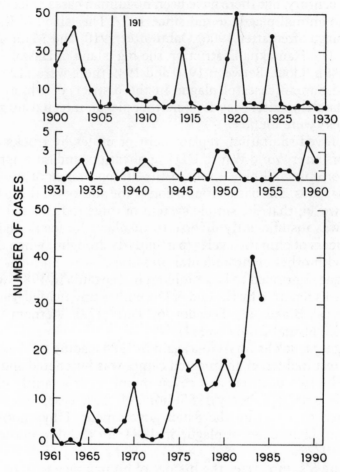

Figure 5 Human Plague in the U.S.A., 1900–1984

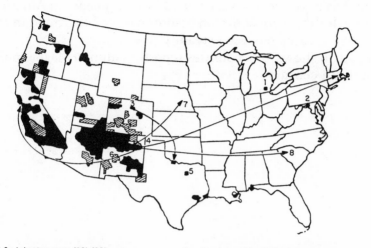

1, 2. Laboratory cases, 1901, 1959
3.   Case imported into Texas from Colorado
4.   Case imported into Massachusetts from New Mexico
5.   Case imported into Texas from Vietnam
6.   Case imported into California from New Mexico
7.   Case imported into Nebraska from New Mexico
8.   Case imported into South Carolina from New Mexico
▨▨▨ New areas of human plague since 1972

Figure 6   Distribution of Human Plague in the U.S.A.

plague resulting from contact with wild rodents averaged only slightly more than one case a year from 1900 to 1964.

In the two parts of the figure covering the second and third quarters of the twentieth century, the vertical scale for the number of cases is different, happily, from that of the first twenty-five years.

From 1925 on, no rat-borne plague was reported in America, and there was a spectacular drop in the level of plague cases. Three or more cases a year were reported only three times in the second quarter-century.

The twenty-five-year period ending in 1975 is again different from the two preceding quarter-centuries. Human plague activity began to pick up in 1958, although the next four-year period was not spectacularly bad by the standards of previous years. Then, in 1964, a distinct change occurred. Since then, there has never been a year free of human plague in America, although they were common before that, and the trend in the number of cases has been steadily upward.

Figure 6 shows U.S. counties reporting human plague in the twentieth century.

20

The Resistance Movement

Yersinia pestis and its familiars are clearly not, in the last years of the twentieth century, in anything like headlong retreat from the forces of technology. This is partly the result of what we might call the resistance movement.

It arises from a basic fact of life: that nearly all creatures on earth at this time are the result of selective evolutionary pressures over millions of years. They exist because they have proved themselves tough and resourceful, able to adapt to new threats to their existence as they appear.

The resistance of wild rodents in plague foci has been mentioned. These animals are presumably distinguished by the presence of specific antibodies in their blood formed in response to plague infection, although young animals may retain maternal antibodies for some months after birth. A second type of resistance comes from genetic selection. In a population of animals continually exposed to violent plague epizootics that kill most of them, some that do survive do so because they have superior defense mechanisms against the plague bacillus. Some offspring of such animals inherit this resistance and survive the next epizootic that kills most of their nonresistant brothers and sisters. In these circumstances the animal population is gradually enriched in plague-resistant individuals. This natural resistance persists even in laboratory rats maintained in protected environments for generations.

The 50 percent lethal dose for the laboratory albino strain of the Norway rat is 50 to 100 *Y. pestis* of the virulent Indian strain known as 195P. Yet of forty-nine ordinary laboratory rats, five survived infection with six thousand or more plague bacilli; one tolerated infection with six hundred thousand. When wild rats from the plague-infected Hamakua area of Hawaii were similarly tested with inoculation of nearly thirteen thousand plague bacilli, ten died of thirty-nine injected; ten of the survivors showed no antibody response.

This sort of resistance to plague infection is important in the survival of plague foci. But the kind of resistance that most concerns us here is resistance to plague-control agents.

Rodenticides, insecticides, and antimicrobial drugs (antimicrobials include both the antibiotics produced by living organisms and the chemically synthesized drugs like the sulfas) have threatened the existence of rats, fleas, and *Y. pestis*, but in some degree, these threats have been turned aside.

Warfarin, for example, has become the cornerstone of rodent control, both urban and rural, because of its effectiveness, ease of use, and relatively low hazard to other animals. Then, in Scotland in 1958, twelve years after the introduction of the anticoagulant, some Norway rats were found to be resistant to it. Further study showed that they were resistant to all other available anticoagulant rodenticides as well. The discovery of warfarin resistance in Scotland was soon confirmed in the Netherlands, Denmark, West Germany, and England. As an official of the British Ministry of Agriculture put it (with stiff upper lip), "We aren't exactly alarmed—the Ministry of Agriculture is never alarmed—but we are working very hard to find an alternative to warfarin."

In 1971 resistant Norway rats were found in a barn near Raleigh, North Carolina, and later elsewhere in the vicinity. As in Europe, the warfarin-resistant rats were also resistant to all other anticoagulants available in the United States. In

Europe the area dominated by resistant rats, both black and Norway varieties, spread rapidly.

A survey of twenty-three U.S. cities, largely in the eastern half of the country, showed that by 1975 over half of them had Norway rats resistant to warfarin. A high proportion of resistant animals (a quarter of those trapped) was found in East Orange, New Jersey, and smaller ratios in three other cities (Hoboken, Jersey City, and Newark) nearby.[1]

The highest concentration of resistant animals in the U.S. survey was found in the Lawndale area of Chicago. Here, over 50 percent of the rats trapped were warfarin-resistant, while along Bates Street in Washington, D.C., about one-fourth of the rats trapped were resistant; Charlotte, North Carolina, had a similar level. Johnson County, North Carolina, the site where resistant U.S. rats were first discovered, had more than 50 percent of its rats warfarin-resistant. Of the rats in Poughkeepsie, New York, and its environs, an area about fifty miles up the Hudson River from New York City, more than a third were resistant.

The problem gets steadily worse. In April 1978 a UPI dispatch told of mice resistant to anticoagulants spreading throughout neighborhoods in Memphis. Exterminators—at least when their bosses were out of earshot—were advising homeowners to get a cat.[2]

Meanwhile, black rats in Liverpool, England, were also found to be resistant, as were mice in San Francisco. Some rats from the Bay Area also proved to be immune to anticoagulants. A United Press report in November 1974 spoke of the difficulties of controlling "superrats" in New York City but offered the hope that they could be poisoned with the "new" rodenticide zinc sulfide (widely used since 1911).

Since the reports of warfarin resistance are comparatively recent, it is not clear how widespread the phenomenon currently is. It is probably a worldwide development of increasing significance. And the resistance movement does not stop with warfarin.

The widespread use of DDT has saved millions of lives. It has been used on a vast scale, primarily for malaria control;

a fringe benefit has been the killing of plague-infected fleas in the same areas. Widespread use of DDT began in 1946. A mere four years later, DDT-resistant *Xenopsylla* were reported from Ecuador. This was no laboratory exercise. Efforts to control this notorious plague transmitter with DDT simply failed. In Greece human fleas were found in 1951 to be DDT-resistant, and the same result was reported in the Palestine refugee camps the following year. Resistant dog fleas were discovered in Florida and elsewhere in the South in 1952, and similar observations were made on the Oriental rat flea in that region, although *X. cheopis* still appeared to be susceptible to DDT throughout most of its range in the United States. Then a decade later, DDT-tolerant *X. cheopis* were found in San Francisco. These fleas survived treatment with about twice the level of DDT required to kill susceptible insects.

Naturally, there was great interest in these observations on the subcontinent of India, where plague was still very much a present fact of life—or death. In 1960, studies on *X. cheopis*, the dominant rat flea in Bombay State, showed that in some areas it was enormously resistant to DDT. The most DDT-insensitive *X. cheopis* in Bombay State were up to five thousand times more resistant to the insecticide than the normal fleas. To make matters worse, the highly DDT-resistant fleas were also resistant to other chlorinated hydrocarbon insecticides with which they had never come in contact. These results led to a nationwide survey in India, with the outcome that rat fleas resistant to DDT were found wherever the insecticide had been used. Control of the flea population with DDT was no longer possible.

Once the fact of DDT resistance in plague-bearing fleas was confirmed, the same result was found elsewhere. In both South Vietnam and Thailand, *X. cheopis* was DDT-resistant.

Plague outbreaks have been stopped by using organophosphorus insecticides, but these have the major disadvantages of being highly toxic to man and other animals and of quickly decomposing in the environment. Repeated application is necessary. They are very useful compounds for combating small, local eruptions of the disease; a large-scale epidemic would require the use of more persistent insecticides.

In various parts of Vietnam no concentration of DDT can now suppress infestations of the Oriental rat flea. The worldwide occurrence of insecticide resistance in plague-carrying insects is especially worrisome because the most convenient and rational means of controlling an outbreak is by flea control. This situation is further complicated by the development of cross-resistance, whereby an insect often becomes immune to other agents when it becomes resistant to the one most frequently encountered. Resistance to DDT commonly carried with it resistance to a large number of chlorinated insecticides, but not to the organophosphorus compounds. On the other hand, resistance to the organophosphorus agents commonly imparts cross-resistance to the two other major classes of insecticides, the chlorinated hydrocarbons and the carbamates. Incredibly, there is evidence that some insects resistant to chemical insecticides also acquire resistance to juvenile hormone analogs, the highly touted "third-generation" insecticides.

In California, by 1972, several species of mosquitos had developed resistance to all available organophosphorus and chlorinated hydrocarbon insecticides. Elsewhere, resistance to DDT and related compounds was followed by resistance to carbamates and organophosphorus compounds.

The development of resistance, especially by the malarial mosquitos in various countries, to the two latter classes of compounds did not result from the use of these agents in health protection but from their extensive application in agriculture, primarily on cotton and rice crops. The crops of the farmers were protected, but the protection of the people against malaria was lost.

Insect resistance to DDT ordinarily becomes a problem after a few years of exposure. There is some comfort in the fact that when the selection pressure of the insecticide is removed, the resistance may be lost nearly as rapidly as it was gained. This is not everywhere the case, however. On the Lamia Plain, some 124 miles (200 kilometers) northwest of Athens near the village and the mountain pass of Thermopylae, DDT spraying to control malaria was discontinued after thirteen years of intensive treatment. In 1973, more than a dozen years later, the malarial mosquitos were still highly resistant to DDT.[3]

The mechanism of warfarin and insecticide resistance seems to be mutation of (usually) one gene in the course of evolution. Mutation occurs continually at an extremely low frequency; the results are expressed more rapidly the greater the multiplication rate of the organism involved. Most mutations are fatal to the cell that bears them, some are harmful though not immediately fatal—these lead to such abnormalities as cancer and some birth defects, for example. A very small percentage are beneficial, and some are neutral, doing neither good nor harm. The neutral mutations are those that lead to resistance of the warfarin or DDT types.

The mutations that make *X. cheopis* resistant to DDT may have occurred fifty thousand or more years ago. It did not matter then, but it was a stable change, and the progeny of the flea in which the mutation took place continued to pass it along from generation to generation. Since DDT did not exist, there was nothing for the mutated gene to do but go along, as it were, for the ride. It was a cure looking for a disease. When *X. cheopis* first encountered DDT, those very occasional fleas that had the altered gene suddenly, after unnumbered millenia, had an immense selective advantage. While other *X. cheopis* were dying like—well, fleas—the unique gene of the resistant insects was making an enzyme that turned DDT into a nontoxic compound. These fleas lived to breed other DDT-resistant fleas while their less fortunate brethren perished. The cure had found its disease.

As expected, a process that takes several generations, a dozen years in a rat and some months in a flea, takes a few hours in a bacterium. But the process basically occurs in the same way. A mutation that confers neither advantage nor disadvantage for eons may suddenly mean the difference between life and death. And life for the bacterium may mean death for its host.

The earliest chemotherapeutic agent used against *Y. pestis* was a sulfonamide. The sulfa drugs were also extensively used in the treatment of gonorrhea. The results with the venereal disease were much more spectacular than with plague. In 1940, 70 percent of all gonorrhea patients could be cured with sulfa drugs. Only four years later the figures were sadly reversed; the gonococcus in 70 percent of the disease victims was resistant to sulfa treatment, and their infection could not be effectively treated with sulfa compounds.

The experience with *Y. pestis* was similar except that the cure rate was never as good as with gonorrhea. Wily *Y. pestis* indifferent to sulfa rapidly evolved, and even this modest weapon against the disease was increasingly blunted by the defenses of plague bacillus.

More formidable weapons were on their way. As we saw earlier, the impact of the discovery of streptomycin on the treatment of plague was striking, truly the beginning of a golden age. But there were ominous signs. In the earliest experiments on the cure of pneumonic plague in guinea pigs with streptomycin, shortly after the drug became available in 1946, nearly all the infected animals made an almost unbelievable recovery from an infection that uniformly killed others not given the drug. But one treated guinea pig showed only a transitory effect of streptomycin injection. Six days after infection, three days after streptomycin treatment had begun, it was dead of pneumonic plague.

When *Y. pestis* was isolated from the spleen of this animal, it was found to be tremendously resistant to the lethal action of the drug. Ordinarily *Y. pestis* would not grow in a medium containing four micrograms of streptomycin per milliliter. The plague bacilli from the spleen of the dead, streptomycin-treated guinea pig grew normally in a medium in which each milliliter contained not four micrograms of streptomycin but twenty-five thousand. The amount of drug tolerated by *Y. pestis* had increased more than six thousand times in seventy-two hours. Plague caused by such an organism could not be treated effectively with streptomycin; no amount of the drug that could reasonably be administered would have the slightest effect.[4]

This was a further example of a neutral mutation of no consequence to *Y. pestis* until it encountered streptomycin.

After that, in the body of an infected animal treated with streptomycin, only the descendants of those few *Y. pestis* that had this mutation could survive. They could not only survive, they could also multiply and infect other animals. Therapy with streptomycin accomplished nothing.

The selection for drug resistance can easily be carried out in the laboratory, and *Y. pestis* resistant to streptomycin, tetracycline, and chloramphenicol can be produced. A strain of *Y. pestis* resistant to streptomycin was isolated from a rat in Vietnam; over 20 percent (one in five) of the strains of *Y. pestis* from a variety of sources were resistant to streptomycin. Other such isolations can be expected as the three major antibiotics against plague are increasingly used against this and other diseases. Isolation of a streptomycin-resistant strain of the plague bacillus from a human case has not yet occurred. When it does, it might not be catastrophic because a neutral mutation causing resistance to streptomycin would not affect the sensitivity of the organism to tetracycline or chloramphenicol, and the likelihood of neutral mutations to two of the drugs appearing in the same organism in nature is infinitely small.

A more frightening story, however, began in Japan in 1955. A woman returned to Japan from Hong Kong and developed a stubborn case of dysentery. The organism causing the disease appeared when isolated to be the usual bacillus involved, a member of the genus *Shigella*; but it was not as ordinary as it looked. It was resistant to streptomycin. The shocking aspect was that it was simultaneously resistant to sulfanilamide, chloramphenicol, and tetracycline (every drug commonly used in the treatment of plague). This sturdy little organism spread all over the islands of Japan in the next few years, bringing with it epidemics of drug-resistant dysentery.

It was a new and awesome phenomenon. As Dr. Louis Weinstein, visiting professor of medicine at Harvard, wrote in 1975, "In some instances resistance develops to so many of the commonly used antimicrobial drugs that the physician may have to resort to the use of more dangerous and less well known drugs or *there may not be an effective agent for the treatment of a particular infection*" (italics added).

The mechanism of this process is fundamentally different from the process of neutral mutation, by which other types of resistance are conferred in an entirely random manner. This process, called infectious drug resistance, involves transfer of factors (R factors, "R" standing for *resistance*) conferring resistance to as many as nine different drugs from one kind of bacteria to another. One of the known recipients of such resistance is *Y. pestis.*

In the laboratory a small number of bacteria, such as the common colon bacillus *Escherichia coli,* which carry the R factors, are added to a culture of drug-sensitive plague bacteria. In about twenty-four hours the plague bacilli become impervious to all drugs for which the transferred R factors confer resistance. The R factors multiply within the previously drug-susceptible bacteria, faster than the bacteria themselves divide. Thus, the R factors can be transferred through a bacterial population with breathtaking speed. The previously susceptible bacteria become "infected" with the resistance-conferring factors—hence the term *infectious drug resistance.*

If this process were confined to the laboratory, there would be no great concern, aside from keeping it there. That it unfortunately occurs in the outside world was demonstrated by the experience of the Japanese woman in 1955 and has been frequently confirmed since. In 1971 the antibiotic gentamycin, a compound related to streptomycin, was introduced. Only a few months after its first use, some bacteria had grown resistant to it. Bacteria from the first patient in whom gentamycin resistance was detected were also resistant to chloramphenicol, sulfonamides, and a synthetic penicillin. Normal intestinal bacteria carrying R factors for *all known antimicrobial compounds* have been isolated in most parts of the world. By 1965, 60 to 70 percent of all common intestinal bacteria isolated in hospitals carried R factors that conferred resistance to three or more antimicrobial drugs. Before 1955 such factors were rarely found.

Colon bacilli carrying R factors are found with increasing frequency in river water. Ingesting such bacilli can transfer drug resistance to other bacteria in the body with which they come into close contact, usually in the lower intestine, especially if antimicrobial drugs are being taken. Transfer could also occur in a plague bubo secondarily infected with an R-factor-bearing, gram-negative organism.

In a study of an English river, 56 percent of the organisms found were resistant to streptomycin; 54 percent, to tetracycline; and 23 percent, to chloramphenicol. Of eight strains resistant to chloramphenicol, all were resistant to streptomycin; five of the eight were also resistant to tetracycline.[5] In Germany, in 1974, tests showed that about a third of all the *Shigella* (dysentery) bacilli tested were resistant to *all known antimicrobials*. In Michigan, about the same time, two-thirds of the *Shigella* isolated were multiply drug-resistant.[6] Researchers in England also showed that if persons whose feces did not contain R-factor-bearing bacteria were fed such organisms, along with an antimicrobial, they continued to secrete resistant bacteria for up to three months.

The common colon bacillus *E. coli* is a frequent inhabitant of surgical wounds. In a survey of a major medical center in 1973, more than half the surgical incisions were contaminated before they were closed, and about one fourth of the patients with contaminated incisions developed wound infections. Thus, there is a real risk of developing multiple-drug resistance in plague victims when a bubo is surgically removed or when unnecessary surgery (for incarcerated hernia or appendicitis) is performed on a plague victim because of misdiagnosis.

The general significance of the phenomenon of drug resistance is seen in a recent study of the causes of death in a large number of U.S. cancer patients. Infection was the principal cause of death. It was the major factor in 36 percent of the fatalities and a contributing cause in another 13 percent. Most of the fatal infections were caused by antimicrobial-resistant organisms.[7]

As the World Health Organization has recently pointed out, antimicrobial resistance is an ever-increasing problem a significant portion of which is due to the completely inappropriate use of antibiotics in the treatment of human illness.[8]

The "neutral" mutations that give rise to single-drug resistance in bacteria are not always neutral. Frequently the bacterial mutants grow less vigorously than the unmutated strain. The bacterium made multiply drug resistant by the transfer of an R factor, however, is entirely normal. Multiple-drug resistance by the transfer of R factors can be produced in *Y. pestis* in the laboratory. Such strains are stable and have the normal infective properties of other plague bacilli. It is inevitable that they will be produced outside the laboratory as well.

The significance of pharyngeal plague as a possible carrier state was discussed in connection with the discoveries made during the Vietnam epidemic. Aside from the question of plague carriers, pharyngeal plague indicates that *Y. pestis* is present in the throats of people without plague symptoms. An obvious consequence is that *Y. pestis* is swallowed by those with the organism in their throats and passes through the digestive tract before being excreted. The real significance of pharyngeal plague may lie in the opportunity it provides for *Y. pestis* to acquire multiple-drug resistance by close contact with R-factor-bearing organisms during its passage through the gut. Such persons may continually enrich the environment in multiply drug-resistant *Y. pestis*, especially if they are given antimicrobials prophylactically.

The more that modern antibiotics are used to combat serious plague infection and protect contacts of plague victims, particularly in the case of pneumonic plague, the more likely it becomes that a multiply drug-resistant strain will arise. Conditions for production of such a strain are enhanced the greater the experience of a given population with a wide variety of antimicrobial compounds. Thus, multiply drug-resistant *Y. pestis* might be expected to develop most rapidly if plague were to break out in an urban center in western Europe or North America.

There is no need to labor the point. It is clear that our most valuable weapons against plague and our last defense of the inner citadel—man himself—could splinter in our hands at the moment when they are most needed. This is partly the result, sadly enough, of the indiscriminant drenching of the human environment with an antibiotic fog.

21

Future Epidemics

Still thou art blest, compared wi' me!
The present only toucheth thee:
But och! I backwards cast my e'e,
    On prospects drear!
An' forward, though I canna see,
    I guess an' fear!
                              —Robert Burns, *To a Mouse*, 1785

Plague's history is one of a series of pandemics, lasting years or centuries, interspersed with periods when the disease withdraws to its permanent foci and waits. In the quiescent periods there are vicious outbreaks that rain terror and death on a relatively limited area, such as Vietnam, but that do not afflict the entire world. We are at present in such a quiescent period.

In any area the quiet can be abruptly shattered by an epidemic that is no less horrifying for being localized. Here we examine ways in which epidemics might be ignited.

The historical association of pestilence with famine, war, and death—the Four Horsemen of the Apocalypse— needs no emphasis. Similarly obvious is the relation between overpopulation and famine. Much has been, and will be, written about the world food-population problem; only a brief summary is needed.

To oversimplify for brevity, there are optimists and pessimists; the latter are sometimes called neo-Malthusians.

The optimists feel that the food-population problem is under

317

control for the next decade but that beyond that the situation is in doubt. The pessimists point out that death rates are already rising in some of the poorest countries of the world and that the situation is grave but not hopeless for the next decade if, and only if, good weather prevails in North America. The only region with substantial grain surpluses, it supplies 90 percent of the grain in world trade.

Pessimists note that since 1891 droughts have withered the crops in the North American grain belt about every twenty years. If bad weather appears in any form, the minuscule grain surplus (presently higher than usual but still less than enough for fifty days of world consumption) will quickly fade away. Then painful decisions must be faced—who lives and who dies. Analogies have been made to an overloaded lifeboat and to a beleaguered battlefield hospital where those who will recover without treatment are left alone to live and hopeless cases are left alone to die so that attention can be concentrated on those who will live only if adequately treated. The latter concept, called triage, comes from the French verb *trier*, meaning "to sort." This "sorting" may be applied to countries if prolonged drought strikes the North American plains.

Both optimists and pessimists agree that famines will occur frequently in the next decade, about one major famine each year somewhere in the world. Currently, at least five hundred million people are undernourished; four million or more, mostly children, will die of starvation this year.

The current African famine is the result of one of the worst and longest droughts in history—it's been going on for three years. In sub-Saharan Africa generally life expectancy is forty-six years, and one child in five dies before its first birthday. Real income per person has been falling and is generally below what it was before independence. In Mozambique 200,000 people may have died of starvation last year and at least that many will die this year, according to the UN Food and Agricultural Organization.[1] In Africa generally, per capita food production in thirty countries fell in 1979 and again in 1980. Worldwide, the grain output per person is barely keeping up and may fall behind before the end of this century. Real per capita income in Latin America has declined three years in a row and is now 10 percent below that in 1980.[2] U.S. leadership in helping to solve the overpopulation problem is nearly totally absent at present.

Malnutrition and starvation are not caused by inadequate total food supply but by maldistribution. The rich and powerful eat well wherever they are. The poor eat poorly. Efforts to feed the poor often only make the wealthy wealthier. Ethiopia is an example. In 1974 between one hundred thousand and two hundred thousand Ethiopians died of starvation, and the Ethiopian military government appealed for emergency relief. But, at the same time, the country's foreign currency reserves were increasing rapidly and it was spending nothing to purchase grain for its people. Ethiopia had, in fact, exported grain in the preceding year at the same time as it was receiving food from the United States. Ten years later the story is nearly the same.

As the UN Food and Agriculture Organization has pointed out, *there are now more people living under worse conditions than ever before in history.* Many live in areas menaced by periodic or endemic plague.

India is the country most closely identified with plague in the twentieth century. Its present position is both precarious and instructive. About one of every seven inhabitants on earth is Indian; their number swells by thirteen million a year (thirty-six thousand a day). India is rich in agricultural land and water and has an innovative and vigorous agricultural research establishment. In an incredible six-year period, India doubled its wheat crop by using the high-yield strains largely adapted to local conditions in Indian laboratories. Such an increase had never before been achieved anywhere in the world. By 1972 the subcontinent was nearly self-sufficient in grain.

Then a series of reverses overcame this great accomplishment. Among these was the increased price of fuel, but corruption, mismanagement, and bad weather played important roles. In 1972 India imported only about half a million tons of grain. By 1975 total imports approached fourteen times that figure. Although India had an excellent grain harvest in 1976, imports are needed to build up her reserves, and because of population growth, the grain supply per capita is still below the 1971 level. The 1976 grain glut caused other problems because of lack of storage capacity. The problem in India is not lack of natural resources but rather developing the organizational ability to use these resources as they must be used to prevent catastrophe.

India is one country that won't stabilize its population in the next century. It is estimated to stabilize in 2141 at 1.8 billion people![3]

One important effect of malnutrition is to cripple the ability of people to resist disease. In the developing countries, communicable diseases are a major cause of sickness and death, as they were in the developing countries at the beginning of this century. Vaccination of people with protein deficiency has a sharply reduced effect, since they do not form antibodies in adequate amounts to protect themselves from illness. Other defenses are similarly weakened. In Mexico the fatality rate from measles is nearly two hundred times that in the United States; in Ecuador it is almost five hundred times higher. Two recent developments illustrate the problem. One is the upsurge of malaria in which insecticide resistance also plays an important role. India had only 125,000 cases of malaria in 1965; in 1976 the total had climbed to about six million, or some twenty-four times the 1965 rate. Sri Lanka (formerly Ceylon) had only 16 new cases of malaria in 1963 but over 500,000 in 1975.

Malaria is not communicable person to person; cholera is. West Africa has not had cholera since the nineteenth century. Then, in August 1970, epidemic cholera exploded, causing 150,000 cases and 20,000 deaths. The following year there were 121 cases in six European countries. Cases confirmed as imported by air were reported in Sweden, France, the United Kingdom, and West Berlin.

The message is clear. Malnutrition and starvation, with the accompanying civil unrest and migration, provide rich soil for the eruption of epidemic disease. And such epidemics can spread rapidly around the world. Famine anywhere in the world is a potential threat to everyone. A more difficult question is, what, if anything, can be done about it?

How do plague epidemics begin? There is a highly speculative idea of the origin and disappearance of plague epidemics that merits brief discussion. *Yersinia pestis* and the organism known as *Y. pseudotuberculosis* (*Y. pseudo-tb.*) are closely related. There is some evidence that, under certain circumstances, *Y. pestis* converts to *Y. pseudo-tb.*, which is widely found in Europe, where *Y. pestis* no longer exists, but also in America, where *Y. pestis* is widely distributed. Human infections with *Y. pseudo-tb.* are common in Europe but rare in the United States.

One explanation for the ebb and flow of epidemic plague is the conversion of *Y. pestis* into *Y. pseudo-tb.* during periods when plague is submerging, and the reverse reaction when it suddenly reappears. It is a fascinating idea. There is little evidence, however, for the conversion of *Y. pseudo-tb.* into *Y. pestis.* This does not mean that it has not, or will not, happen.

There are at least four well-established routes to epidemic plague. One is a flaring up of the disease in, or near, plague foci because of ecological disruption that displaces man and plague-bearing rodents from their normal habitat into contact more intimate than usual. An example is Vietnam. A future example may be the Rocky Mountain West.

The eight states of this region contain 4 percent of the U.S. population but about 50 percent of its energy reserves. The inevitable mining of these reserves (for the extensive utilization of the vast oil shale reservoir, for example), will devastate the habitats of wild animals subject to enzootic plague. This will probably be accompanied by the creation of instant slums to accommodate the sudden influx of power plant constructions worker and miners. The ravaging of the Rocky Mountain West has a potential for stimulating epidemic plague. The handful of people involved in plague control in America, despite their skill and dedication, might be powerless to prevent it.

Another potential epidemic seed is the introduction into a plague-free region of infected fleas or animals; yet another is

the arrival of infected people still in the symptomless incubation period of the disease; a fourth is the deliberate introduction of plague, as in biological warfare. We shall explore
each in turn.

That infected rats and fleas can travel long distances is obvious from the history of plague. This was true at the beginning of this century, when the Third Pandemic spread worldwide
through the agency of the iron steamship. It is even more true
with the advent of jet passenger and cargo aircraft, whose
routes knit the world into a small epidemiological bundle.

Military cargo has brought both rats and fleas from Vietnam
into the United States. Fortunately, no epidemic has resulted,
and beginning belatedly in 1969, more stringent controls were
established to reduce the number of such incidents. In 1970,
however, 16 rodents and 134 fleas were found in planes and
ships returning from Southeast Asia. Fortunately, none was
plague-infected.

There is also the subsidiary danger that efficient plague
carriers that do not now exist in the United States may be
brought into the country and thrive here. A leading candidate
for this role is the tiny Polynesian rat, the principal rodent
brought in from Vietnam.

Commercial flights also transport both rodents and insects,
even in passenger aircraft. Insects not native to the country
of destination are frequently found on jet planes—African
mosquito larvae in a Kansas airport, for example—in spite of
the International Sanitary Regulations, which dictate that both
cabins and landing gear be sprayed with insecticide when a
plane is ready to depart from an airport where disease-bearing
insects are common. Although many airline passengers from
the Far East can testify to having the cabin sprayed with insecticides before takeoff, the procedure is not always carried
out. It is disliked by both passengers and crew, and it is sometimes done perfunctorily, if at all.[4]

Infected animals or insects may travel in containerized cargo.
These truck-sized shipments are packaged at their point of
origin and transported intact to their final destination. A shipment of weapons from the burgeoning arms industry of plague-

infected Brazil might be unopened before it reached the interior of Israel or Iran. Such containers offer infected animals, especially fleas, an almost impregnable fortress. WHO has developed effective methods for killing insects in containerized cargo before it is sealed for shipping, but it is a formidable challenge to see that the procedures are used.

Reasonable cooperation may be expected in treating passenger aircraft, cargo planes, ships, and containerized freight. The transportation of illegal cargo is quite a different problem. This consists mainly of drugs, weapons, and people, and, as is well known, the traffic frequently moves from plague-infected to relatively plague-free areas.

That people, even in the course of ordinary travel, can carry plague for long distances during its incubation period is attested by recent events. Donna Delattre, whose tragic story opens this book, is one example. The young soldier who brought plague from Vietnam to Dallas is another; the geologist who carried the disease from Santa Fe to Boston, the boy who brought plague from Albuquerque to San Francisco, and a Korean soldier who carried it from Vietnam to South Korea illustrate the principle.

There is also the possible spread of the disease from person to person. Fortunately, bubonic plague is not highly contagious, although it is not so innocuous as sometimes described. Victims of the disease may excrete plague bacilli in their urine and feces and may also carry the organism in their sputum. An infectious aerosol capable of causing pneumonic plague infection can be created by the agitating water of a toilet flush that ejects droplets into the air.

Nevertheless, transfer of bubonic plague person to person is rare. Much more alarming is the potentially highly contagious pneumonic form of the disease, capable of spreading rapidly under suitable conditions. It is this form that holds the greatest potential for an epidemic in a major city; it is also the most effective form in which the disease could be used in biological warfare.

If a pneumonic plague victim begins coughing, plague bacilli may be sprayed into the air and inhaled by another person.

This can trigger *primary* pneumonic plague in which *Y. pestis* is transmitted directly from person to person. The involvement of rodents or other animals is no longer necessary to propagate the disease.

Pneumonic plague spreads by "droplet infection," which is really a combination of infection by liquid droplets themselves and the material that remains when the droplet dries. When a person with *Y. pestis* in his lungs coughs, sneezes, shouts, or sometimes simply speaks, he may eject a fine cloud of liquid droplets into the air around him, very like the cloud of fog droplets into which breath condenses on a cold day. Like the fog droplets of breath, the fluid droplets from the lungs of a pneumonic plague victim rapidly evaporate. They leave only a tiny, invisible flake of protein containing plague bacilli and other materials from the lung. These tiny infectious flakes (called droplet nuclei) may be airborne for hours. Even after they settle to the ground or floor, they may be swept up again on air currents generated by movement or a sudden draft. These flakes are easily inhaled by other people. Some of the smallest infiltrate the lower reaches of the lung.

If a room contains more than one or two persons, everyone takes in some dried flakes from other people's throats with every breath. The infectious particles can spread throughout a subway car, a plane, a train, or a building on random currents of air. If a building or vehicle is air-conditioned, the spread is liable to be much more efficient, since the filters in such systems do not remove particles as small as those involved in the transmission of droplet infection, yet the air is vigorously circulated.

Transoceanic air travel in which people are confined for some hours in a space in which all the air is recirculated every three to five minutes offers a particularly good environment for a single infectious pneumonic plague victim to expose other people to a virulent fog of *Y. pestis.* Such a plague victim—for example, on a business trip from Asia to Los Angeles via New York—could expose several hundred people. Passengers might enter and leave the plane in Cairo, Rome, Paris, London, and Chicago, in addition to New York. Many would board other planes en route to their final destination. By this mechanism pneumonic plague could suddenly erupt in cities all over the world in the space of just a few days. The individual epidemics would probably be small; the psychological effect might be immense.

Once a person has pneumonic plague, treatment must begin within fifteen hours of the onset of fever and cough if the patient is to be saved. This is much easier said than done, since the disease is exceptionally difficult to differentiate from influenza or a variety of bacterial and viral pneumonias. It is characterized chiefly by its precipitous course. By the time that is clearly established it is often too late for treatment.

Were pneumonic plague to strike a large city in the United States or in western Europe, it would probably not be diagnosed correctly until some days after the outbreak began. Once the symptoms began to recur frequently, the balance would swing in the opposite direction. Then the malady would be overdiagnosed, so that every case of influenza or simple pneumonia would be liable to be treated as plague, with the resultant strain both on the medical facilities and on the drug supply.

Droplet (or droplet nuclei) infection is not unique to pneumonic plague. It is the principal route by which many respiratory viral and bacterial infections are spread. One may easily forget that the decline in the incidence of infectious disease has been because of the decline in maladies like cholera, typhus, and yellow fever. Respiratory diseases occur at an undiminished—and probably at a growing—rate as humans live in cities of ever-increasing size and as the number of very vulnerable immunosuppressed patients (recipients of organ transplants or cancer chemotherapy, for example) likewise increases.

In the United States at the moment the total number of hospital days accumulated by patients with respiratory infections is nearly three times higher than days for cancer, heart disease, and stroke combined. As René Dubos put it,

Most clinicians, public health officers, epidemiologists, and microbiologists felt justified in proclaiming during the 1950s that the conquest of infectious disease had finally been achieved. . . . Despite so much oratory on the conquest of microbial diseases, the paradox is that the percentage of hospital beds occupied by patients suffering from infection is now as high as it was 50 years ago.[5]

Smallpox, like measles and influenza, is a virus disease caused by an organism hundreds of times smaller but less rugged than *Y. pestis* and spread by droplet infection. Smallpox was imported into western Europe on twenty-eight different occasions between 1960 and 1970 and caused nearly four hundred secondary cases. One of the worst outbreaks occurred in the United Kingdom in 1966 where one case of introduced smallpox led to seventy-one additional victims.

One of the most fascinating of these savage little epidemics took place in Saint Walburga's Hospital in the town of Meschede, about sixty-two miles (one hundred kilometers) east of Düsseldorf, in West Germany.[6] A young carpenter, just returned from Karachi (where smallpox was then still present) was hospitalized in the infectious-disease ward on the ground floor of a three-story building. On Wednesday he developed a rash; by Friday his disease was confirmed as smallpox. The man was then bundled up completely inside a plastic bag, like a gigantic head of lettuce, and transferred to a recently constructed isolation hospital.

As soon as the diagnosis of smallpox was made, all staff and patients in the building were isolated and immunized with killed smallpox vaccine. Some were later given both immune globulin (the active fraction of smallpox antiserum) and live vaccine as well. The Meschede hospital staff took all possible measures against spreading the disease.

Nevertheless, six days after the young man was transferred to another hospital, three persons developed fever; two later had the typical rash of smallpox. One victim was a patient on the floor above the isolation ward; one was a patient one floor higher; the third was a young nurse who also worked on the top floor. There had been *no contact* of any of these people with the infected man. Two of these cases ended in full recovery; the nurse died.

From then on, cases were frequent among nurses and patients in the hospital, although few had been in contact with the young carpenter. By the end of the month there were thirteen cases in all; three were fatal. Only three of the eighteen victims had been in the isolation ward. One was a visitor who was in a hallway around the corner from the isolation ward for *only fifteen minutes.* Later, there were two secondary cases in the hospital with one death, a total of twenty cases.

A smoke generator was placed in the closed room where the carpenter had been confined to trace the path of infection. A dense cloud entered the corridor and the rooms adjoining his, then spread down the hallway to the stairwell. The smoke ascended the stairwell and spread partway down the halls of the two floors above. If the window of the young man's former room was opened slightly, the smoke flowed out the window and up along the wall into open windows on the floors above. The path of the cloud was the path followed by the infecting droplet nuclei of smallpox. The transfer of infection could only have taken place in a period of slightly more than forty-eight hours. It was fortunate that the young man had smallpox. It might have been pneumonic plague.

Two diseases with which everyone has had experience are also often spread by droplet infection, namely influenza and the common cold. Influenza is also a reasonable model for some aspects of the spread of plague. It, like plague, tends to occur in the form of pandemics that originate in the Far East, then spread quickly around the world.

Measles is another common disease spread by droplet infection. Not long ago a measles epidemic swept through a school in upstate New York.[7] Beginning with a second-grade girl, twenty-eight additional cases were initially produced in fourteen different classrooms. Two infection generations later sixty children had been infected by the organisms recirculated through the ventilation system of the school.

The most recent influenza pandemic began in the summer

of 1968. Its progress is worth reviewing as a model of how a pneumonic plague epidemic might spread.

On Friday, July 12, the *Times* of London reported the outbreak of acute respiratory disease in southeastern China. The Wednesday following the *Times* announcement, the disease broke out in Hong Kong. By the end of August, the disease had appeared in Singapore, the Philippines, Taiwan, Vietnam, and Malaysia. In September it broke out in Thailand, India, and Australia.

On September 2 the first Hong Kong–influenza virus was isolated at the CDC in Atlanta from a Marine Corps major just returned from Vietnam. About the same time the disease broke out in a Marine Corps drill instructors' school in San Diego. Scattered cases appeared in all fifty states.

By mid-October nearly all of California reported the disease. Two weeks later Hawaii, Alaska, Puerto Rico, and four western states were generally infected. In mid-December only Idaho in the West; Louisiana, Arkansas, Oklahoma, and North Carolina in the South and Southwest; and New Hampshire in the East were free of the ailment. In two more weeks every state in the Union was infected.

The disease spread over western Europe, beginning a little later than in the United States, and lasted until April. It struck Poland in mid-January, and later that year the southern hemisphere was attacked. From Hong Kong the disease had spread by droplet infection to cover every state in the U.S. in five months and most of Europe in a few months more.

An influenza epidemic stops when about half the people in a community have been infected because an attack confers immunity against that strain of the virus for about three years. After an illness of a week or more the influenza victim returns to the general population and continues soaking up his share of the virus in circulation. In a recovered patient, however, the virus encounters a dead end. Thus, that virus is removed from the environment. When the proportion of such people reaches 50 percent or a bit less, the epidemic dies out.

Pneumonic plague spreads by the same mechanisms except that *Y. pestis* remains alive some fifteen times longer in the form of fine aerosol droplets than does the influenza virus. The epidemiology of pneumonic plague is also different. Infected plague patients do not return to the active population to help quench the epidemic by providing a dead end for some of the circulating organisms. If the patients are not treated very promptly and properly they die. If they are treated in time with potent antibiotics, they probably acquire no immunity and may return to the population as suceptible to the disease as when they left it. They may even have the disease a second time. If they were ill long enough to develop immunity, they would not return to the population in time to have much effect in quenching the epidemic. Thus, although pneumonic plague has the same, or greater, potential for spread as does influenza, its onslaught does not have the self-limiting character of an influenza epidemic. One may expect a much higher attack rate with pneumonic plague, under suitable circumstances, than with influenza. What circumstances favor the spread of pneumonic plague are, however, unclear. There has been no direct human-to-human transmission of the disease in the U.S. since 1925, but it is not clear why.

The increasing concentration of people into cities; the crowding of buses, trains, and buildings; and increased air pollution provide more fertile ground for the spread of respiratory illness, as the increasing frequency of influenza epidemics suggests. In addition widespread cigarette smoking is a comparatively recent development, and it is well known that cigarette smoke along with other air pollutants inhibits the ability of the human lungs to defend themselves against infection. An epidemic of pneumonic plague might effectively reduce cigarette consumption by removing its most ardent enthusiasts who are, increasingly, women and the poor, despite the impression that cigarette advertising attempts to convey.

Prevention of a pneumonic plague epidemic requires that infected people be diagnosed and isolated before they can transmit the disease. This is not presently possible. Use of the various vaccines may have some effect on the outcome if a vaccinated person contracts the pneumonic form of the disease. Fatal or very serious cases of pneumonic plague have occurred, however, in people extensively vaccinated. Mass protection, in the sense that polio or smallpox vaccination is used, is out of the question for pneumonic plague. The induction of immunity to plague—when it occurs—takes too long and lasts far too short a time to be practical in time of epidemic.

Another route to a plague epidemic is deliberate homicidal attack. It is not a new idea. There were the plague-infected corpses flung over the walls of Jaffa in 1347 by the besieging Tatars. There was also the fantastic case known as the Pakur murder, which took place in Bengal early in this century.[8]

The protagonists were two half brothers, Benoyendra and Amarendra Pandey, joint heirs to an estate. One day, as Amarendra was waiting in the railway station in Calcutta (probably to go to a town called Pakur), his half brother unexpectedly appeared to see him off. In the hustle and bustle of the crowded station, Amarendra was jostled and felt something like a pinprick on his arm. Eight days later he was dead. A blood culture revealed *Y. pestis*, and he had an ulcerated puncture wound in his arm. It was later revealed that his half brother had tried to take out a large life insurance policy on him and then conspired with a renegade bacteriologist to obtain a culture of *Y. pestis*. His accomplice injected the culture into Amarendra's arm in the railway station. Both the surviving half brother and his collaborator were found guilty of murder.

Although Benoyendra Pandey showed a certain flair, he was in the wrong place at the wrong time. Plague was then a common disease in India and the cause of his brother's death was immediately recognized. The same trick would work much better now in most of the world's large cities.

The psychoses of nations are more dangerous than those of individuals; thus, the large-scale uses of the plague bacillus in warfare or terrorist attack are a more pressing concern. Except for Janibeg khan, these uses have been largely the work of the Japanese army from 1930 to the end of 1945.

The airing of a television documentary by the Tokyo Broadcasting System on Japanese biological warfare during World

War II was the beginning of the story as it became generally known in the West, although there had been at least one previous report in a Japanese newspaper of the dropping of infected rats and voles by air and of flea nurseries capable of the rapid production of millions of fleas.

As reported by John Saar in the *Washington Post* of November 19, 1976, the film alleges that the Japanese killed at least three thousand Chinese prisoners in bacteriological warfare experiments, some of which involved packing plague-infected fleas in heat-resistant bomb casings and then dropping these bombs near prisoners tied to trees. The members of Unit 731, as it was called, were said to have escaped prosecution by turning their findings over to American occupation forces. Further information was given in an excellent article in the *Bulletin of the Atomic Scientists* in October 1981.[9]

Unit 731 was the main station and was located a few miles from Harbin, Manchuria. Two other units were Unit 100 near Changchun and the Tama Detachment in Nanjing. An undetermined number of American soldiers were among the human guinea pigs.

In 1931, soon after the Japanese occupation of Manchuria, a Japanese Army surgoen, Ishii Shiro, later a lieutenant general, suggested that biological warfare was immensely cost effective. He built the facilities used by Unit 731. The production capacity of his plant was eight tons (wet weight) of bacteria, including *Y. pestis*, each month.

A top secret "memorandum for the record" from U.S. Army Headquarters in Tokyo dated May 6, 1947, noted that

> Documentary immunity from "war crimes" given to higher echelon personnel involved (in Unit 731) will result in exploiting twenty years experience of the director, former General Ishii, who can insure complete cooperation of his former subordinates, indicate the connection of the Japanese General Staff and provide tactical and strategic information.

A memo by Dr. Edward Wetter and Mr. H. I. Stubblefield dated July 1, 1947, for restricted circulation to military and State Department officials pointed out that

This Japanese information is the only known source of scientifically controlled experiments showing the direct effect of BW (biological warfare) agents on man . . . evaluation (from animal experiments) is inconclusive and far less complete than results obtained from certain types of human experimentation.

Cecil F. Hubbert, a member of the State, War, Navy Coordinating Committee responded to the Wetter-Stubblefield memo a week later agreeing with its conclusions but warning that the United States "is at present prosecuting leading German scientists and medical doctors at Nuremburg for offenses which included experiments on human beings which resulted in the suffering and death of most of those experimented upon." He went on to suggest, incredibly, that "the data on hand (concerning Unit 731) does not appear . . . to constitute a basis for sustaining a war crimes charge against Ishii and/or his associates."

In December 1949 a Soviet court at Khabarovsk produced massive evidence supporting the charge by the Chinese government of eleven cities subjected to BW attacks between 1940 and 1944. Twelve Japanese airmen were tried and found guilty of participating in these attacks.

The Tokyo Broadcasting System television documentary "A Bruise—Terror by the 731 Corps" was shown on November 2, 1976. It was produced by Yoshinaga Haruka and has subsequently been shown in Europe but not in the U.S. Several of the Japanese officers involved testified in the documentary that they wrote reports for the U.S. Army on the condition that the army would protect them from the Soviets. Later, General Ishii went to America and, according to ex-flight engineer Kumamoto, "took his research data and begged for remission for us all." He was apparently successful.

In the first edition of this book I ridiculed the Chinese reports of biological warfare carried out by American Air Force planes at three locations in North Korea during the Korean War as well as attacks by the Japanese against Nationalist Chinese targets during World War II. On the basis of the more recent evidence I may have been mistaken.

Although there are rumors of increased Soviet interest in

biological warfare, and of the construction or enlargement of production facilities for biological weapons in the cities of Zagorsk, Omutninsk, and Sverdlovsk [I've discussed the situation in Sverdlovsk in more detail elsewhere],[10] the governments of nations usually have some forces acting to restrain their ferocity in dealing with other countries. Little groups of psychotics like the Provisional Irish Republican Army find in a twisted patriotism a convenient cloak for their homicidal tendencies. And biological weapons are, in some ways, much more accessible to terrorists than, for example, nuclear weapons.

A terrorist organization can buy or lease a large fermentor and grow all the *Y. pestis* it wishes. A garage is big enough, and the investment, even for the most modern equipment is about $100,000. The biggest technical problem is that of stabilizing the plague bacillus in an aerosol. The necessary information is not readily available, but it can be obtained. The remaining requirement is for a large-scale aerosol generator and something to mount it on.

In 1969 consultants to WHO calculated the results of a modest attack on a modern city of half a million population in an industrialized country.[11] The assumptions include dispersal of dried powder containing *Y. pestis* and stabilizing agents in a cloud a bit more than a mile long (two kilometers) on the windward edge of a city. About 110 pounds (50 kilograms) of powder are required. The most favorable circumstances are a clear midwinter night between 1:00 and 3:00 A.M., with a wind velocity of about five miles (nine kilometers) per hour and a moderate temperature and relative humidity, about 41°F (5°C) and 65 percent or more, respectively. Dispersal of the cloud of organisms could be made from an aerosol generator mounted in a plane, boat, or truck.

About 95 percent of the plague bacilli are lost during aerosolization. Either they are killed or they are trapped in droplets too large either to reach the city or to reliably produce pneumonic plague if inhaled. The remaining 5 percent of the organisms, if they are not inhaled by inhabitants of the city, are dead by the time the cloud has moved some five miles from its point of origin.

The results of such a cloud passing over the city of half a million are conservatively estimated at 27,000 pneumonic plague cases and 6,500 deaths initially. Another 3,000 cases and 750 deaths later result from person-to-person transmission of the disease.

This prediction (only 6 percent of the population infected) assumes that the disease is instantly recognized and treated and that every inhabitant of the city is given prophylactic antibiotic treatment to stop its spread. From 20 to 30 percent of the population is expected to flee the city, in spite of efforts to prevent an exodus. This causes secondary epidemics in neighboring cities, but these are relatively small and easily controlled.

A city of five hundred thousand persons should have about four thousand hospital beds within the city and another eight hundred in the surrounding area, assuming a total metropolitan population of about seven hundred thousand. At the time of the attack, 10 percent of the hospital beds are vacant; another 30 percent can be vacated by discharging all but the most seriously ill patients. This makes nearly two thousand beds available. Utilizing boarding schools, hotels, and so on doubles this number.

Pneumonic plague appears within about forty-eight hours after the attack and reaches a peak in another two or three days. If antibiotic therapy is given promptly, perhaps only 50 percent of the cases need to be hospitalized over a period of a few days, but there are only four thousand beds available. The hospital stay for the victims would be two or three weeks, while secondary cases should begin to present themselves for treatment beginning about a week after the attack. The result is that beds could be provided for less than one-third of the initial victims and half the secondary cases. After the first week this situation could be partly relieved through the setting up of mobile units like the Package Disaster Hospitals (PDH) of the U.S. Public Health Service and the Mobile Army Surgical Hospitals. *Mobile* is a relative term. The PDH con-

sists of nearly five hundred large crates; the intravenous solutions alone weigh seven tons.[12]

The estimates of case numbers in this attack assume prompt
antibiotic treatment of the victims and prophylactic administration of antibiotics to protect the people not yet infected.
WHO's consultants did not calculate the quantity of drugs
required. If we take a figure of thirty grams of tetracycline or
chloramphenicol to treat a pneumonic plague victim (three
grams a day for ten days) and six grams (one gram a day for
six days) given prophylactically to all other inhabitants, the
total antibiotic requirement is about thirty-eight hundred kilograms (eight thousand four hundred pounds). With the number of people requiring treatment, and the short time available,
the drugs must be given orally. Thus, streptomycin (which
must be injected) could be used only for those who could not
tolerate the oral drugs.

The quantity of drugs needed is enormous. No such amount
will be immediately available. Here we consider only the tetracyclines and ignore chloramphenicol, which is produced in
relatively small quantities (less than 1 percent of the amount
of the tetracyclines).

Total tetracycline production in the United States in 1976
(and probably in Europe and Japan as well) amounted to a bit
fewer than twelve grams a year for every man, woman, and
child in the nation (ignoring the agricultural use). If 10 percent
of a year's supply is on hand at the time of the attack, this is
some 1.2 grams per person. Tetracycline is sold in solutions
for injection, in eyedrops, and in salves. If 80 percent of the
stock is on hand in the form of tablets or syrups, the amount
available for the treatment of plague is one gram per person,
500 kilograms in all—about 13 percent of what is needed.

Additional tetracycline could be brought in from outside.
But from where? The surrounding areas are having plague epidemics and would be reluctant to surrender their drug supplies until their own needs were clearer. Drugs could, and
would, be sent in from cities farther away, but this would take
time, a day or two at least.

Some cases would be hospitalized before the physicians of

the afflicted community realized that they were dealing with a pneumonic plague epidemic. In the United States the Public Health Service's expertise in plague is largely concentrated at the CDC laboratory in Fort Collins, Colorado. But CDC can send in personnel only if they are invited by the city or state health department or if the disease crosses state lines. If a health department refuses to ask the CDC for help—and this has occurred with human cases of plague—the Public Health Service cannot act. Here, as in many parts of the world, perhaps in most, the recognition of plague might be a long time coming. And the onset of the disease, especially in a terrorist attack, would be frighteningly abrupt.

Suppose that on the day the illness is recognized, perhaps four days after the attack, and forty-eight hours after the first cases have appeared, there are fifteen thousand cases requiring treatment. First claim on the available drugs must go to those already stricken with the disease. If they each receive three grams of tetracycline, their requirement on the first day is forty-five kilograms of the drug. Second priority must go to protecting those who are essential to care for the sick, dispose of the dead, and maintain essential services.

In a community of five hundred thousand there should be one thousand doctors, and about six thousand nurses and nurse's aides. All must be given prophylactic treatment. Beyond this, ambulance drivers and attendants, hospital orderlies, morticians, and some firemen and police must be protected. If these medical and other essential personnel number ten thousand in all, their demand on the tetracycline supply is ten kilograms a day (for six days).

Third priority in an intelligent defense plan must go to the contacts (immediate family, friends, and close co-workers) of those already ill with pneumonic plague. They must be protected to prevent explosive spread of the disease. If each diagnosed case has ten contacts (and recent U.S. cases have often had over a hundred contacts before they were diagnosed), 150 kilograms of antibiotics are needed each day to prevent spread of the disease to those at high risk. The arithmetic is simple.

To treat those already sick and to protect those at highest

risk of exposure and those necessary to maintain essential services requires over two hundred kilograms of tetracycline *every day* for at least the first week. But the community's total supply is exhausted in sixty hours, even if the number of cases does not increase. Even an adequate supply for sixty hours is only available if two inhabitants of every three *are denied protective treatment* during this critical period. If no one were given prophylactic treatment and the tetracycline available were used only to treat actual and suspected cases the drug supply would last eleven days and the risk of producing drug-resistant *Y. pestis* would be correspondingly reduced. This, however, is at variance with current practice.

When all twenty-seven thousand expected cases are in treatment at once, the stricken city's antibiotic requirement will be 361 kilograms *each day*, assuming prophylaxis for the three high-priority groups. Fortunately, this level of demand continues for only a few days. After that, large numbers of the earliest patients will begin to die (the assumed mortality is optimistically about one in four), and the number of new cases appearing will diminish sharply.

Under optimal conditions—that is, the rapid organization of an airlift, good flying weather, an efficient system for locating the needed drugs and arranging their shipment and distribution—there will be a period of several days when most of the citizens of the infected city will receive no preventive treatment, even though the possible fate of the untreated is everywhere before their eyes. What are the results?

Flight, for one. Some people (perhaps a third of the total) will leave the city, frantically seeking elsewhere the protection they are denied at home. Another sequel is a desperate attempt by those remaining behind to get drugs by any means available. For the beleaguered pharmacist, there will be great temptation to hold out some of his supply for himself, his family and friends, and those who offer fantastic sums for only a few grams of the life-saving compounds. Unscrupulous people will sell any substance, from street drugs to horse-worming pills, to those made gullible by fear.

Finally, those people unable to pay what the market will

bear may riot, steal, or both. The emotional reactions will not be very different from those of A.D. 542, 1348, or 1665.

Within a week, with reasonably good fortune, the situation should be under control. The facilities for storing, embalming, and burying the dead are flooded with corpses, but that problem gradually will be solved. The disease may also pass to other animals. Pneumonic plague is a nearly universal ailment of warm-blooded creatures. The result is a corresponding slaughter among pets and the probable passage of the disease into commensal, then into wild, animals. A new inveterate plague focus might result from such an attack.

The tactical result of this attack is not very impressive. The casualty rate is assumed to be low, and although there is a period of bedlam and chaos, the overall effect is rather insignificant, except as a preview of what might be expected were a full-scale assault to be launched in the future. In achieving the terrorist's goal of sowing distrust and dissension by slaughtering the innocent, it might be considered a modest success.

Our example is from an industralized country. What is the effect of such an attack on a city of the same size in a less developed nation?

There are important differences. The number of physicians is about one-fourth; the total nursing staff is smaller still— two hundred instead of about six thousand. There are fewer hospital beds, and a greater proportion of them are occupied, mostly by those critically ill. Drugs of all sorts are in short supply. Under these circumstances, the total number of people requiring treatment is estimated by WHO at one hundred thousand, but there are only one thousand beds available. Of the one hundred thousand stricken in the first wave of infection, not fewer than fifty-five thousand will die. The wave of secondary infection person to person results in an additional twenty-five thousand cases and thirteen thousand deaths. The social consequences of even a small-scale and unsophisticated attack under these conditions are devastating.

Pneumonic plague introduced into a major city by whatever means has an immense capacity for destruction if conditions are suitable for its spread. The calculations of the WHO committee are conservative. The mortality rate for pneumonic plague is taken as 25 percent in a developed country and 55 percent in an undeveloped one. In the United States in recent years, the mortality rate from pneumonic plague has been close to 50 percent; previously it was nearer 75.

In this description of a deliberate assault, the use of multiply drug-resistant *Y. pestis* as the infecting agent was not considered. If such organisms are used, more than 95 percent of all cases of pneumonic plague would be fatal. There is no protection for medical personnel or for contacts through prophylactic treatment. Inadequate supplies of antibiotics are of no moment. Our community of half a million souls, nestled securely in a highly developed country in the last quarter of the twentieth century, suddenly resembles Florence or Siena when those cities groaned under the burden of the incurable Black Death.

22

Watchman,
What of the Night?

Plague retains its power to attack modern cities, leaving a tangle of death and devastation. We may reasonably ask, who shields us from epidemic plague? How strong are our defenses?

The threat of importation of plague-infected insects or rodents increases with the volume of international travel, and at best the International Sanitary Regulations on insect control are often ignored, or if heeded, then only perfunctorily.

The medically trained inspector scanning international airline passengers for possible illness is a casualty of the huge increase in air travel (in the U.S., both domestic and international traffic have more than doubled since 1970), coupled with declining budgets for public health. Immigration officers now get cursory training in disease recognition. The most they usually do is to hand incoming passengers from overseas a yellow card called a Health Alert Notice. The card is to be held for six weeks and given to a physician should the traveler become ill in that time. The notice reminds the physician that plague must be reported to local health officials and by telephone to the CDC, Atlanta. For pneumonic plague cases, the physician is asked to supply the date and place of arrival in the United States and the airline flight number or other identification of the mode of entry. These cards are mostly left on the floor of the Customs and Immigration buildings after a planeload of passengers has departed—a fact that offers convincing testimony to the indifference toward infectious disease even among a relatively sophisticated segment of the population.

The chance is slight that a person in the early infective stage of pneumonic plague would be recognized as such in passing through the usual entry procedures of any international airport. Were the disease identified later, the task of alerting the victim's fellow passengers is nearly hopeless. Public health officials have urged that all passengers from overseas receive a card on which to list their itineraries, and where they can be reached, for several weeks after arrival. Airline managers have refused to consider this suggestion, claiming that it would be too great an infringement on their cabin attendants' time. Since no lists of passengers are retained by the airlines for very long, people infected by a plague-stricken fellow traveler would announce their locations only by their sudden prostration from the disease, and perhaps by their celebrity as the focus of a modest (we may hope) epidemic.

Human plague acquired in the United States is more likely to be detected, but preventive measures against plague are still unimpressive. The steady decline continues of personnel and funds for plague research specifically, and of public health work generally.

The WHO's Weekly Epidemiological Report for April 3, 1973, contains a five-page guide to plague surveillance in permanent foci. The goal is to study carefully and over a long period of time the flora and fauna of each plague focus and to monitor the sentinel animals whose infections signal an epizootic. Then steps can be taken to protect humans. This required surveillance is the responsibility of public health personnel, largely at the federal and state levels.

At the federal level, particularly since 1972, financial support for all aspects of public health has fallen sharply. Allowing for inflation, the budget for the U.S. Public Health Service Center for Disease Control fell by one-third between 1972 and

President Ford's budget for the fiscal year ending in September 1976. In President Carter's budget for 1978, the amount for the CDC was reduced yet another 2 percent below that of the 1976 fiscal year. In recognition of these realities, for every four persons leaving the CDC in the coming years only three will be replaced.

The figure of $416 million proposed for the CDC for fiscal year 1985 (beginning October 1, 1984) represents the major portion of funds available to defend the United States against the importation of epidemic disease. For defense against our human enemies, real or imagined, the Pentagon will spend $800 million every day of 1985 (approximately a 10 percent increase over the preceding year), yet plague alone has killed more people than all the wars in history.

At the state level, of the fourteen states in the plague focus, six have no state personnel involved in plague surveillance. They rely wholly on the staff of the plague branch of the CDC in Fort Collins, Colorado. Five of the remaining states have a single person in charge of plague surveillance, but that person has many other responsibilities as well, often including such complex issues as the disposal of nuclear wastes. These states also depend on the CDC branch for help in controlling the disease.

Yet, financially, the plague branch has fared even worse than its parent organization. Between 1968 and 1977, CDC's plague branch lost two-thirds of its staff. Half that loss came in the 1970s when human plague was burgeoning in the United States.

In the U.S. carrying out the surveillance program recommended by WHO is hopeless with the few people available, even if their only responsibility were plague control, which it is not. In America the "sentinel animal" too often is man; a human infection signals the presence of the disease.

The effectiveness of the dwindling number of people involved in plague research and surveillance is unfortunately still further diminished by petty rivalries that may effectively stifle cooperation among people at various governmental levels.

Although our defenses are flaccid everywhere, the most frightening deficiencies are in our ability to detect and combat a possible terrorist attack that would use plague as a weapon against civilians.

In the 1960s the potential for biological warfare between nations was a popular topic in magazines, newspapers, and books. This interest was stimulated by the announcement, in February 1956 (by Marshall G. K. Zhukov, then defense minister of the Soviet Union), that both chemical and biological weapons would be employed in future conflicts as weapons of mass destruction. This statement was repeated seventy-two hours later by the commander-in-chief of the Soviet navy. The natural consequence was a flurry of activity in the Pentagon that was later reflected in the communications media. (The U.S. Army had actually begun a massive expansion of its biological warfare capabilities after the beginning of the Korean War in June 1950, but this buildup was not publicized.) Even earlier (October 1948) a Defense Department committee had stressed the United States's susceptibility to biological warfare and the utility of biological warfare agents for subversive (or terrorist) activities.

Public and military interest in biological warfare then waned. It does seem clear that those countries with the technological sophistication to launch large-scale biological attacks can destroy human civilization much more efficiently with nuclear weapons.

In late 1969, public outrage over U.S. use of chemical warfare in Vietnam forced President Nixon to outlaw the possession or use of biological weapons by American forces. All biological weapons were reportedly destroyed by mid-April 1973 (except for those held by the Central Intelligence Agency, which defied the presidential order). An unintended effect of the destruction of U.S. biological weapons was the subsidiary dismantling of the research organization that was knowledgeable concerning the defense against such weapons, and that portion of the intelligence community that watched for signs of such weapon development overseas. Only fifteen years later is some effort being made to redress these deficiencies in part because of the publicity surrounding the possible use of biological warfare agents in Afghanistan and Southeast Asia.

Terrorist organizations have much to admire in *Y. pestis* as a weapon. Part of its appeal to such twisted minds is that the United States and other countries lie helpless before it. In the preface to a report on the U.S. Army Biological Warfare Programs (presented to Senator Edward M. Kennedy's Subcommittee on Health and Scientific Resources on March 8, 1977) the authors comment, "The problems of biological defense are far greater today than at any time in the past because of the technological advances in the biological sciences."

Who defends American cities against attack by clouds of *Y. pestis?* The answer apparently is no one!

The U.S. Army, with great experience in such matters, has elaborate plans to defend its own installations (the army spent some $9 million for research in this area in 1977), but it has no plans for defending civilian populations. This charge was made by Jack Anderson in his column of April 7, 1977; he also pointed out that the U.S. Public Health Service likewise had no program for detecting such attacks or for defending American cities against them, although the ease and effectiveness of biological warfare as a terrorist weapon was established with frightening clarity by the army's mock attacks on subways and public buildings.

Detection and defense against plague aerosols is possible, although very difficult at present. Outdoor air usually contains one bacterium per liter. In a deliberate attack with a cloud of *Y. pestis,* this level would soar a million or more times as the infective mist passed over the air-sampling detectors. Detection could trigger release of a disinfectant counteraerosol and stimulate defensive measures such as the issuing of military gas masks to essential personnel (most respirators and hospital gauze masks would be nearly useless), or ordering people into shelters with suitably protected ventilation systems—if such shelters existed.

Moreover, such detectors would permit isolation of the organisms (tentative identification could be made in a few hours in the most favorable situation, or in minutes with methods being developed in the Life Sciences Division at Los Alamos by my colleagues and me).[1] Testing of their antibiotic sensitivity, if any, could be possibly done in a few hours more. Thus the infection agent could be characterized early in the epidemic, perhaps even before the first cases appeared.

Such an early warning network, coupled with regional, national, and international plans to send medical supplies and drugs to any suddenly infected area, could save thousands of lives at comparatively modest cost. Yet no such network exists.

Even without the possibility of terrorist attack, the problem of plague breaking out in a modern city remains a serious one. Late in 1971 Dr. William C. Reeves, dean of the School of Public Health of the University of California, Berkeley, gave his presidential address to the American Society of Tropical Medicine and Hygiene. Its title was "Can the War to Contain Infectious Disease Be Lost?" He explained,

> I have chosen a broad theme, namely that we face serious problems in our continuing effort to control the infectious diseases that prevail in both tropical and temperate regions. I fear that society and the scientific community have become complacent with the advances made in research and their relative freedom from epidemics. I contend that while we have won many battles in our research effort the long range and bigger war to contain certain infectious disease can still be lost.

Later, with respect to plague and the multiplying problems of its control, he said, "Thus, we again have the situation where new research developments for control are needed and intelligence and surveillance must be kept high or we could be back in a war to control plague in an urban center."

Since 1971, however, the amount of research on plague control has declined precipitously, along with the level of surveillance.

It bears repeating that, worldwide, more people now live under worse conditions than ever before in history. The threat of war and famine is constantly present. Permanent plague foci exist on every inhabited continent except Australia, and jet aircraft interlace the world into a global community in which most points can be easily reached in a day's journey. All the ingredients for a Fourth Pandemic are at hand. The tinder lies waiting for the spark.

We still have, moreover, only a feeble understanding of the many complex cycles that must fall into step to generate a plague pandemic. Our theories of the ebb and flow of the great plagues of the past are a pastiche of conjecture, confusion, and wishful thinking. Our defenses against plague—rodenticides, insecticides, antimicrobials, surveillance—fail to inspire the confidence they did twenty or thirty years ago.

In short, plague remains what it has always been—a lurking threat to humanity everywhere. Wily *Y. pestis*, the vicious bacillus, has never really been tamed.

Notes

The references for the first edition of this book numbered about 700 and take up some five feet of shelving. New references for the second edition probably add at least another 100. I would be pleased to answer questions concerning sources from anyone, but it seems pointless to list all the references used in a book intended for the general public. Hence I have chosen to give a limited number of sources here for the various chapters to lead the interested reader into the literature.

Chapter 1

1. Philip Ziegler, *The Black Death* (Harmondsworth, England: Penguin Books Ltd., 1970). An excellent book used extensively by me and by Barbara Tuchman (see below). Barbara W. Tuchman, *A Distant Mirror: The Calamitous 14th Century* (New York: Knopf, 1978), pp. 92–125. Dr. Tuchman's book came out about six months after the first edition of *Plague!* There are errors in her treatment of plague, but the book shines, as usual in her work, with the distinguishing intelligence, style, and scholarship of its author. William L. Langer, "The Black Death," *Scientific American* 210 (1964): 114–21. Charles Creighton, *History of Epidemics in Britain* A.D. *664–1666* (Cambridge: Cambridge University Press, 1891), 144–45. John Norris, "East or West? The Geographical Origin of the Black Death," *Bulletin of the History of Medicine* 51 (1977): 1–23. Arturo Castiglioni, *A History of Medicine*, transl. by E. B. Krumbharr (New York: Knopf, 1947), 353–62.

2. Daniel Defoe, *A Journal of the Plague Year* (Harmondsworth, England: Penguin Books, Ltd., 1966), originally published in 1722. C. V. Edgeworth, "When Black Death Stalked in London," *New York Times Magazine* (September 12, 1964): 92–98. "Nathaniel Hodges (1629–1688), Physician of the Great Plague," *Journal of the American Medical Association* 190 (1964): 133. Archibald W. Sloan, "Medical and Social Aspects of the Great Plague of London," *South African Medical Journal* 17 (February 1973): 270–76. Walter George Bell, *The Great Plague in London in 1665* (London, England: John Lane, The Bodley Head Ltd., 1924).

3. Albert Camus, *The Plague*, transl. by Stuart French (New York: Knopf, 1969), 278.

Chapter 2

1. Ziegler, *The Black Death*, 92–125.
2. Defoe, *A Journal of the Plague Year*.
3. Percy B. Green, *A History of Nursery Rhymes* (London: Greening & Co., Ltd., 1899), 44–50.
4. D. Wolfers, "A Plaguey Piper," *The Lancet* (April 13, 1965): 756–57.
5. Fielding H. Garrison, *An Introduction to the History of Medicine* (Philadelphia: W. B. Saunders, 1929), 305–6.

Chapter 3

1. Madagascar is listed by the World Health Organization as a "probable" plague focus (see Frontispiece). After over eighty-five years of annual plague deaths this designation seems absurd. Madagascar is clearly a plague focus.
2. P. A. Earnshaw, "Unwept, Unhonour'd and Unsung," *Medical Journal of Australia* (March 12, 1966): 427–36.

Chapter 4

1. Victor H. Hass, "When Bubonic Plague Came to Chinatown," *American Journal of Tropical Medicine and Hygiene* 8 (1964): 141–47. Loren G. Lipson, "Plague in San Francisco in 1900," *Annals of Internal Medicine* 77 (1972): 303–10. Silvio J. Onesti, Jr., "Plague, Press, and Politics," *Stanford Medical Bulletin* 13 (1955): 1–10. L. S. McClung and K. F. Meyer, "Beginnings of Bacteriology in Cali-

fornia," *Bacterilogical Review* 38 (1974): 251–71. Vernon B. Link, *A History of Plague in the United States of America*, Public Health Monograph No. 26 (Washington, D.C.: U.S. Government Printing Office, 1955), 3–11.

Chapter 5

1. Louis Pasteur had just developed the first rabies vaccine. A group of Russian men severely mauled by a rabid wolf had been sent to Paris for vaccine treatment. Yersin, as a senior medical student, performed an autopsy on one of the Russians who died of rabies and, as not infrequently happens, cut himself on a sharp bone spur during examination of the body. He was sent to Roux's laboratory to receive the vaccine and, over the course of the injections, became so enthralled with the work being done there that he became Roux's assistant.

2. J. E. Moseley, "Travels of Alexandre Yersin: Letters of a Pastorian in Indochina, 1890–1894," *Perspectives in Biology and Medicine* (Summer 1981): 607–17.

3. E. Lagrange, "Concerning the Discovery of the Plague Bacillus," *Journal of Tropical Medicine and Hygiene* 29 (1926): 299–303. A. G. Millott Severn, "A Note Concerning the Discovery of the Bacillus Pestis," *Journal of Tropical Medicine and Hygiene* 30 (1927): 208–9. Norman Howard-Jones, "Was Shibasaburo Kitasato the Co-discoverer of the Plague Bacillus?," *Perspectives in Biology and Medicine* (Winter 1973): 292–307. Norman Howard-Jones, "Kitasato, Yersin, and the Plague Bacillus," *Clio Medica* 10 (1975): 23–27. David J. Bibel and T. H. Chen, "Diagnosis of Plague: An Analysis of the Yersin-Kitasato Controversy," *Bacteriological Review* 40 (1976): 633–51.

4. J. Lowe, "A Note on the Work of Dr. P. L. Simond on the Transmission and Epidemiology of Plague," *Indian Medical Gazette* (July 1942): 418–21.

Chapter 6

1. S. A. Barnett, "Rats," *Scientific American* 216 (1967): 79–85. Anthony Barnett, "The Wild Rat," *Natural History* (1959): 532–37.

2. Ernest Schwartz, "Classification, Origin and Distribution of Commensal Rats," *World Health Organization Bulletin* (1959): 411–15. J. Chaline, "Rodents, Evolution, and Prehistory," *Endeavor* 1 (1977): 44–51.

3. "The Black Rat in Britain," *Nature* 281 (1979): 101.

4. "Rats Eat Government Files While Indian Cats Stand By," *Albuquerque Journal,* March 3, 1984.

5. "Rats Resisting Man's Most Aggressive Efforts at Eradication," *Los Angeles Times,* October 18, 1979.

6. "Cleveland Confronted by Rampaging Rodents," Associated Press, October 20, 1978.

7. "Woman Flees Following Rat Attack," *Los Angeles Times,* May 12, 1979.

8. "Frightened Family Flees Apartment Infested by Rats," United Press International, June 5, 1978.

9. "Rats Fleeing Exterminators Invade New York's 5th Avenue," Associated Press, October 18, 1979.

Chapter 7

1. R. Pollitzer, *Plague* (Geneva: WHO, 1954): 315–408. David Hendin, "Year of the Flea," *Saturday Review* (August 5, 1972): 30–31. Miriam Rothschild, Y. Sclein, K. Parker, C. Neville, and S. Sternberg, "The Flying Leap of the Flea," *Scientific American* 229 (1973): 92–100.

2. The World Health Organization is presently considering changing the name for reasons that would take us too deeply into the thickets of bacterial nomenclature. The proposed change will probably not (and should not) occur.

3. R. Pollitzer, *Plague,* 71–113.

4. Solomon Kadis, Thomas C. Montie, and Samuel Ajl, "Plague Toxin," *Scientific American* 220 (1969). Thomas C. Montie and Samuel J. Ajl, "Nature and Synthesis of Murine Toxins of Pasteurella Pestis," *Microbial Toxins* 3: 1–37.

Chapter 8

1. "Quake Toll Worse Than Thought," Knight-Ridder Newspapers, May 13, 1984.

2. Vernon B. Link, *A History of Plague in the United States of America,* Public Health Monograph No. 26 (Washington, D.C.: U.S. Government Printing Office, 1955), 12–23.

3. James G. Cumming, "The Plague: A Laboratory Case Report," *Military Medicine* (1963): 435–39.

4. Link, *A History of Plague in the United States of America,* 24–26.

Chapter 9

1. Martin I. Goldenberg, Stuart F. Quan, and Bruce W. Hudson, "The Detection of Inapparent Infection with Pasteurella Pestis in a Microtus Californicus Population in the San Francisco Bay Area," *Zoonoses Research* 3 (1964): 1–13. Bruce W. Hudson, Martin L. Goldenberg, and Thomas J. Quan, "Serological and Bacteriological Studies on the Distribution of Plague Infection in a Wild Rodent Plague Pocket in the San Francisco Bay Area of California," *Journal of Wildlife Diseases* 8 (1972): 278–86.

2. Link, *A History of Plague in the United States of America*, 27–42. Illar Muul, "Mammalian Ecology and Epidemiology of Zoonoses," *Science* 170 (1970): 1275–83.

3. Judith H. Meyers and Charles J. Krebs, "Population Cycles in Rodents," *Scientific American* 230 (1974): 38–46.

4. James H. Rust, Jr., Dan C. Cavanaugh, Roy O'Shita, and John D. Marshall, "The Role of Domestic Animals in the Epidemiology of Plague, I: Experimental Infection of Dogs and Cats," *Journal of Infectious Diseases* 124 (1971): 522–26.

5. M. Baltazard, "The Conservation of Plague in Inveterate Foci," *Journal of Hygiene, Epidemiology, Microbiology, and Immunology* 8 (1964): 409–21.

Chapter 10

1. Priscilla A. Campbell, "Immunocompetent Cells in Resistance to Bacterial Infections," *Bacteriological Reviews* 40 (1976): 284–313. Thomas P. Stossel, "Phagocytosis (First of Three Parts)," *New England Journal of Medicine* 290 (1974): 717–23. The two succeeding parts are in the next two issues of the journal.

2. Eugene D. Weinberg, "Iron and Susceptibility to Infectious Disease," *Science* 184 (1974): 952–56. Akira Wake, Hidemi Morita, and Makoto Yamamoto, "The Effect of an Iron Drug on Host Response to Experimental Plague Infection," *Japanese Journal of Medical Science and Biology* 25 (1972): 75–84.

3. Arthur C. Guyton, M.D., *Textbook of Medical Physiology* (Philadelphia: W. B. Saunders, 1976), 397.

Chapter 11

1. Richard Lurz, "An Epidemic of Plague on Kilimanjaro in 1912," transl. by C. A. W. Guggisberg from *Archivs der Schiffs- und Tro-*

penhygiene 17 (1913), 593–99. *East African Medical Journal* 11 (1967): 215–20.

2. David van Zwangenberg, "The Last Epidemic of Plague in England? Suffolk 1906–1918," *Medical History* 14 (1970): 63–74. "The Plague's Last Visit?" *The Lancet* (March 14, 1970): 558.

3. Link, *A History of Plague in the United States of America*, 43–53.

4. Ibid., 35–36.

5. Ibid., 54–56.

6. Ibid., 57–64.

7. Arthur J. Veseltear, "The Pneumonic Plague Epidemic of 1924 in Los Angeles," *Yale Journal of Biology and Medicine* 1 (1974): 40–54.

Chapter 12

1. Karl Paul Link, "The Discovery of Dicumarol and Its Sequels," *Circulation* 19 (1959): 97–107.

2. Thomas Jukes, "DDT," *Journal of the American Medical Association* 229 (1974): 571–73.

3. Meir Yoeli, "A Portrait of Waldemar M. Haffkine in Global Public Health," *American Journal of Medical Science* 267 (1974): 202–12.

4. K. F. Meyer, "Effectiveness of Live or Killed Plague Vaccines in Man," *World Health Organization Bulletin* 42 (1970): 653–66. Peter J. Barteiloni, John D. Marshall, and Dan C. Cavanaugh, "Clinical and Serological Responses to Plague Vaccine U.S.P.," *Military Medicine* (November 1973): 720–22.

5. A. F. Hallet, Margaretha Isaäcson, and K. F. Meyer, "Pathogenicity and Immunogenic Efficacy of a Live Attenuated Plague Vaccine in Vervet Monkeys," *Infection and Immunity* 8 (1973): 876–81. T. H. Chen, Sanford S. Elberg, and Daniel M. Eisler, "Immunity in Plague: Protection of the Vervet (*Cercopithecus aethiops*) Against Pneumonic Plague by the Oral Administration of Live Attenuated Yersinia Pestis," *Journal of Infectious Diseases* 135 (1977): 289–93.

6. Gilbert B. Forbes and Grace M. Forbes, "An Historical Note on Chemotherapy of Bacterial Infections," *American Journal of Diseases of Children* 119 (1970): 6–11.

7. K. F. Meyer and S. F. Quan, "Plague," in Selman A. Waksman (ed.) *Streptomycin* (Baltimore: Williams & Wilkins Co., 1949): 394–407.

8. Ibid.

Chapter 13

1. R. K. Chandrahas, A. K. Krishnaswami, and C. K. Rao, "Studies on the Epidemiology of Plague in a South Indian Plague Focus," *Indian Journal of Medical Research* 7 (1974): 1089–1103.

2. F. LaForce, I. L. Archarya, Gordon Stott, Philip S. Brachman, Arnold F. Kaufman, Richard F. Class, and N. K. Shah, "Clinical and Epidemiological Observations on an Outbreak of Plague in Nepal," *World Health Organization Bulletin* 45 (1971): 693–706.

3. B. Velimirovic, V. Zikmund, and J. Herman, "Plague in the Lake Edward Focus: The Democratic Republic of Congo, 1960–1966," *Zeitschrift für Tropenmedicin und Parasitologie* 20 (1969): 373–87.

4. M. Bahmanyar, "Human Plague Episode in the District of Khawlan, Yemen," *American Journal of Tropical Medicine and Hygiene* 20 (1971): 123–28.

Chapter 14

1. R. Betts and F. Denton, *An Evaluation of Chemical Crop Destruction in Vietnam*, Memorandum RM-5446-1-ISA/ARPA, October 1967 (Santa Monica, Ca: Rand). J. Russo, *A Statistical Analysis of the U.S. Crop Spraying Program in South Vietnam*, Memorandum RM-5450-1-ISA/ARPA (Santa Monica, Ca: Rand).

2. Boris Velimirovic, "Untersuchungen über die Epidemiologie und Bekämpfung der Pest in Südvietnam, Teil I und II," *Zentralblatt für Bakteriologie und Hygiene*, I. Abteilung, Originale A. 228 (1974): 482–532.

3. E. J. Feely and J. J. Kriz, "Plague Meningitis in an American Serviceman," *Journal of the American Medical Association* 191 (1965): 412–13.

4. Richard J. Cohen and Joe L. Stockard, "Pneumonic Plague in an Untreated Plague-Vaccinated Individual," *Journal of the American Medical Association* 202 (1967): 217–18.

5. P. Trong, T. Q. Nhu, and J. D. Marshall, "A Mixed Pneumonic Plague Outbreak in Vietnam," *Military Medicine* (February 1967): 93–97.

6. Fred G. Conrad, Frank R. LeCocq, and Robert Krain, "A Recent Epidemic of Plague in Vietnam," *Archives of Internal Medicine* 123 (1968): 193–98.

7. C. G. Reiley and E. D. Kates, "The Clinical Spectrum of Plague in Vietnam," *Archives of Internal Medicine* 126 (1970): 990–94.

8. J. R. Cantey, "Plague in Vietnam," *Archives of Internal Medicine* 133 (1974): 280–93.

9. Llewellyn J. Legters, Andrew J. Cottingham, Jr., and Donald H. Hunter, "Clinical and Epidemiological Notes on a Defined Outbreak of Plague in Vietnam," *American Journal of Tropical Medicine and Hygiene* 19 (1970): 639–52.

Chapter 15

1. R. W. Burmeister, W. D. Tigert, and E. L. Overholt, "Laboratory-acquired Pneumonic Plague: Report of a Case and Review of Previous Cases," *Annals of Internal Medicine* 56 (1962): 789–800.

2. Richard N. Collins, Albert R. Martin, Leo Kartman, Robert L. Brutsche, Bruce W. Hudson, and H. Gordon Doran, "Plague Epidemic in New Mexico, 1965," *Public Health Reports* 82 (1967): 1077–99.

3. Jack Schwade and Jay P. Sanford, "Hepatic Granulomata due to 'Benign' Plague Imported from Vietnam," *Military Medicine* (July 1974): 554–56.

4. Berton Roueché, "Annals of Medicine: A Small Apprehensive Child," *New Yorker* 47 (1971): 70–90. Bruce W. Hudson, Martin I. Goldenberg, J. Douglas McCluskie, Harvard E. Larson, C. David McGuire, Allan M. Barnes, and Jack C. Poland, "Serological and Bacteriological Investigations of an Outbreak of Plague in an Urban Tree Squirrel Population," *American Journal of Tropical Medicine and Hygiene* 20 (1971): 255–63.

5. W. P. Reed, D. C. Palmer, R. C. Williams, Jr., and A. L. Kisch, "Bubonic Plague in the Southwestern United States: A Review of Recent Experience," *Medicine* 49 (1970): 465–86.

Chapter 16

1. J. E. Williams, B. W. Hudson, R. W. Turner, J. Sulianti Saroso, and D. E. Cavanaugh, "Plague in Central Java, Indonesia," *World Health Organization Bulletin* 58 (1980): 459–68.

2. B. Velimirovic, "Reappearance of Plague in Khymer Republic" *Zeitschrift für Tropenmedicin und Parasitologie* 24 (1973): 265–70.

3. Margaretha Isaäcson, D. Levy, J. Te W. N. Pienarr, Hazel D. Bubb, J. A. Louw, and D. K. Genis, "Unusual Cases of Human Plague in Southern Africa," *South African Medical Journal* (10 November 1973): 2109–13.

4. C. R. Almeida, A. R. Almeida, J. B. Vieira, U. Guida, and T. Butler, "Plague in Brazil During Two Years of Bacteriological and Serological Surveillance," *World Health Organization Bulletin* 59 (1981): 591–97.

Chapter 17

1. William P. Reed, Eppie Rael, and Ulton G. Hodgin, Jr., "The Cure of Plague—Two Viewpoints," *Journal of the American Medical Association* 216 (1971): 1197–98.

2. A. M. Jones, J. Mann, and R. Braziel, "Human Plague in New Mexico: Report of Three Autopsied Cases," *Journal of Forensic Science* 24 (1979): 26–38.

3. J. B. Coopes, "Bubonic Plague in Pregnancy," *Journal of Reproductive Medicine* 25:91–5.

4. M. E. White, R. J. Rosenbaum, T. M. Canfield, and J. D. Poland, "Plague in a Neonate," *American Journal of Diseases of Children* 135 (1981): 418–19.

5. A. M. Jones, J. Mann, and R. Braziel, *Human Plague in New Mexico: Report of Three Autopsied Cases.*

6. J. M. Mann, W. J. Martone, J. M. Boyce, A. F. Kaufman, A. M. Barnes, and N. S. Weber, "Endemic Human Plague in New Mexico, Risk Factors Associated with Infection," *Journal of Infectious Diseases* 140 (1979): 397–401.

7. A. F. Kaufman, J. M. Boyce, and W. J. Martone, "Trends in Human Plague in the United States," *Journal of Infectious Diseases* 141 (1980): 522–24.

Chapter 19

1. A. F. Kaufman, J. M. Mann, T. M. Gardiner, F. Heaton, J. D. Poland, A. M. Barnes, and G. O. Maupin, "Public Health Implications of Plague in Domestic Cats," *Journal of the American Veterinary Medical Association* 179 (1981): 875–78. D. J. Rollag, M. R. Skeels, L. J. Nims, J. P. Thielsted, and J. M. Mann, "Feline Plague in New Mexico: Report of Five Cases," *Journal of the American Veterinary Medical Association* 179 (1981): 1381–83.

2. J. M. Mann, G. P. Schmidt, P. A. Stoesz, M. D. Skinner, and A. F. Kaufman, "Peripatetic Plague," *Journal of the American Medical Association* 247 (1982): 47–48.

3. J. M. Mann, L. Shandler, and A. H. Cushing, "Pediatric Plague," *Pediatrics* 69 (1982): 762–67.

4. S. B. Werner, C. E. Weidmer, B. C. Nelson, G. S. Nygaard, R. M. Goethals, and J. D. Poland, "Primary Plague Pneumonia Contracted from a Domestic Cat at South Lake Tahoe, Calif.," *Journal of the American Medical Association* 251 (1984): 929–31.

5. "Health Officials Call Plague Impossible to Stamp Out," Associated Press, November 11, 1981.

6. A. M. Jones, J. Mann, and R. Braziel, "Human Plague in New Mexico: Report of Three Autopsied Cases," 26–38.

7. "Village to Attack Plague Problem with Cleanup Drive," *Albuquerque Journal*, October 9, 1981.

8. D. D. Hopkins and R. A. Gresbrink, "Surveillance of Sylvatic Plague in Oregon by Serotesting Carnivores," *American Journal of Public Health* 72 (1982): 1295–97.

9. B. G. Weniger, A. J. Warren, V. Forseth, G. W. Shipps, T. Creelman, J. Gorton, and A. M. Barnes, "Human Bubonic Plague Transmitted by a Domestic Cat Scratch," *Journal of the American Medical Association* 251 (1984): 927–28.

10. "Plague—South Carolina," *Morbidity and Mortality Weekly Report*, Centers for Disease Control, August 19, 1983, 418.

11. Mann et al., "Pediatric Plague."

12. "Boy, 13, Becomes Third Plague Fatality; Case Called Most Severe Yet," *Albuquerque Journal*, August 16, 1983.

13. P. Q. Tomich, A. M. Barnes, W. S. Devich, H. H. Higa, and G. E. Haas, "Evidence for the Extinction of Plague in Hawaii," *American Journal of Epidemiology* 119 (1984): 261–73.

Chapter 20

1. William B. Jackson, Joe E. Brooks, Alan M. Bowerman, and Dale E. Kaukeinen, "Anticoagulant Resistance in Norway Rats in U.S. Cities," *Pest Control* (April 1973): 56–64.

2. "'Mighty Mice' Foiling Efforts at Capture," United Press International, April 6, 1978.

3. R. Pal, "The Present Status of Insecticide Resistance in Anopheline Mosquitos," *Journal of Tropical Medicine and Hygiene* 77 (1974): 28–41.

4. Selman A. Waksman, ed., *Streptomycin* (Baltimore: Williams & Wilkens Co., 1949), 394–407.

5. Colin Hughes and G. G. Meynell, "High Frequency of Antibiotic-resistant Enterobacteria in the River Stour, Kent," *The Lancet* (August 23, 1974): 451–53.

6. Ralph C. Gordon, Theodore R. Thompson, William Carlson, John W. Dyke, and Lynne I. Stevens, "Antimicrobial Resistance of Shigellae Isolated in Michigan," *Journal of the American Medical Association* 231 (1975): 1159–61.

7. "What is Cancer? What Form Does it Take? How Does it Kill?," *Science* 183 (1974): 1068–69.

8. WHO Scientific Working Group, "Antimicrobial Resistance," *World Health Organization Bulletin* 61 (1983): 383–94.

Chapter 21

1. Tad Szulc, "One Person Too Many?," *Parade Magazine* (April 29, 1984): 16.

2. "Third World's Ills Worsening," United Press International, March 26, 1984.

3. Ted Szulc, "One Person Too Many?"

4. R. B. Highton and E. C. C. van Someren, "The Transportation of Mosquitos between International Airports," *World Health Organization Bulletin* 42 (1970): 334–35.

5. René Dubos, *Man Adapting* (New Haven: Yale University Press, 1965): 163–64.

6. P. F. Wehrle, J. Posch, K. H. Richter, and D. A. Henderson, "An Airborne Outbreak of Smallpox in a German Hospital and Its Significance with Respect to Other Recent Outbreaks in Europe," *World Health Organization Bulletin* 43 (1970): 669–79.

7. E. C. Riley, G. Murphy, and R. L. Riley, "Airborne Spread of Measles in a Suburban Elementary School," *Journal of Epidemiology* 107 (1978): 421–32.

8. "Homicide by Means of Plague Bacilli," *Bulletin of the New York Academy of Medicine* 43 (1967): 850–51.

9. "Japan's Biological Weapons: 1930–45," *Bulletin of the Atomic Scientists* 37 (1981): 43–53.

10. Charles T. Gregg, *A Virus of Love and Other Tales of Medical Detection*, reprint ed. (Albuquerque: University of New Mexico Press, 1985): 113–34.

11. *Health Aspects of Chemical and Biological Weapons: Report of a WHO Group of Consultants* (Geneva: WHO, 1970): 98–99, 107–9.

12. Robert L. Price, "Use of the Packaged Disaster Hospital in Nigeria," *Public Health Reports* 85 (1970): 659–65.

Chapter 22

1. C. T. Gregg, D. M. McGregor, W. K. Grace, and G. C. Salzman, "Rapid Microbial Identification by Circular Intensity Differential Scattering," in *Rapid Methods and Automation in Microbiology and Immunology* (Heidelberg: Springer Verlag, in press).

Bibliography

Boccaccio, Giovanni. *The Decameron*. Transl. by G. H. McWilliam. Middlesex, England: Penguin Books Ltd., 1970.

Burnet, McFarlane, and David O. White. *Natural History of Infectious Disease*, 4th ed. Cambridge: Cambridge University Press, 1972.

Butler, Thomas. *Plague and Other Yersinia Infections*. New York: Plenum Medical Book Company, 1983.

Davis, D. H. S., A. F. Hallet, and Margaretha Isaäcson. "Plague." In W. T. Hubbert, W. F. McCulloch, and P. R. Schnurrenberges, eds., *Diseases Transmitted from Animals to Man*. Springfield, Ill., Charles C. Thomas, 1975.

Ecke, D. H., C. W. Johnson, V. I. Miles, M. J. Wilcomb, and J. V. Irons. *Plague in Colorado and Texas*. Public Health Monograph No. 6. Washington, D.C.: Government Printing Office, 1952.

Hirst, L. F. *The Conquest of Plague*. Oxford, England: Clarendon Press, 1953.

Lehane, B. *The Compleat Flea*. New York: Viking, 1969.

McNeil, William H. *Plagues and Peoples*. New York: Anchor Press/Doubleday, 1976.

Pollitzer, R. *Plague and Plague Control in the Soviet Union*. New York: Institute of Contemporary Russian Studies, Fordham University, 1966.

Shrewsbury, J. F. D. *A History of Bubonic Plague in the British Isles*. Cambridge: Cambridge University Press, 1970.

Zinsser, H. *Rats, Lice, and History*. Boston: Little, Brown and Co., 1941.

Index

Index

X5904X